Say It in
Spanish

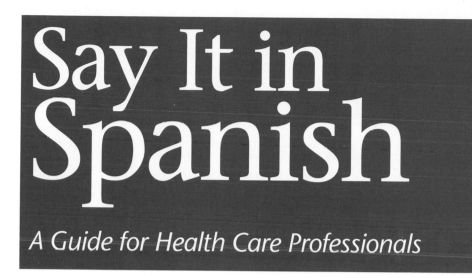

Say It in Spanish

A Guide for Health Care Professionals

Third Edition

Esperanza Villanueva Joyce, EdD, CNS, RN

Dean and Professor
Our Lady of the Lake College
Division of Nursing
Baton Rouge, Louisiana

Maria Elena Villanueva, MD

Mexico City, D.F.

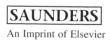

SAUNDERS

An Imprint of Elsevier

SAUNDERS

An Imprint of Elsevier

11830 Westline Industrial Drive
St. Louis, Missouri 63146

Say It in Spanish: A Guide for Health Care Professionals   ISBN 0-7216-0424-2
Copyright © 2004, Elsevier Science (USA). All rights reserved.

Previous editions copyrighted 2000, 1996

Library of Congress Cataloging-in-Publication Data

Joyce, Esperanza Villanueva.
    Say it in Spanish : a guide for health care professionals / Esperanza Villanueva Joyce,
Maria Elena Villanueva.—3rd ed.
    p. ; cm.
    Includes bibliographical references.
    ISBN 0-7216-0424-2
    1. Medicine—Dictionaries.   2. Spanish language—Conversation and phrase books
(for medical personnel).   3. Spanish language—Dictionaries—English.   I. Villanueva,
Maria Elena.   II. Title.
    [DNLM: 1. Medicine—Phrases—English.   2. Medicine—Phrases—Spanish.
W 15 J89s 2004]
R121.J69 2004
468.2'421'02461–dc22

                                                                           2003061706

Acquisitions Editor: Jeanne Wilke
Developmental Editor: Rebecca Swisher
Publishing Services Manager: Pat Joiner
Project Manager: Karen M. Rehwinkel
Designer: Julia Dummitt
Cover Art: MW Design

Printed in the United States of America

Last digit is the print number: 9   8   7   6   5   4   3   2   1

I want to thank Raymond Joyce, for his perseverance in retyping the same chapters many times. He also carefully edited each chapter and provided feedback that was not only useful but very practical. Thanks to the contributors and to the hospitals that provided consent forms (Our Lady of the Lake Regional Medical Center, Baton Rouge, Louisiana and East Houston Regional Medical Center, Houston, Texas). My gratitude to all the health professionals who have bought this textbook. They are indeed increasing their quality of practice through communication.

E. V. Joyce

Special thanks to my daughter Claudia, who consistently helped by reading the translations multiple times, and José, my husband, who contributed with his kind support.

M. E. Villanueva

Preface

I am pleased to present you with the third edition of *Say It in Spanish: A Guide for Health Care Professionals*. The idea for this text grew from multiple observations in clinical settings where the frustrations of non-Spanish-speaking health care providers are evident. These frustrations stem from the lack of control providers feel when they are not in command of the language of their patients and must depend on translators for data collection. My bicultural background and my bilingualism have afforded me the opportunity to translate for many Spanish-speaking patients. This has allowed me to appreciate the predicament that Spanish-speaking patients find themselves in when they require medical care. The communication of simple facts can be difficult, and miscommunication can have lethal consequences.

As a faculty member in schools of nursing I was often amused by my students' comments: "Don't assign me a Spanish-speaking patient," or "I don't know how to speak Spanish." I had little choice, since 52 percent of the large medical centers' patient population was Hispanic. For many years I taught Spanish courses for nurses in academic and clinical centers. Evaluations confirmed that the courses helped students provide better care to their Spanish-speaking patients. Students were able to interact with families, collect data, and make meaningful contributions to their patients' care. In those settings, it was clear that the opportunities gained by knowledge of a second language were invaluable!

APPROACH

Say It in Spanish is designed primarily to meet the needs of health care professionals and students who anticipate contact with Spanish-speaking patients. Health providers in hospitals, clinics, physician's offices, outpatient and community centers, as well as students in nursing and allied health schools, can benefit from the use of this textbook. This text can also be used as a self-instructional program for those whose occupations bring them into daily contact with patients whose primary language is Spanish. To facilitate the self-instructional approach, all translations are accompanied by their pronunciation.

Over the past decade there has been a growing recognition in health care settings of the importance of communicating with Spanish-speaking patients. Clinicians who can communicate with their patients will be able to assess more effectively the success of the treatment they are providing. The Spanish expressions used in this book are primarily those used in Spanish-speaking countries close to the United States and Spanish communities within the United States. The term "Hispanic" includes persons from Mexico, South America, Central America, Puerto Rico, Cuba, and other countries where Spanish is the primary language. Note that each Spanish-speaking group has a distinct number of regional dialects and it would be difficult to capture each of them in any one book. In addition, this textbook does not contain pure Castillian language, since the majority of the Spanish-speaking persons living in the United States do not speak it.

This text provides an introduction to the Spanish language, but it is not a comprehensive grammar textbook. The intent is to present practical language that can be used in clinical settings in which intervention with a Spanish-speaking patient may be short term or long term. Those who use this text will be able to express in simple Spanish what they need to say. Special emphasis is placed on the use of meaningful medical vocabulary. Medical situations mentioned in the text are those experienced in everyday life.

NEW TO THIS EDITION

Much of the content from the second edition has been rearranged, some chapters have been combined, and three new chapters have been added. In addition, two audio CDs are included with the text. The CDs allow the clinician to listen to Chapter 5, "Physical Exam" and Chapter 28, "Greetings and Common Expressions." Each phrase is introduced in English and then in Spanish. The Spanish is repeated twice to increase familiarity with the pronunciation.

Chapter 7, "Consent to Procedures/Treatment," was added to this edition because in our litigious society it is of utmost importance that the patient understands the type of procedure, surgery, or treatment that he is agreeing to have. Patients who can read the form in Spanish will feel less apprehensive of surgical interventions.

Chapter 8, "Discharging a Patient," deals specifically with activities that the health care provider must focus on when discharging a patient from the hospital or an outpatient setting. Ideally, discharge planning ensures continuity of care. When communication occurs in a language that the patient is familiar with, the intention of discharge planning is validated.

Chapter 11, "Home Health/Hospice Care," will help with essential information that the health care provider must give to and elicit from the patient. Information about medications, activities of daily living, hazards in the environment, and follow-up are included in the chapter.

FEATURES OF THE TEXT

For the convenience of the health provider, Chapters 1 through 42 include English-Spanish usage. This bilingual text eliminates the time-consuming process of looking up words in the dictionary.

The questioning techniques presented have been selected to elicit **"yes"** or **"no"** answers. These will assist those providers who have a limited knowledge of Spanish.

Dialogues are presented as situations with corresponding appropriate basic vocabulary. The dialogues deal with familiar situations in the medical setting, and they are simple and interesting, so the provider has the opportunity to use repetition that will enhance retention.

Scenes are illustrated using basic vocabulary. This will help health providers to link the object with its Spanish equivalent without reference to English.

English phrases are not always translated literally; instead, the most common Spanish words have been selected and presented.

Tables in the chapters help the provider review key words, ideas, and concepts. A cultural perspective that increases the awareness of the health care provider for the needs of the Spanish-speaking population is included.

ORGANIZATION

The text is comprised of chapters organized to present a patient's usual movement from the community to the hospital setting. The first four chapters focus on practical language skills that are used in first aid, pre-hospital care, and emergency situations. The use of short dialogues that will elicit "yes" or "no" answers will facilitate data collection essential for immediate care. Chapters 5 through 9 provide essential information needed to perform a physical assessment, admit, interview, secure consents, and discharge a patient. Chapters 10 through 22 focus on specialties reflecting current health care emphasis. Chapter 11 will assist home health care workers to ask pertinent questions related to the health status of family members. Chapters 23 through 27 emphasize the most common vocabulary used in various hospital departments, such as pharmacy, laboratory, and radiology. The health provider can refer quickly to the appropriate chapter, thus increasing his or her communication skills and not delaying treatment while waiting for a translator.

The discussion of physical assessment (Chapter 5) specifically relates to internal and external parts of the body. Chapters 28 through 30 provide specific content related to greetings and common expressions that will assist in creating a welcoming environment for the patient. The chapters on phrases and commands will facilitate the completion of a physical assessment.

Chapters 32 through 35 present the terminology of numbers, time, colors, days, and months. These sections have been selected to enhance the health provider's knowledge of everyday terms that will be useful in the clinical setting.

Chapters 36 through 42 present an overview of the most essential grammatical concepts. The pronunciation and spelling of Spanish sounds are explained in detail. Most of the Spanish sounds are similar to sounds in English and therefore are easy to learn. These chapters provide the basis for appropriate use of the language and also serve as a quick reference.

The last two chapters describe cultural variations among Spanish-speaking groups, as well as the common health beliefs and popular health cures practiced by each group. The intent in this unit is to increase the health provider's awareness of cultural differences in the health perceptions of Spanish-speaking patients.

The English-Spanish index is divided into two sections: a phrase and sentence index and a word index. The unique phrase and sentence index is a useful tool that will save the health care worker time when determining which question to ask.

Difficult terms, important terms, and useful vocabulary are highlighted in tables that appear throughout the book.

Esperanza Villanueva Joyce

Contents

Unit 3 *Interacting with Health Care Providers*, 115
Unidad 3 *Comunicándose con Proveedores de la Salud*

Unit 4 *The Hospital Setting*, 197
Unidad 4 *En el Hospital*

Unit 5 *General Vocabulary*, 243
Unidad 5 *Vocabulario General*

Say It in
Spanish

Unit 1

Assessing, Admitting, and Discharging a Patient

Unidad 1

Evaluando, Admitiendo, y Dando de Alta al Paciente

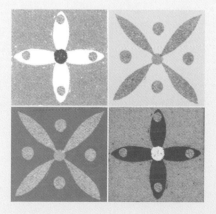

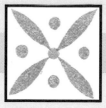

CHAPTER ONE
First Aid

CAPITULO UNO
Primeros Auxilios

Injury or sudden illness becomes an emergency when life is threatened. Injured persons depend on others for their well-being. Health providers must communicate accurately and in a language a patient can understand. In an emergency, there is no time for lengthy conversation. Use short phrases that elicit either a "yes" or "no" response.

Una herida o enfermedad repentina se convierte en una emergencia cuando la vida corre peligro. Las personas que han sufrido daños dependen de otros para sobrevivir. Los proveedores de la salud deben comunicarse con exactitud para darse a entender por el paciente. En un caso de emergencia, no hay tiempo para conversar. Use frases cortas para que las respuestas sean "sí" o "no".

Excuse me.	**Con permiso.**
	(Kohn pehr-mee-soh)
Let me go through.	**Déjeme pasar.**
	(Deh-heh-meh pah-sahr)
I need to see the injured.	**Necesito ver al accidentado.**
	(Neh-seh-see-toh behr ahl ahk-see-dehn-tah-doh)
Make some room!	**¡Haga lugar!**
	(Ah-gah loo-gahr)
Stay away!	**¡Hágase a un lado!**
	(Ah-gah-seh ah uhn lah-doh)
Don't touch anything!	**¡No toque nada!**
	(Noh toh-keh nah-dah)

Do not move the patient!

¡No mueva al paciente!
(Noh moo-eh-bah ahl pah-see-ehn-teh)

I have to assess first.

Necesito evaluar primero.
(Neh-seh-see-toh eh-vah-loo-ahr pree-meh-roh)

Other EMS staff ask questions if there are witnesses.

Otros empleados de servicios de emergencia hacen preguntas si hay testigos.

Who saw the accident?

¿Quién vió el accidente?
(Kee-ehn bee-oh ehl ahk-see-dehn-teh)

What kind of accident?

¿Qué tipo de accidente?
(Keh tee-poh deh ahk-see-dehn-teh)

How many cars crashed?

¿Cuántos carros chocaron?
(Koo-ahn-tohs kah-rohs choh-kah-rohn)

How many people were in the car/bus/truck?

¿Cuántas personas estaban en el carro/el autobús/la camioneta?
(Koo-ahn-tahs pehr-soh-nahs ehs-tah-bahn ehn ehl kah-roh/ehl ahoo-toh-boohs/lah kah-mee-oh-neh-tah)

Was the victim on the road?

¿Estaba la víctima en el camino?
(Ehs-tah-bah lah beek-tee-mah ehn ehl kah-mee-noh)

How did you move the victim?

¿Cómo movió a la víctima?
(Koh-moh moh-bee-oh ah lah beek-tee-mah)

Was the victim alive/dead?

¿Estaba la víctima con vida/muerta?
(Ehs-tah-bah lah beek-tee-mah kohn bee-dah/moo-ehr-tah)

Was the victim unconscious?

¿Estaba la víctima inconsciente?
(Ehs-tah-bah lah beek-tee-mah een-kohn-see-ehn-teh)

Use your hands when talking, pantomime, point, use facial expressions! There are several expressions you can use to get someone's attention (Table 1-1).

Use las manos al hablar, haga pantomimas, apunte, ¡use expresiones faciales! Hay varias expresiones que puede usar para atraer la atención (Tabla 1-1).

TABLE 1-1	Attention-Getting Phrases	
TABLA 1-1	Frases Para Atraer Atención	
English	**Spanish**	**Pronunciation**
Mr.	Señor	*seh-nyohr*
Mrs.	Señora	*seh-nyoh-rah*
Miss	Señorita	*seh-nyoh-ree-tah*
Listen!	¡Oiga!	*Oh-ee-gah*
Excuse me!	¡Perdón!	*Pehr-dohn*
young man/woman	joven	*hoh-behn*
boy/girl	muchacho(a)	*moo-chah-choh/moo-chah-chah*
boy/girl	niño(a)	*nee-nyoh/nee-nyah*

Miss	señorita
	(seh-nyoh-ree-tah)
Mrs.	señora
	(seh-nyoh-rah)
Mr.	señor
	(seh-nyohr)
Hello!	¡Hola!
	(Oh-lah)
Can you hear me?	¿Puede oírme?
	(Poo-eh-deh oh-eer-meh)
Can you talk?	¿Puede hablar?
	(Poo-eh-deh ah-blahr)
Can you breathe?	¿Puede respirar?
	(Poo-eh-deh rehs-pee-rahr)
What is your name?	¿Cómo se llama?
	(Koh-moh seh yah-mah)
Do you know where you are?	¿Sabe dónde está?
	(Sah-beh dohn-deh ehs-tah)
Do you know the day?	¿Qué día es hoy?
	(Keh dee-ah ehs oh-ee)
Please don't move.	Por favor, no se mueva.
	(Pohr fah-bohr noh seh moo-eh-bah)
I need to see if you are hurt.	Necesito ver si está lastimado.
	(Neh-seh-see-toh behr see ehs-tah
	lahs-tee-mah-doh)

Unless an emergency is life threatening, a person needs to participate in his/her own care to maintain a sense of control. Ask the patient to speak slowly when speaking Spanish and remind him/her to respond with "yes" or "no" as much as possible. Table 1-2 shows a list of common commands you can use.

A menos que esté en peligro la vida, una persona necesita participar en su cuidado para mantener el sentido de control. Pídale al paciente que hable despacio cuando hable en español y recuérdele que responda "sí" o "no" lo más posible. La Tabla 1-2 le muestra una lista de mandatos comunes que puede usar.

Open your eyes.	Abra los ojos.
	(Ah-brah lohs oh-hos)
Don't turn.	No voltee.
	(Noh bohl-teh-eh)
Where does it hurt?	¿Dónde le duele?
	(Don-deh leh doo-eh-leh)
Point.	Apunte/señale.
	(Ah-poon-teh/seh-nyah-leh)
Did you fall?	¿Se cayó?
	(Seh kah-yoh)
Were you hit by a car?	¿Le golpeó un carro?
	(Leh gohl-peh-oh oon kah-roh)
Did you lose consciousness?	¿Perdió el conocimiento?
	(Pehr-dee-oh ehl koh-noh-see-mee-ehn-toh)
Where do you live?	¿Dónde vive?
	(Dohn-deh bee-beh)

TABLE 1-2   Pronunciation of Commands
TABLA 1-2   Pronunciación de Mandatos

English	Spanish	Pronunciation
Sit!	¡Siéntese!	*See-ehn-teh-seh*
Move!	¡Mueva!	*Moo-eh-bah*
Don't move!	¡No se mueva!	*Noh seh moo-eh-bah*
Breath!	¡Respire!	*Rehs-pee-reh*
Speak!	¡Hable!	*Ah-bleh*
Open!	¡Abra!	*Ah-brah*
Turn!	¡Voltée!	*Bohl-teh-eh*
Be still!	¡Quieto!	*Kee-eh-toh*
Point!	¡Apunte!	*Ah-poon-teh*
	¡Señale!	*Seh-nyah-leh*
Bend!	¡Doble!	*Doh-bleh*

Do you remember the street?	¿Recuerda la calle? *(Reh-koo-ehr-dah lah kah-yeh)*
Where were you going?	¿A dónde iba? *(Ah dohn-deh ee-bah)*
Your leg is broken.	Tiene la pierna quebrada/ fracturada. *(Tee-eh-neh lah pee-ehr-nah keh- brah-dah/frahk-too-rah-dah)*
I need to cut the pants.	Necesito cortar el pantalón. *(Neh-seh-see-toh kohr-tahr ehl pahn- tah-lohn)*
I am going to put a splint on the leg.	Voy a ponerle una tablilla en la pierna. *(Boy ah poh-nehr-leh oo-nah tah- blee-yah ehn lah pee-ehr-nah)*
Do not bend your leg!	¡No doble la pierna! *(Noh doh-bleh lah pee-ehr-nah)*
Keep the leg straight.	Mantenga la pierna derecha. *(Mahn-tehn-gah lah pee-ehr-nah deh-reh-chah)*
I am going to cover you.	Lo voy a cubrir. *(Loh boy ah koo-breer)*
I will put you on the stretcher.	Voy a ponerlo en la camilla. *(Boy ah poh-nehr-loh ehn lah kah- mee-yah)*
We are going to the hospital.	Vamos al hospital. *(Bah-mohs ahl ohs-pee-tahl)*
We are going in the ambulance.	Vamos en la ambulancia. *(Bah-mohs ehn lah ahm-boo-lahn- see-ah)*
It takes 10 minutes.	Se toma diez minutos. *(Seh toh-mah dee-ehs mee-noo-tohs)*
Have you been a patient before?	¿Ha sido paciente antes? *(Ah see-doh pah-see-ehn-teh ahn-tehs)*
Have you had any accidents?	¿Ha tenido algún accidente? *(Ah teh-nee-doh ahl-goon ahk-see- dehn-teh)*

While traveling to the Emergency Room and if the patient's condition is stable, ask for more information. This helps the staff to complete forms and decrease delays in calling family or friends (Table 1-3).

Mientras que viaja al cuarto de emergencias y si la condición del paciente es estable, haga más preguntas. Esto ayuda a los empleados a completar las formas y disminuye la demora en llamar a la familia o a los amigos (Tabla 1-3).

TABLE 1-3   Other Important Questions
TABLA 1-3   Otras Preguntas Importantes

English	Spanish	Pronunciation
Did you faint?	¿Se desmayó?	*Seh dehs-mah-yoh*
Do you feel nauseated?	¿Siente náuseas?	*See-ehn-teh nah-oo-seh-ahs*
Do you feel weak?	¿Se siente débil?	*Seh see-ehn-teh deh-beel*
Do you feel dizzy?	¿Se siente mareado?	*Seh see-ehn-teh mah-reh-ah-doh*
Are you cold?	¿Tiene frío?	*Tee-eh-neh free-oh*
Are you hot?	¿Tiene calor?	*Tee-eh-neh kah-lohr*

What kind?
¿Qué clase?
(Keh klah-seh)

Have you had anything broken?
¿Ha tenido algo quebrado?
(Ah teh-nee-doh ahl-goh keh-brah-doh)

How long ago?
¿Hace cuánto tiempo?
(Ah-seh koo-ahn-toh tee-ehm-poh)

Were you hospitalized?
¿Lo hospitalizaron?
(Loh ohs-pee-tah-lee-sah-rohn)

Do you know the hospital name?
¿Sabe el nombre del hospital?
(Sah-beh ehl nohm-breh dehl ohs-pee-tahl)

The doctor will see you in the Emergency Room.
Lo verá el doctor en el cuarto de emergencia.
(Loh beh-rah ehl dohk-tohr ehn ehl koo-ahr-toh deh eh-mehr-hehn-see-ah)

The doctor will give you something for the pain.
El doctor le dará algo para el dolor.
(Ehl dohk-tohr leh dah-rah ahl-goh pah-rah ehl doh-lohr)

The nurse will ask how you feel.
La enfermera le preguntará como se siente.
(Lah ehn-fehr-meh-rah leh preh-goon-tah-rah koh-moh seh see-ehn-teh)

They will let you talk to your family.	Le dejarán hablar con su familia. *(Leh deh-hah-rahn ah-blahr kohn soo fah-mee-lee-ah)*
Do you have a phone?	¿Tiene teléfono? *(Tee-eh-neh teh-leh-foh-noh)*
Give it to the clerk.	Déselo a la secretaria. *(Deh-seh-loh ah lah seh-kreh-tah-ree-ah)*
Is your family in town?	¿Está su familia en la ciudad? *(Ehs-tah soo fah-mee-lee-ah ehn lah see-oo-dahd)*

Add *es* to a singular noun that ends in a consonant *z* to make it a plural. In words ending in *z*, change the *z* to *c* before adding *es*. Add *s* to a singular noun that ends in a vowel to make it a plural noun. Table 1-4 lists examples of singular and plural nouns and articles.

Añada *es* al nombre singular que termina en una consonante para hacerlo plural. Si la palabra termina en *z*, cambie la *z* a *c* antes de agregar *es*. Añada *s* al nombre singular que termina en una vocal para hacerlo plural. La Tabla 1-4 da una lista de ejemplos de nombres y artículos singulares y plurales.

TABLE 1-4   Singular and Plural
TABLA 1-4   Singular y Plural

Singular		Plural	
the girl	la niña *(lah nee-nyah)*	the girls	las niñas *(lahs nee-nyahs)*
the boy	el niño *(ehl nee-nyoh)*	the boys	los niños *(lohs nee-nyohs)*
the doctor	el doctor *(ehl dohk-tohr)*	the doctors	los doctores *(lohs dohk-toh-rehs)*
the hospital	el hospital *(ehl ohs-pee-tahl)*	the hospitals	los hospitales *(lohs ohs-pee-tah-lehs)*
a heart	un corazón *(oon koh-rah-sohn)*	some hearts	unos corazones *(oo-nohs koh-rah-sohn-ehs)*
a table	una mesa *(oo-nah meh-sah)*	some tables	unas mesas *(oo-nahs meh-sahs)*
a pencil	un lápiz *(oon lah-pees)*	some pencils	unos lápices *(oo-nohs lah-pee-sehs)*

Do you have any children?	¿Tiene niños? *(Tee-eh-neh nee-nyohs)*
How many?	¿Cuántos? *(Koo-ahn-tohs)*
How many boys/girls?	¿Cuántos niños/Cuántas niñas? *(Koo-ahn-tohs nee-nyohs/Koo-ahn-tahs nee-nyahs)*
How old are they?	¿Cuántos años tienen? *(Koo-ahn-tohs ah-nyohs tee-eh-nehn)*
Do all go to school?	¿Todos van a la escuela? *(Toh-dohs bahn ah lah ehs-koo-eh-lah)*
What is the name of the school?	¿Cómo se llama la escuela? *(Koh-moh seh yah-mah lah ehs-koo-eh-lah)*
Do you have a husband/wife?	¿Tiene esposo/esposa? *(Tee-eh-neh ehs-poh-soh/ehs-poh-sah)*
Is he/she at work?	¿Está trabajando? *(Ehs-tah trah-bah-hahn-doh)*
Do you know his/her phone number?	¿Sabe su teléfono? *(Sah-beh soo teh-leh-foh-noh)*
Do you have brothers/sisters?	¿Tiene hermanos/hermanas? *(Tee-eh-neh ehr-mah-nohs/ehr-mah-nahs)*
Do they live close to you?	¿Viven cerca de usted? *(Bee-behn sehr-kah deh oos-tehd)*
What do you do?	¿Qué hace usted? *(Keh ah-seh oos-tehd)*
Are you employed?	¿Trabaja usted? *(Trah-bah-hah oos-tehd)*
Where do you work?	¿Dónde trabaja? *(Dohn-deh trah-bah-hah)*
Do you know the street name?	¿Sabe el nombre de la calle? *(Sah-beh ehl nohm-breh deh lah kah-yeh)*
Do you work every day?	¿Trabaja todos los días? *(Trah-bah-hah toh-dohs lohs dee-ahs)*
How many hours do you work?	¿Cuántas horas trabaja? *(Koo-ahn-tahs oh-rahs trah-bah-hah)*
Who can take care of the children?	¿Quién puede cuidar a los niños? *(Kee-ehn poo-eh-deh koo-ee-dahr ah lohs nee-nyohs)*

You will need a cast.	Necesitará un yeso.
	(Neh-seh-see-tah-rah oon yeh-soh)
You can walk on crutches.	Puede caminar con muletas.
	(Poo-eh-deh kah-mee-nahr kohn moo-leh-tahs)
Keep your leg elevated.	Mantenga la pierna elevada.
	(Mahn-tehn-gah lah pee-ehr-nah eh-leh-bah-dah)
Can you take off work?	¿Puede faltar al trabajo?
	(Poo-eh-deh fahl-tahr ahl trah-bah-hoh)
Are you on vacation?	¿Está de vacaciones?
	(Ehs-tah deh bah-kah-see-ohn-ehs)
Can you take vacation?	¿Puede tomar vacaciones?
	(Poo-eh-deh toh-mahr bah-kah-see-ohn-ehs)
Do you have another car?	¿Tiene otro carro?
	(Tee-eh-neh oh-troh kah-roh)
Do you have car insurance?	¿Tiene seguro de carro?
	(Tee-eh-neh seh-goo-roh deh kah-roh)
Do you have hospital insurance?	¿Tiene seguro de hospital?
	(Tee-eh-neh seh-goo-roh deh ohs-pee-tahl)
Do you have help at home?	¿Tiene ayuda en casa?
	(Tee-eh-neh ah-yoo-dah ehn kah-sah)
Will you need help?	¿Va a necesitar ayuda?
	(Bah ah neh-seh-see-tahr ah-yoo-dah)
Call your friends.	Llame a sus amigos.
	(Yah-meh ah soos ah-mee-gohs)
They can help clean.	Pueden ayudar a limpiar.
	(Poo-eh-dehn ah-yoo-dahr ah leem-pee-ahr)
Try to calm down.	Trate de calmarse.
	(Trah-teh deh kahl-mahr-seh)
You will get help.	Se le ayudará.
	(Seh leh ah-yoo-dah-rah)

We know the gender of a Spanish word by its ending. If the word ends in *a* usually it is feminine. If the word ends in *o* usually it is masculine (Table 1-5).

Se determina el género de la palabra en español al ver su terminación. Si la palabra termina en *a* es femenina. Si la palabra termina en *o* es masculina (Tabla 1-5).

| TABLE 1-5 | Nouns and Articles |
| TABLA 1-5 | Sustantivos y Artículos |

Nouns ending in *a, d, ión,* or *z* are feminine. Female nouns are feminine.		Nouns ending in *o, or, al,* or *dor* are masculine. Male nouns are masculine even though the noun may end in *a*.	
the	la (feminine) (lah)	the	el (masculine) (ehl)
a *or* an	una (feminine) (oo-nah)	a *or* an	un (masculine) (oon)
the house	la casa (lah kah-sah)	the man	el hombre (ehl ohm-breh)
a door	una puerta (oo-nah poo-ehr-tah)	an author	un autor (oon ah-oo-tohr)
the daughter	la hija (lah ee-hah)	the son	el hijo (ehl ee-hoh)
the friend	la amiga (lah ah-me-gah)	the friend	el amigo (ehl ah-mee-goh)
the woman	la mujer (lah moo-hehr)	the hospital	el hospital (ehl ohs-pee-tahl)
the health	la salud (lah sah-lood)	the month	el mes (ehl mehs)

IMPORTANT EXCEPTION:
the hand *la mano.* Note the ending *o,* yet *la mano* is FEMININE.
The days of the week, months of the year, and the names of languages are masculine.

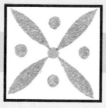

CHAPTER TWO
Pre-Hospital Care

CAPITULO DOS
Cuidados Pre-Hospitalarios

Emergency Medical Technicians (EMTs) are trained to provide efficient and immediate care to persons who have sustained injuries or trauma.

Los Técnicos de Cuidados de Emergencia están entrenados para proveer cuidado inmediato y eficiente a personas que han tenido daños o trauma.

Typical EMT questions when the patient is conscious may include those in Table 2-1. See below for additional questions.

Preguntas típicas que hacen los técnicos cuando el paciente está consciente pueden incluir las palabras en la tabla 2-1. Vea abaja para preguntas adicionales.

Are you from this area?

¿Es usted de esta área?
(Ehs oos-tehd deh ehs-tah ah-reh-ah)

Are you under a doctor's care?

¿Está bajo el cuidado de un doctor?
(Ehs-tah bah-hoh ehl koo-ee-dah-doh deh uhn dohk-tohr)

At what hospital have you been treated?

¿En qué hospital lo han tratado?
(Ehn keh ohs-pee-tahl loh ahn trah-tah-doh)

Did you take medications today? When?

¿Tomó sus medicinas hoy? ¿Cuándo?
(Toh-moh soos meh-dee-see-nahs oh-ee) (Koo-ahn-doh)

Do you have any symptoms: nausea, dizziness, other unusual feelings?

¿Tiene algún síntoma como: náuseas, vértigo, otra sensación rara?
(Tee-eh-neh ahl-goon seen-toh-mah koh-moh nah-oo-seh-ahs, behr-tee-goh, oh-trah sehn-sah-see-ohn rah- rah)

Do you have allergies?

¿Tiene alergias?
(Tee-eh-neh ah-lehr-ghee-ahs)

Do you have medical problems:

¿Tiene problemas médicos:
(Tee-eh-neh proh-bleh-mahs meh-dee-kohs)

Cardiac problems?

¿Problemas cardíacos?
(proh-bleh-mahs kahr-dee-ah-kohs)

Respiratory problems?

¿Problemas respiratorios?
(proh-bleh-mahs rehs-pee-rah-toh-ree-ohs)

Renal problems?

Problemas renales?
(proh-bleh-mahs reh-nah-lehs)

Do you live here?

¿Vive aquí?
(Bee-beh ah-kee)

Do you take medications?

¿Toma medicinas?
(Toh-mah meh-dee-see-nahs)

Which ones?

¿Cuáles?
(Koo-ah-lehs)

Does the pain move from one place to another?

¿El dolor se mueve de un lugar a otro?
(Ehl doh-lohr seh moo-eh-beh deh oon loo-gahr ah oh-troh)

Does the pain get better if you stop and rest?

¿Se mejora el dolor si se detiene y descansa?
(Seh meh-hoh-rah ehl doh-lohr see seh deh-tee-eh-neh oh dehs-kahn-sah)

Did anyone treat you prior to our arrival?

¿Lo trató alguien antes de nuestra llegada?
(Loh trah-toh ahl-gee-ehn ahn-tehs deh noo-ehs-trah yeh-gah-dah)

Has this problem happened before?

¿Le ha pasado antes este problema?
(Leh ah pah-sah-doh ahn-tehs ehs-teh proh-bleh-mah)

Has the pain gotten worse or gotten better?

¿Se ha puesto el dolor peor o mejor?
(Seh ah poo-ehs-toh ehl doh-lohr peh-ohr oh meh-hohr)

	TABLE 2-1	Typical Questions
	TABLA 2-1	Preguntas Típicas

English	Spanish	Pronunciation
Do you have a doctor?	¿Tiene un doctor?	Tee-eh-neh oon dohk-tohr
What hospital do you go to?	¿A qué hospital va?	Ah keh ohs-pee-tahl bah
Do you take medicines?	¿Toma medicinas?	Toh-mah meh-dee-see-nahs
What do you feel?	¿Qué siente?	Keh see-ehn-teh
Do you have pain?	¿Tiene dolor?	Tee-eh-neh doh-lohr
Are you nauseated?	¿Está nauseado?	Ehs-tah nah-oo-seh-ah-doh
Do you have medical problems?	¿Tiene problemas medicos?	Tee-eh-neh proh-bleh-mahs meh-dee-kohs
Has this happened to you before?	¿Le ha pasado esto antes?	Leh ah pah-sah-doh ehs-toh ahn-tehs
What were you doing?	¿Qué estaba haciendo?	Keh ehs-tah-bah ah-see-ehn-doh
What caused the accident?	¿Qué causó el accidente?	Keh kah-oo-soh ehl ahk-see-dehn-teh

Did you take drugs or alcohol in the last 3 hours?	¿Tomó drogas o alcohol en las últimas tres horas?
	(Toh-moh droh-gahs oh ahl-kohl ehn lahs ool-tee-mahs trehs oh-rahs)
How much medicine did you take?	¿Cuánta medicina tomó?
	(Koo-ahn-tah meh-dee-see-nah toh-moh)
How old are you?	¿Cuántos años tiene?
	(Koo-ahn-tohs ah-nyohs tee-eh-neh)
How often do you have the pain?	¿Qué tan seguido tiene el dolor?
	(Keh tahn seh-gee-doh tee-eh-neh ehl doh-lohr)
How severe is the pain?	¿Qué tan severo es el dolor?
	(Keh tahn seh-beh-roh ehs ehl doh-lohr)

On a scale from 1 (insignificant) to 10 (unbearable):	En una escala del uno (insignificante) al diez (intolerable): *(Ehn oo-nah ehs-kah-lah dehl oo-noh [een-seeg-nee-fee-kahn-teh] ahl dee-ehs [een-toh-leh-rah-bleh])*
Is the pain there all the time, or does it come and go?	¿Está el dolor allí todo el tiempo, o va y viene? *(Ehs-tah ehl doh-lohr ah-yee toh-doh ehl tee-ehm-poh, oh bah ee bee-ehn-eh?)*
Tell me, have you ever had a heart attack?	Dígame, ¿A tenido alguna vez un ataque cardíaco? *(Dee-gah-meh, Ah teh-nee-doh ahl-goo-nah behs oon ah-tah-keh kahr-dee-ah-koh)*
What is bothering you the most?	¿Qué es lo que más le molesta? *(Keh ehs loh keh mahs leh moh-lehs-tah)*
What caused the pain?	¿Qué causó el dolor? *(Keh kah-oo-soh ehl doh-lohr)*
What did you do that caused the pain?	¿Qué hacía cuando apareció el dolor? *(Keh ah-see-ah koo-ahn-doh ah-pah-reh-see-oh ehl doh-lohr)*
What makes the pain better?	¿Qué hace mejorar el dolor? *(Keh ah-seh meh-hoh-rahr ehl doh-lohr)*

Get close to the patient if he is responsive and appears to be alert. It will help ease his fear. Ask questions clearly and at a normal rate. Do not say such things as, "Everything will be OK," or "Take it easy." The patient knows differently. He may have little confidence in you if you use such phrases. Typical questions asked of witnesses are found in Table 2-2.

Acérquese al paciente si responde y parece estar alerta. Esto ayuda a disminuir el miedo. Haga preguntas claras y de manera normal. No le diga cosas como "Todo estará bien" o "Tómelo con calma." El paciente sabe lo contrario y tendrá menos confianza en usted si usa frases semejantes. Preguntas típicas que se hacen a los testigos se encuentran en la Tabla 2-2.

Were you knocked down, did you fall, or were you thrown?	¿Se golpeó, se cayó o lo lanzó el impacto? *(Seh gohl-peh-oh, seh kah-yoh, oh loh lahn-soh ehl eem-pahk-toh)*

| TABLE 2-2 | Typical Questions to Witnesses | |
| TABLA 2-2 | Preguntas Típicas a Testigos | |

English	Spanish	Pronunciation
Did you see how the accident happened?	¿Vió cómo pasó el accidente?	Bee-oh koh-moh pah-soh ehl ahk-see-dehn-teh
Are you related?	¿Es pariente?	Ehs pah-ree-ehn-teh
Do you know him/her?	¿Lo/la conoce?	Loh/lah koh-noh-seh
Who moved him/her?	¿Quién lo/la movió?	Kee-ehn loh/lah moh-bee-oh
Was the car burning?	¿Estaba el carro en llamas?	Ehs-tah-bah ehl kah-roh ehn yah-mahs
Was he/she conscious?	¿Estaba conciente?*	Ehs-tah-bah kohn-see-ehn-teh
How did he/she fall?	¿Cómo se cayó?*	Koh-moh seh kah-yoh
From what height did he/she fall?	¿De qué altura cayó?*	Deh keh ahl-too-rah kah-yoh

*Note that there is no need to repeat the article for the person (he/she) in Spanish. It is understood.

Did you hit the windshield/ steering wheel?	¿Se pegó contra el parabrisas/ volante? (Seh peh-goh kohn-trah ehl pah-rah-bree-sahs/boh-lahn-teh)
Has this happened before?	¿Pasó esto antes? (Pah-soh ehs-toh ahn-tehs)
How did this injury happen?	¿Cómo ocurrió esta lesión? (Koh-moh oh-koo-ree-oh ehs-tah leh-see-ohn)
Were you thrown forward/backward?	¿Fué lanzado hacia adelante/ hacia atrás? (Foo-eh lahn-sah-doh ah-see-ah ah-deh-lahn-teh/ah-see-ah ah-trahs)
I have to call your parents.	Tengo que llamar a sus padres. (Tehn-goh keh yah-mahr ah soos pah-drehs)
Is there numbness/a tingling sensation/burning in your leg/arm/foot/hand?	¿Está entumecido/adormecido/ tiene ardor en su pierna/ brazo/pie/mano? (Ehs-tah ehn-too-meh-see-doh/ah-dohr-meh-see-do/tee-eh-neh ahr- dohr ehn soo pee-ehr-nah/brah-soh/pee-eh/mah-noh)

Were you thrown from the car?	¿Fué lanzado fuera del carro?
	(Foo-eh lahn-sah-doh foo-eh-rah dehl kah-roh)
What is wrong?	¿Qué pasa?
	(Keh pah-sah)
Is there any pain?	¿Tiene algún dolor?
	(Tee-eh-neh ahl-goon doh-lohr)
What problems do you have?	¿Qué problema tiene?
	(Keh proh-bleh-mah tee-eh-neh)
Where can I reach your mother or father?	¿Dónde puedo localizar a su mamá o su papá?
	(Dohn-deh poo-eh-doh loh-kah-lee-sahr ah soo mah-mah oh soo pah-pah)

As part of the assessment, EMTs must frequently give commands to the patients. Some commands are found in Table 2-3.

Como parte de la evaluación, los Técnicos de Cuidados de Emergencia dan órdenes a los pacientes. Algunos mandatos se encuentran en la Tabla 2-3.

The following are typical commands.

Las siguientes son órdenes comunes.

Breathe in.	Respire.
	(Rehs-pee-reh)
Breathe out.	Saque el aire.
	(Sah-keh ehl ah-ee-reh)
Hold your breath.	Sostenga la respiración.
	(Sohs-tehn-gah la rehs-pee-rah-see-ohn)
Open your mouth.	Abra la boca.
	(Ah-brah lah boh-kah)
Open your eyes.	Abra los ojos.
	(Ah-brah lohs oh-hohs)
Follow my finger.	Siga mi dedo.
	(See-gah mee deh-doh)
Don't move.	No se mueva.
	(Noh seh moo-eh-bah)
Push down with your feet against my hands.	Empuje los pies contra mis manos.
	(Ehm-poo-heh lohs pee-ehs kohn-trah mees mah-nohs)
Relax your leg.	Relaje la pierna.
	(Reh-lah-heh lah pee-ehr-nah)
Relax your arm.	Relaje el brazo.
	(Reh-lah-heh ehl brah-soh)
Squeeze my hand.	Apriete mi mano.
	(Ah-pree-eh-teh mee mah-noh)

TABLE 2-3   Typical Commands
TABLA 2-3   Mandatos Típicos

English	Spanish	Pronunciation
Open your eyes!	¡Abra los ojos!	Ah-brah lohs oh-hohs
Do not move!	¡No se mueva!	Noh seh moo-eh-bah
Move carefully!	¡Muévase con cuidado!	Moo-eh-bah-seh kohn koo-ee-dah-doh
Open your mouth!	¡Abra la boca!	Ah-brah lah boh-kah
Listen!	¡Escuche!	Ehs-koo-cheh
	¡Oiga!	Oh-ee-gah
Keep moving!	¡Siga moviéndose!	See-gah moh-bee-ehn-doh-seh
Push!	¡Empuje!	Ehm-poo-heh
Squeeze my hand!	¡Apriete mi mano!	Ah-pree-eh-teh mee mah-noh

Squeeze the fingers of each of my hands.

Apriete cada uno de los dedos de mi mano.
(Ah-pree-eh-teh kah-dah oo-noh deh lohs deh-dohs deh mee mah-noh)

Stick your tongue out.

Saque la lengua.
(Sah-keh lah lehn-goo-ah)

Tell me if this hurts.

Dígame si esto le duele.
(Dee-gah-meh see ehs-toh leh doo-eh-leh)

Patients have a variety of responses when questions are asked about their condition or accident.

Los pacientes dan una variedad de respuestas cuando se les pregunta acerca de su condición o su accidente.

The following are some examples of responses.

Los siguientes son unos ejemplos de respuestas.

I was just sitting, watching television when the pain started.

Sólo estaba sentado, viendo televisión cuando comenzó el dolor.
(Soh-loh ehs-tah-bah sehn-tah-doh, bee-ehn-doh teh-leh-bee-see-ohn koo-ahn-doh koh-mehn-soh ehl doh-lohr)

I was doing nothing.

No estaba haciendo nada.
(Noh ehs-tah-bah ah-see-ehn-doh nah-dah)

Nothing seems to make it better or worse.	Nada parece hacerlo peor o mejor. *(Nah-dah pah-reh-seh ah-sehr-loh peh-ohr oh meh-hohr)*
The pain is sharp.	El dolor es agudo. *(Ehl doh-lohr ehs ah-goo-doh*
The pain starts here (beneath the sternum) and goes to my jaw.	El dolor comienza aquí(abajo del esternón) y se va a la mandíbula. *(Ehl doh-lohr koh-mee-ehn-sah ah-kee [ah-bah-hoh dehl ehs-tehr-nohn] ee seh bah ah lah mahn-dee-boo-lah)*
The pain is constant.	El dolor es constante. *(Ehl doh-lohr ehs kohns-tahn-teh)*
The pain has gotten worse.	El dolor ha empeorado. *(Ehl doh-lohr ah ehm-peh-oh-rah-doh)*
The pain starts here and travels down my left arm.	El dolor comienza aquí y se recorre por el brazo izquierdo. *(Ehl doh-lohr koh-mee-ehn-sah ah-kee ee seh reh-koh-reh pohr ehl brah-soh ees-kee-ehr-doh)*
The pain is cutting.	El dolor es cortante. *(Ehl doh-lohr ehs kohr-tahn-teh)*
The pain started two hours ago.	El dolor comenzó hace dos horas. *(Ehl doh-lohr koh-mehn-soh ah-seh dohs oh-rahs)*
The pain is throbbing.	El dolor es punzante. *(Ehl doh-lohr ehs poon-sahn-teh)*

Dialogue between a paramedic and a patient.
Diálogo entre un paramédico y un paciente.

Paramedic: Hello, I'm John Goodguy.	*Paramédico: (Pah-rah-meh-dee-koh)* Hola, soy John Goodguy. *(Oh-lah, soh-ee John Goodguy)*
I'm a paramedic.	Soy paramédico. *(Soh-ee pah-rah-meh-dee-koh)*
What happened here?	¿Qué pasa aquí? *(Keh pah-sah ah-kee)*
Patient: The kids left their skates on the stairs and I fell over them.	*Paciente: (Pah-see-ehn-teh)* Los niños dejaron los patines en las escaleras y me tropecé. *(Lohs nee-nyohs deh-hah-rohn lohs pah-tee-nehs ehn lahs ehs-kah-leh-rahs ee meh troh-peh-seh)*

Paramedic:
I guess this wasn't a planned activity for today!

Paramédico: (Pah-rah-meh-dee-koh)
¡Supongo que esta actividad no estaba planeada para hoy!
(Soo-pohn-goh keh ehs-tah ahk-tee-bee-dahd noh ehs-tah-bah plah-neh-ah-dah pah-rah oh-ee)

Patient:
That is for sure!

Paciente: (Pah-see-ehn-teh)
¡Délo por seguro!
(Deh-loh pohr seh-goo-roh)

Paramedic:
Tell me your name

How old are you?

Paramédico: (Pah-rah-meh-dee-koh)
Dígame su nombre.
(Dee-gah-meh soo nohm-breh)
¿Cuántos años tiene?
(Koo-ahn-tohs ah-nyohs tee-eh-neh)

Patient:
My name is Mr. Badluck

I'm 53.

Paciente: (Pah-see-ehn-teh)
Mi nombre es señor Badluck.
(Mee nohm-breh ehs seh-nyohr Badluck)
Tengo cincuenta y tres años.
(Tehn-goh seen-koo-ehn-tah ee trehs ah-nyos)

Paramedic:
Tell me where it hurts, Mr. Badluck.

Paramédico: (Pah-rah-meh-dee-koh)
Dígame dónde le duele señor Badluck.
(Dee-gah-meh dohn-deh leh doo-eh-leh, seh-nyohr Badluck)

Patient:
My left leg hurts.

I think it is broken.

Paciente: (Pah-see-ehn-teh)
Me duele la pierna izquierda.
(Meh doo-eh-leh lah pee-ehr-nah ees-kee-ehr-dah)
Creo que está rota.
(Kreh-oh keh ehs-tah roh-tah)

Paramedic:
Well, it is possible.

What is the pain like?

Paramédico: (Pah-rah-meh-dee-koh)
Pues, es posible.
(Poo-ehs ehs poh-see-bleh)
¿Qué tipo de dolor tiene?
(Keh tee-poh deh doh-lohr tee-eh-neh)

Patient:
Right now it is throbbing like a bad toothache.

Paciente: (Pah-see-ehn-teh)
Ahora está punzando, como un mal dolor de muelas.
(Ah-oh-rah ehs-tah poon-sahn-doh, koh-moh oon mahl doh-lohr deh moo-eh-lahs)

Paramedic:
How bad is it?

Patient:
It is not as bad when I stay
   still, but it hurts a lot if I
   try to move the leg.

Paramedic:
Is there anything else
   bothering you?

Patient:
No, not that I know of.

Well, I do have a tingling
   feeling in my left foot. It
   must have gone to sleep.

Paramedic:
I see.

Patient:
Also, I have a headache.

I never have headaches!

Paramedic:
Are you under a doctor's care,
   Mr. Badluck?

Patient:
Yes, Dr. Fellow at Juan Sealy
   General. He keeps track of my
   cholesterol.

Paramédico: (Pah-rah-meh-dee-koh)
¿Qué tan mal está?
(Keh tahn mahl ehs-tah)
Paciente: (Pah-see-ehn-teh)
No está tan mal cuando estoy
   quieto, pero me duele mucho si
   trato de mover la pierna.
*(Noh ehs-tah tahn mahl koo-ahn-
   doh ehs-toh-ee kee-eh-toh, peh-
   roh meh doo-eh-leh moo-choh see
   trah-toh deh moh-behr lah pee-
   ehr-nah)*
Paramédico: (Pah-rah-meh-dee-koh)
¿Hay otra cosa que le moleste?
*(Ah-ee oh-trah koh-sah keh leh
   moh-lehs-teh?*
Paciente: (Pah-see-ehn-teh)
No, que yo sepa.
(Noh, keh yoh seh-pah)
Pues, tengo picazón en el pie
   izquierdo. Se me durmió.
*(Poo-ehs, tehn-goh pee-kah-sohn
   ehn ehl pee-eh ees-kee-ehr-doh.
   Seh meh duhr-mee-oh)*
Paramédico: (Pah-rah-meh-dee-koh)
Ya veo.
(Yah beh-oh)
Paciente: (Pah-see-ehn-teh)
También, tengo dolor de cabeza.
*(Tahm-bee-ehn, tehn-goh doh-
   lohr deh kah-beh-sah)*
¡Nunca tengo dolor de cabeza!
*(Noon-kah tehn-goh doh-lohr deh
   kah-beh-sah)*
Paramédico: (Pah-rah-meh-dee-koh)
¿Está bajo el cuidado de un
   doctor, Señor Badluck?
*(Ehs-tah bah-hoh ehl koo-ee-
   dah-doh deh oon dohk-tohr, Seh-
   nyohr Badluck)*
Paciente: (Pah-see-ehn-teh)
Sí, el doctor Fellow en Juan
   Sealy General. El me controla
   el colesterol.
*(See. Ehl dohk-tohr Fellow ehn Juan
   Sealy General. Ehl meh kohn-troh-
   lah ehl koh-lehs-teh-rohl)*

Paramedic:
Besides your cholesterol, are there any other medical problems?

Patient:
None.

Paramedic:
Do you take any medication?

Patient:
Lescol for the cholesterol and naproxin for my aches.

Paramedic:
Are you allergic to anything?

Patient:
Nothing that I have ever known of.

Paramedic:
OK Mr. Badluck, my partner and I are going to put the leg in a splint to keep it from moving around on the way to the hospital.

Paramédico: (Pah-rah-meh-dee-koh)
Además de su colesterol, ¿tiene otros problemas médicos?
(Ah-deh-mahs deh soo koh-lehs-teh-rohl, tee-eh-neh oh-trohs proh-bleh-mahs meh-dee-kohs)

Paciente: (Pah-see-ehn-teh)
Ninguno.
(Neen-goo-noh)

Paramédico: (Pah-rah-meh-dee-koh)
¿Toma alguna medicina?
(Toh-mah ahl-goo-nah meh-dee-see-nah?

Paciente: (Pah-see-ehn-teh)
Lescol para el colesterol y Naproxeno para mis dolores.
(Lehs-kohl pah-rah ehl koh-lehs-teh-rohl ee nah-prohx-eh-noh pah-rah mees doh-loh-rehs)

Paramédico: (Pah-rah-meh-dee-koh)
¿Es alérgico a alguna cosa?
(Ehs ah-lehr-hee-koh ah ahl-goo-nah koh-sah)

Paciente: (Pah-see-ehn-teh)
A nada que yo sepa.
(Ah nah-dah keh yoh seh-pah)

Paramédico: (Pah-rah-meh-dee-koh)
OK señor Badluck, mi compañero y yo vamos a entablillar la pierna para no moverla mucho en el viaje al hospital.
(OK seh-nyohr Badluck, mee kohm-pah-nyeh-roh ee yoh bah-mohs ah ehn-tah-blee-yahr lah pee-ehr-nah pah-rah noh moh-behr-lah moo-choh ehn ehl bee-ah-heh ahl ohs-pee-tahl)

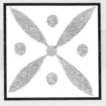

CHAPTER THREE
Emergency Care

CAPITULO TRES
Cuidado de Urgencia
(Emergencia)

Emergency rooms are frequently very busy. There is a tendency to rush through procedures. When possible, take a few extra minutes to attempt to communicate so your diagnosis is accurate. This saves time in the long run.

Los cuartos de urgencia (emergencia) frecuentemente están ocupados. Hay una tendencia a apurarse en los procedimientos. Cuando le sea posible, tome unos minutos adicionales para intentar la comunicación para que su diagnóstico sea exacto. Esto ahorra tiempo a la larga.

While taking the vital signs, the triage nurse observes the patient's breathing. She checks the carotid and peripheral pulses. She next checks for uncontrolled bleeding and shock. Finding no immediate problems, she begins a systematic assessment.

Mientras toma los signos vitales, la enfermera del área del triage observa la respiración del paciente. Ella revisa los pulsos de la carótida y los periféricos. Después verifica si hay sangrados y choque. Al no encontrar problemas inmediatos, inicia una evaluación sistemática.

The words in Table 3-1 will help you with common emergency terms.

Las palabras en la Tabla 3-1 le ayudarán con los términos de emergencia comúnes.

May I help you?	¿Puedo ayudarlo?
	¿Poo-eh-doh ah-yoo-dahr-loh?
—I have been sick all morning.	—Me he sentido mal toda la mañana.
	(Meh eh sehn-tee-doh mahl toh-dah lah mah-nyah-nah)

Are you having problems
 breathing?

¿Tiene problemas al respirar?
*(Tee-eh-neh proh-bleh-mahs ahl
 rehs-pee-rahr)*

—I have noticed some difficulty
 for the last two days.

—Me he dado cuenta de alguna
 dificultad para respirar en los
 últimos dos días.
*(Meh eh dah-doh koo-ehn-tah deh
 ahl-goo-nah dee-fee-kuhl-tahd
 pah-rah rehs-pee-rahr ehn lohs
 ool-tee-mohs dohs dee-ahs)*

Have you had any hard blows to
 your head or chest?

¿Se ha golpeado fuerte la
 cabeza o el tórax?
*(Seh ah gohl-peh-ah-doh foo-
 ehr-teh lah kah-beh-zah oh ehl
 toh-rahx)*

—No.

—No.
(Noh)

Have you had any bleeding,
 swelling, or bruising?

¿Ha tenido sangrados, hinchazón,
 o moretones?
*(Ah teh-nee-doh sahn-grah-dohs,
 een-chah-sohn oh moh-reh-toh-
 nehs)*

—No, I have not noticed any.

—No, no me he dado cuenta
 de ninguna cosa.
*(Noh, noh meh eh dah-doh koo-
 ehn-tah deh neen-goo-nah koh-
 sah)*

Your skin color looks good.

El color de su piel es normal.
*(Ehl koh-lohr deh soo pee-ehl
 ehs nohr-mahl)*

Fever?

¿Fiebre?
(Fee-eh-breh)

—About 99 degrees today.

—Cerca de noventa y nueve
 grados hoy.
*(Sehr-kah deh noh-behn-tah ee
 noo-eh-beh grah-dohs oh-ee)*

—I feel dizzy.

Me siento mareado.
(Meh see-ehn-toh mah-reh-ah-doh)

Have you had neck pain?

¿Ha tenido dolor en el cuello?
*(Ah teh-nee-doh doh-lohr ehn
 ehl koo-eh-yoh)*

—Once in a while.

—De vez en cuando.
(Deh behs ehn koo-ahn-doh)

Stay sitting here.

Quédese sentado aquí.
(Keh-deh-seh sehn-tah-doh ah-kee)

TABLE 3-1	**Pronunciation of Selected Words**	
TABLA 3-1	Pronunciación de Palabras Selectas	

English	Spanish	Pronunciation
airway	vía aérea	*bee-ah ah-eh-reh-ah*
arrest	arresto	*ah-rehs-toh*
cardiopulmonary	cardiopulmonar	*kahr-dee-oh-pool-moh-nahr*
choking	ahogar	*ah-oh-gahr*
dizzy	mareado	*mah-reh-ah-doh*
hyperthermia	hipertermia	*ee-pehr-tehr-mee-ah*
obstruction	obstrucción	*ohb-strook-see-ohn*
respiratory	paro	*pah-roh rehs-pee-rah-*
arrest	respiratorio	*toh-ree-oh*
anaphylactic	choque	*choh-keh ah-nah-fee-*
shock	anafilático	*lah-tee-koh*
traumatic	traumático	*trah-oo-mah-tee-koh*
swelling	hinchazón	*een-chah-sohn*
swollen	hinchado	*een-chah-doh*
temperature	temperatura	*tehm-peh-rah-too-rah*

I am going to get a wheelchair.	**Voy a traer una silla de ruedas.** *(Boh-ee ah trah-ehr oo-nah see-yah deh roo-eh-dahs)*

Mrs. Vargas, a pregnant 30-year-old woman was involved in a car accident. She just arrived at the emergency room.

La señora Vargas, una mujer embarazada que tiene 30 años de edad, estuvo en un accidente automovilístico. Acaba de llegar al cuarto de urgencias (emergencias).

Hello, Mrs. Vargas.	**Hola, señora Vargas.** *(Oh-lah, seh-nyoh-rah Bahr-gahs)*
I am going to ask you questions.	**Voy a hacerle preguntas.** *(Boh-ee ah ah-sehr-leh preh-goon-tahs)*
What is your name?	**¿Cómo se llama?** *(Koh-moh seh yah-mah)*
What is your last name?	**¿Cuál es su apellido?** *(Koo-ahl ehs soo ah-peh-yee-doh)*
Answer "yes" or "no."	**Conteste "sí" o "no".** *(Kohn-tehs-teh "see" oh "noh")*

Did you lose consciousness?	¿Perdió el conocimiento/Se desmayó? *(Pehr-dee-oh ehl koh-noh-see-mee-ehn-toh/Seh dehs-mah-yoh)*
Do you know where you are?	¿Sabe dónde está? *(Sah-beh dohn-deh ehs-tah)*
Do you know the day of the week?	¿Sabe el día de la semana? *(Sah-beh ehl dee-ah deh lah seh-mah-nah)*
Are you nauseated?	¿Tiene náuseas? *(Tee-eh-neh nah-oo-seh-ahs)*
Are you bleeding?	¿Está sangrando? *(Ehs-tah sahn-grahn-doh)*
How many months pregnant?	¿Cuántos meses tiene de embarazo? *(Koo-ahn-tohs meh-sehs tee-eh-neh deh ehm-bah-rah-soh)*
When was your last normal period?	¿Cuándo tuvo su última menstruación normal? *(Koo-ahn-doh too-boh soo ool-tee-mah mehns-troo-ah-see-ohn nohr-mahl)*
Is your water bag broken?	¿Se reventó su bolsa de agua? *(Seh reh-behn-toh soo bohl-sah deh ah-goo-ah)*
When?	¿Cuándo? *(Koo-ahn-doh)*
Did you feel warm water run out of your vagina?	¿Sintió que salió agua tibia de su vagina? *(Seen-tee-oh keh sah-lee-oh ah-goo-ah tee-bee-ah deh soo bah-hee-nah)*

In an emergency situation, the objective is to obtain as much information as correctly as possible. Get to the point!

En una situación urgente, el objetivo es obtener información lo más correcta posible. ¡Sea breve!

Have you eaten?	¿Ha comido? *(Ah koh-mee-doh)*
At what time?	¿A qué hora? *(Ah keh oh-rah)*
What did you eat?	¿Qué comió? *(Keh koh-mee-oh)*

Mrs. Vargas, I need to help you change clothes.	**Señora Vargas, necesito ayudarle a cambiar la ropa.** *(Seh-nyoh-rah Bahr-gahs, neh-seh-see-toh ah-yoo-dahr-leh ah kahm-bee-ahr lah roh-pah)*
I have a gown.	**Tengo una bata.** *(Tehn-goh oo-nah bah-tah)*
I am going to examine you.	**Voy a examinarla.** *(Boh-ee ah ehx-ah-mee-nahr-lah)*

Some words are difficult to pronounce because they are too long. Don't hurry, make a pause (Table 3-2).

Algunas palabras son difíciles de pronunciar porqué son muy largas. Tome su tiempo, haga una pausa (Tabla 3-2).

How far apart are your contractions?	**¿Cada cuánto tiempo tiene las contracciones?** *(Kah-dah koo-ahn-toh tee-ehm-poh tee-eh-neh lahs kohn-trahk-see-ohn-ehs)*
Tell me when you feel a contraction!	**¡Dígame cuando sienta una contracción!** *(Dee-gah-meh koo-ahn-doh see-ehn-tah oo-nah kohn-trahk-see-see-ohn)*
We need to count them.	**Tenemos que contarlas.** *(Teh-neh-mohs keh kohn-tahr-lahs)*
Are you cold?	**¿Tiene frío?** *(Tee-eh-neh free-oh)*

TABLE 3-2	**Pronunciation of Selected Words**	
TABLA 3-2	Pronunciación de Palabras Selectas	

English	Spanish	Pronunciation
ambulance	ambulancia	*ahm-boo-lahn-see-ah*
consciousness	conocimiento	*koh-noh-see-mee-ehn-toh*
contractions	contracciones	*kohn-trahk-see-ohn-ehs*
pregnant	embarazada	*ehm-bah-rah-sah-dah*
him/you examine (m)	examinarlo	*ehx-ah-mee-nahr-loh*
her/you examine (f)	examinarla	*ehx-ah-mee-nahr-lah*
receptionist	recepcionista	*reh-sehp-see-ohn-ees-tah*
bleeding	sangrando	*sahn-grahn-doh*
temperature	temperatura	*tehm-peh-rah-too-rah*

Are you hot?	¿Tiene calor?
	(Tee-eh-neh kah-lohr)
Where were you hit?	¿Dónde se golpeó?
	(Dohn-deh seh gohl-peh-oh)
Point!	¡Apunte!/¡Señale!
	(Ah-poon-teh/Seh-nyah-leh)
Do you have pain?	¿Tiene dolor?
	(Tee-eh-neh doh-lohr)
Where?	¿Dónde?
	(Dohn-deh)
Pain at the waist?	¿Dolor en la cintura?
	(Doh-lohr ehn lah seen-too-rah)
Back pain?	¿Dolor de espalda?
	(Doh-lohr deh ehs-pahl-dah)
Is the pain sharp?	¿El dolor es agudo?
	(Ehl doh-lohr ehs ah-goo-doh)
Is the pain in one place?	¿El dolor es fijo?
	(Ehl doh-lohr ehs fee-hoh)
Does it come and go?	¿Va y viene?
	(Bah eeh bee-eh-neh)
Are you feeling a contraction?	¿Está sintiendo una contracción?
	(Ehs-tah seen-tee-ehn-doh oo-nah kohn-trahk-see-ohn)
Tell me when!	¡Dígame cuando!
	(Dee-gah-meh koo-ahn-doh)
I am going to listen to the baby's heart beat.	Voy a escuchar el latido del corazón del bebé.
	(Boh-ee ah ehs-koo-chahr ehl lah-tee-doh dehl koh-rah-sohn dehl beh-beh)
Please breathe normally.	Por favor, respire normal.
	(Pohr fah-bohr, rehs-pee-reh nohr-mahl)
It sounds good.	Se oye bien
	(Seh oh-yeh bee-ehn)
Do you have allergies?	¿Tiene alergias?
	(Tee-eh-neh ah-lehr-hee-ahs)
To foods/dust/medicines?	¿A comidas/polvo/medicinas?
	(Ah koh-mee-dahs/pohl-boh/meh-dee-see-nahs)
How old are you?	¿Cuántos años tiene?
	(Koo-ahn-tohs ah-nyohs tee-eh-neh)
How many pregnancies have you had?	¿Cuántos embarazos ha tenido?
	(Koo-ahn-tohs ehm-bah-rah-sohs ah teh-nee-doh)

How many children do you have?	¿Cuántos niños tiene? *(Koo-ahn-tohs nee-nyohs tee-eh-neh)*
Have you had an abortion?	¿Ha tenido abortos? *(Ah teh-nee-doh ah-bohr-tohs)*
How many?	¿Cuántos? *(Koo-ahn-tohs)*
When was the last one?	¿Cuándo fue el último? *(Koo-ahn-doh foo-eh ehl ool-tee-moh)*
Did you have a miscarriage?	¿Tuvo un niño nacido muerto? *(Too-boh oon nee-nyoh nah-see-doh moo-ehr-toh)*
Did you have an ectopic (tubal) pregnancy?	¿Tuvo un embarazo fuera de la matriz o en las trompas? *(Too-boh oon ehm-bah-rah-soh foo-eh-rah deh lah mah-trees oh ehn lahs trohm-pahs)*
Are you working also?	¿Trabaja también? *(Trah-bah-hah tahm-bee-ehn)*
Are you a housewife?	¿Es ama de casa? *(Ehs ah-mah deh kah-sah)*
What kind of work do you do?	¿Qué clase de trabajo hace? *(Keh klah-seh deh trah-bah-hoh ah-seh)*
How many pounds have you gained?	¿Cuántas libras a aumentado? *(Koo-ahn-tahs lee-brahs ah ah-oo-mehn-tah-doh)*
Do you smoke?	¿Fuma usted? *(Foo-mah oos-tehd)*
Do you drink alcohol?	¿Toma bebidas alcohólicas? *(Toh-mah beh-bee-dahs ahl-koh-lee-kahs)*
Do you drink coffee?	¿Toma café? *(Toh-mah kah-feh)*
Do you take any medicines?	¿Toma algunas medicinas? *(Toh-mah ahl-goo-nahs meh-dee-see-nahs)*
What medicines do you take?	¿Qué medicinas toma? *(Keh meh-dee-see-nahs toh-mah)*
For what reason?	¿Cuál es la razón? *(Koo-ahl ehs lah rah-sohn)*

Do you take any narcotics?	¿Toma narcóticos?
	(Toh-mah nahr-koh-tee-kohs)
Do you take drugs from habit?	¿Tiene vicio de tomar drogas?
	(Tee-eh-neh bee-see-oh deh toh-mahr droh-gahs)
Are you married/single?	¿Está casada o es soltera?
	(Ehs-tah kah-sah-dah oh ehs sohl-teh-rah)
Do you live with your husband?	¿Vive con su esposo?
	(Bee-beh kohn soo ehs-poh-soh)
Where is your husband?	¿Dónde está su esposo?
	(Dohn-deh ehs-tah soo ehs-poh-soh)
Do you have relatives/friends?	¿Tiene parientes/amigos?
	(Tee-eh-neh pah-ree-ehn-tehs/ah-mee-gohs)
Thank you!	¡Gracias!
	(Grah-see-ahs)

Table 3-3 will help you with pronunciation of selected words.
La Tabla 3-3 le ayudará con pronunciación de palabras selectas.

The nurse approaches Mrs. Vargas.
La enfermera se acerca a la señora Vargas.

TABLE 3-3   Pronunciation of Selected Words
TABLA 3-3   Pronunciación de Palabras Selectas

English	Spanish	Pronunciation
last name	apellido	*ah-peh-yee-doh*
you know	sabe	*sah-beh*
week	semana	*seh-mah-nah*
nausea	náusea	*nah-oo-seh-ah*
where	dónde	*dohn-deh*
how many	cuántos	*koo-ahn-tohs*
thank you	gracias	*grah-see-ahs*
blood	sangre	*sahn-greh*
you need	necesita	*neh-seh-see-tah*
question	pregunta	*preh-goon-tah*

Hello Mrs. Vargas. I need to take your temperature and blood pressure.	Hola, señora Vargas. Necesito tomarle la temperatura y la presión de la sangre. *(Oh-lah, seh-nyoh-rah Bahr-gahs. Neh-seh-see-toh toh-mahr-leh lah tehm-peh-rah-too-rah ee lah preh-see-ohn deh lah sahn-greh)*
I also need a urine sample.	También necesito una muestra de orina. *(Tahm-bee-ehn neh-seh-see-toh oo-nah moo-ehs-trah deh oh-ree-nah)*
Don't get up!	¡No se levante! *(Noh seh leh-bahn-teh)*

Supportive measures include ensuring privacy and accepting various reactions to fear and pain. Explain all procedures, even when you think the patient does not understand the language. Try to demonstrate the procedure you are about to perform and what you expect. Commonly used commands are found in Table 3-4.

Las medidas que dan apoyo incluyen el asegurar una área privada y aceptar varias reacciones al miedo y al dolor. Explique todos los procedimientos, aún cuando usted piense que el paciente no entienda el lenguaje. Trate de demostrar el procedimiento que va a hacer y lo que se espera del paciente. Los mandatos que se usan comúnmente están en la Tabla 3-4.

TABLE 3-4	Common Commands	
TABLA 3-4	**Mandatos Comúnes**	
English	**Spanish**	**Pronunciation**
Bend!	¡Doble!	*Doh-bleh*
Call!	¡Llame!	*Yah-meh*
Choose!	¡Escoja!	*Ehs-koh-hah*
Get!	¡Consiga!	*Kohn-see-gah*
Get out!	¡Fuera!	*Foo-eh-rah*
Get up!	¡Levantese!	*Leh-bahn-teh-seh*
Lower!	¡Baje!	*Bah-heh*
Pull!	¡Jale!	*Hah-leh*
Tell me!	¡Dígame!	*Dee-gah-meh*
Wake-up!	¡Despierte!	*Dehs-pee-ehr-teh*

I have the bedpan.	Tengo el bacín/pato. *(Tehn-goh ehl bah-seen/pah-toh)*
Bend your knees!	¡Doble las piernas! *(Doh-bleh lahs pee-ehr-nahs)*
Pull up your hips!	¡Levante la cadera! *(Leh-bahn-teh lah kah-deh-rah)*
Do you have pain?	¿Tiene dolor? *(Tee-eh-neh doh-lohr)*
Where?	¿Dónde? *(Dohn-deh)*
Here is the toilet paper.	Aquí está el papel del baño/ higiénico. *(Ah-kee ehs-tah ehl pah-pehl dehl bah-nyoh/ee-hee-eh-nee-koh)*
Lower your legs.	Baje las piernas. *(Bah-heh lahs pee-ehr-nahs)*
Rest.	Descanse. *(Des-kahn-seh)*
Later on, they will take x-rays.	Más tarde, le van a tomar rayos X. *(Mahs tahr-deh leh bahn ah toh- mahr rah-yohs eh-kees)*
Then they will take blood samples.	Luego le van a tomar muestras de sangre. *(Loo-eh-goh leh bahn ah toh- mahr moo-ehs-trahs deh sahn- greh)*
Here is the bell.	Aquí está la campana. *(Ah-kee ehs-tah lah kahm-pah-nah)*
Call if you need help.	Llame si necesita ayuda. *(Yah-meh see neh-seh-see-tah ah-yoo-dah)*

In the waiting area, Mr. Vargas speaks to the receptionist.
En la sala de espera, el señor Vargas habla con la recepcionista.
See Table 3-5 for pronunciation of selected words.
Vea la Tabla 3-5 para la pronunciación de palabras selectas.

I am going to ask you some questions.	Voy a hacerle unas preguntas. *(Boh-ee ah ah-sehr-leh oo-nahs preh-goon-tahs)*
What is your address?	¿Cuál es su dirección? *(Koo-ahl ehs soo dee-rehk-see-ohn)*
The name of the street . . .	El nombre de la calle . . . *(Ehl nohm-breh deh lah kah-yeh)*

| TABLE 3-5 | Pronunciation of Selected Words | |
| TABLA 3-5 | Pronunciación de Palabras Selectas | |

English	Spanish	Pronunciation
address	dirección	*dee-rehk-see-ohn*
number	número	*noo-meh-roh*
health	salud	*sah-lood*
work	trabajo	*trah-bah-hoh*
insurance	seguro	*seh-goo-roh*
you sign	firme	*feer-meh*
here	aquí	*ah-kee*

Telephone number?

Number of:

  Health insurance?

  Medicaid?

  Social Security?

Where do you work?

Work phone number?

What is the phone number?

Sign here, please.

Thank you!

¿Número de teléfono?
(Noo-meh-roh deh teh-leh-foh-noh)
Número de:
(Noo-meh-roh deh)
  ¿Seguro de salud?
(Seh-goo-roh deh sah-lood)
  ¿Medicaid?
(Meh-dee-keh-eed)
  ¿Seguro Social?
(Seh-goo-roh Soh-see-ahl)
¿Dónde trabaja?
(Dohn-deh trah-bah-hah)
¿Teléfono del trabajo?
(Teh-leh-foh-noh dehl trah-bah-hoh)
¿Cuál es el número de teléfono?
*(Koo-ahl ehs ehl noo-meh-roh
deh teh-leh-foh-noh)*
Firme aquí, por favor.
(Feer-meh ah-kee, pohr fah-bohr)
¡Gracias!
(Grah-see-ahs)

Memorization of numbers is helpful when you are asking for addresses or phone numbers (Table 3-6).

Memorizar los números le ayuda cuando pide direcciones o números de teléfono (Tabla 3-6).

TABLE 3-6	Helpful Numbers		
TABLA 3-6	Números Útiles		

Number	English	Spanish	Pronunciation
1	one	uno	*oo-noh*
2	two	dos	*dohs*
3	three	tres	*trehs*
4	four	cuatro	*koo-ah-troh*
5	five	cinco	*seen-koh*
6	six	seis	*seh-ees*
7	seven	siete	*see-eh-teh*
8	eight	ocho	*oh-choh*
9	nine	nueve	*noo-eh-beh*
10	ten	diez	*dee-ehs*
15	fifteen	quince	*keen-seh*
20	twenty	veinte	*beh-een-teh*
30	thirty	treinta	*treh-een-tah*
40	forty	cuarenta	*koo-ah-rehn-tah*
50	fifty	cincuenta	*seen-koo-ehn-tah*
60	sixty	sesenta	*seh-sehn-tah*
70	seventy	setenta	*seh-tehn-tah*
80	eighty	ochenta	*oh-chehn-tah*
90	ninety	noventa	*noh-behn-tah*
100	one hundred	cien	*see-ehn*

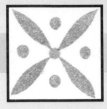

CHAPTER FOUR
In the Hospital

CAPITULO CUATRO
En el Hospital

When someone asks you for directions in Spanish, knowing key words is essential. Do not hesitate to use your hands or draw a map that the patient can use as a guide. He will appreciate it. Table 4-1 will help you with pronunciation of selected words.

Cuando alguien le pide direcciones en español, es esencial saber palabras claves. No vacile en usar las manos o dibujar un mapa que el paciente puede usar como guía. El lo apreciará. La Tabla 4-1 le ayudará con la pronunciación de palabras selectas.

Good morning!	¡Buenos días! *(Boo-eh-nohs dee-ahs)*
Is this _____ Hospital?	¿Es este el Hospital _____? *(Ehs ehs-teh ehl ohs-pee-tahl _____)*
I need to go to the surgery clinic.	Necesito ir a la clínica de cirugía. *(Neh-seh-see-toh eer ah lah klee-nee- kah deh see-roo-hee-ah)*
Can you give me directions?	¿Me puede dar direcciones? *(Meh poo-eh-deh dahr dee-rek-see- ohn-ehs)*
Yes, go to the end of the hall.	Sí, vaya al final del pasillo. *(See, bah-yah ahl feen-ahl dehl pah- see-yoh)*
Can you see the fire extinguisher?	¿Ve el extinguidor de fuego? *(Beh ehl ehx-teen-ghee-dohr deh foo- eh-goh)*

English	Spanish	Pronunciation
administration	administración	*ahd-mee-nee-strah-see-ohn*
arrow	flecha	*fleh-chah*
building	edificio	*eh-dee-fee-see-oh*
cafeteria	cafetería	*kah-feh-teh-ree-ah*
clinic	clínica	*klee-nee-kah*
directions	direcciones	*dee-rehk-see-ohn-ehs*
elevator	elevador	*eh-leh-bah-dohr*
fire escape	escape de fuego	*ehs-kah-peh deh foo-eh-goh*
hesitate	vacilar	*bah-see-lahr*
laboratory	laboratorio	*lah-boh-rah-toh-ree-oh*
lobby	vestíbulo	*behs-tee-boo-loh*
stairs	escalera	*ehs-kah-leh-rah*
surgery	cirugía	*see-roo-hee-ah*
tower	torre	*toh-reh*

TABLE 4-1 Pronunciation of Selected Words
TABLA 4-1 Pronunciación de Palabras Selectas

It's in the middle of the wall. — Está a la mitad de la pared. *(Ehs-tah ah lah mee-tahd deh lah pah-rehd)*

When you get there, turn right. — Cuando llegue ahí, dé vuelta a la derecha. *(Koo-ahn-doh yeh-gheh ah-ee, deh boo-ehl-tah ah lah deh-reh-chah)*

You will pass the cafeteria. — Va a pasar la cafetería. *(Bah ah pah-sahr lah kah-feh-teh-ree-ah)*

Go to the glass doors. — Vaya a las puertas de vidrio. *(Bah-yah ah lahs poo-ehr-tahs deh bee-dree-oh)*

The clinic is in another building. — La clínica está en otro edificio. *(Lah klee-nee-kah ehs-tah ehn oh-troh eh-dee-fee-see-oh)*

You may wish to memorize single words that will help you with directions. Table 4-2 has key words.

Puede memorizar palabras que le ayudarán con las direcciones. La Tabla 4-2 tiene palabras clave.

| TABLE 4-2 | Key Words | |
TABLA 4-2	Palabras Clave	
English	Spanish	Pronunciation
above	arriba	*ah-ree-bah*
below	abajo	*ah-bah-hoh*
blocks	cuadras	*koo-ah-drahs*
corner	esquina	*ehs-kee-nah*
hallway	pasillo	*pah-see-yoh*
left	izquierda	*ees-kee-ehr-dah*
right	derecha	*deh-reh-chah*
sign	letrero	*leh-treh-roh*
straight	derecho	*deh-reh-choh*
wall	pared	*pah-rehd*

You have to cross the street.
Tiene que cruzar la calle.
(Tee-eh-neh keh kroo-sahr lah kah-yeh)

Walk two blocks.
Camine dos cuadras.
(Kah-mee-neh dohs koo-ah-drahs)

Then, turn to the left.
Luego dé vuelta a la izquierda.
(Loo-eh-goh deh boo-ehl-tah ah lah ees-kee-ehr-dah)

The building has beige brick.
El edificio tiene ladrillo crema.
(Ehl eh-dee-fee-see-oh tee-eh-neh lah-dree-yoh kreh-mah)

It is a six-story building.
Es un edificio de seis pisos.
(Ehs oon eh-dee-fee-see-oh deh seh-ees pee-sohs)

Take the elevator to the sixth floor.
Tome el elevador al sexto piso.
(Toh-meh ehl eh-leh-bah-dohr ahl sehx-toh pee-soh)

The elevators are slow.
Los elevadores son lentos.
(Lohs eh-leh-bah-doh-rehs sohn lehn-tohs)

Exit to the right.
Salga a la derecha.
(Sahl-gah ah lah deh-reh-chah)

You will see the sign on the wall.
Verá el letrero en la pared.
(Beh-rah ehl leh-treh-roh ehn lah pah-rehd)

Follow the red arrows.
Siga las flechas rojas.
(See-gah lahs fleh-chahs roh-hahs)

There is a front desk.	Hay un escritorio al frente.
	(Ah-ee oon ehs-kree-toh-ree-oh ahl frehn-teh)
Ask the receptionist for a number.	Pídale un número a la recepcionista.
	(Pee-dah-leh oon noo-meh-roh ah lah reh-sehp-see-ohn-ees-tah)
Wait in the lobby.	Espere en el vestibulo.
	(Ehs-peh-reh ehn ehl behs-tee-boo-loh)
You have to wait your turn.	Tendrá que esperar su turno.
	(Tehn-drah keh ehs-peh-rahr soo tuhr-noh)
Do you want to take the stairs?	¿Quiére tomar la escalera?
	(Kee-eh-reh toh-mahr lah ehs-kah-leh-rah)
They are around the corner.	Están alrededor de la esquina.
	(Ehs-tahn ahl-reh-deh-dohr deh lah ehs-kee-nah)
You can't miss them!	¡No tiene pierde!
	(Noh tee-eh-neh pee-ehr-deh)
The stairs will take you.	La escalera lo llevará.
	(Lah ehs-kah-leh-rah loh yeh-bah-rah)

Sometimes you will only remember a few words. No problem! Verbs usually come in handy because they are the essence of a sentence. You can help the patients if you recognize some useful verbs (Table 4-3).

Algunas veces sólo recordará pocas palabras. ¡No hay problema! Los verbos vienen a la mano porque son lo escencial de una oración. Puede ayudar a los pacientes si reconoce unos verbos útiles (Tabla 4-3).

You can cross at the walkway.	Puede cruzar por el pasillo sobre la calle.
	(Poo-eh-deh kroo-sahr pohr ehl pah-see-yoh soh-breh lah kah-yeh)
I don't think so.	No lo creo.
	(Noh loh kreh-oh)
I am hurting a lot.	Tengo mucho dolor.
	(Tehn-goh moo-choh doh-lohr)
If it is far, could I drive?	Si está lejos, ¿podría manejar?
	(See ehs-tah leh-hohs, poh-dree-ah mah-neh-hahr)
Is there a policeman?	¿Hay un policía?
	(Ah-ee oon poh-lee-see-ah)

TABLE 4-3	Useful Verbs
TABLA 4-3	Verbos Útiles

English	Spanish	Pronunciation
to see	ver	*behr*
to give	dar	*dahr*
to take	tomar	*toh-mahr*
to ask	preguntar	*preh-goon-tahr*
to tell	decir	*deh-seer*
to wait	esperar	*ehs-peh-rahr*
to hurt	doler	*doh-lehr*
to turn	voltear/dar vuelta	*bohl-teh-ahr/dahr boo-ehl-tah*
to follow	seguir	*seh-geer*
to cross	cruzar	*kroo-sahr*

I need better directions.
Necesito mejores direcciones.
(Neh-seh-see-toh meh-hoh-rehs dee-rehk-see-ohn-ehs)

I am afraid to get lost.
Tengo miedo de perderme.
(Tehn-goh mee-eh-doh deh pehr-dehr-meh)

This is a large place.
Este es un lugar grande.
(Ehs-teh ehs oon loo-gahr grahn-deh)

I will not find the street.
No encontraré la calle.
(Noh ehn-kohn-trah-reh lah kah-yeh)

What is the name?
¿Cuál es el nombre?
(Koo-ahl ehs ehl nohm-breh)

Can you write the name?
¿Puede escribir el nombre?
(Poo-eh-deh ehs-kree-beer ehl nohm-breh)

I have a piece of paper.
Tengo un pedazo de papel.
(Tehn-goh oon peh-dah-soh deh pah-pehl)

But I don't have a pencil.
Pero no tengo lápiz.
(Peh-roh noh tehn-goh lah-pees)

I don't have a pen either.
Tampoco tengo una pluma.
(Tahm-poh-koh tehn-goh oo-nah ploo-mah)

Since you are sensitive to the patient's needs, you decide that he is going to need more help than just writing the directions to the clinic. Reassurance sometimes does not help.

Como usted es sensitivo a las necesidades del paciente, decide que él necesita más ayuda que sólo escribir las direcciones a la clínica. El volverlo a asegurar a veces no ayuda.

Sit here and wait.	Siéntese aquí y espere. *(See-ehn-teh-seh ah-kee ee ehs-peh-reh)*
I'll call for a wheelchair.	Pediré una silla de ruedas. *(Peh-dee-reh oo-nah see-yah deh roo-eh-dahs)*
This is an employee.	Este es un empleado. *(Ehs-teh ehs oon ehm-pleh-ah-doh)*
He will take you.	El lo llevará. *(Ehl loh yeh-bah-rah)*
Sit down, please.	Siéntese, por favor. *(See-ehn-teh-seh, pohr fah-bohr)*
Place your feet here.	Ponga los pies aquí. *(Pohn-gah lohs pee-ehs ah-kee)*
Over the stool.	Sobre el taburete. *(Soh-breh ehl tah-boo-reh-teh)*
We have to go far.	Tenemos que ir lejos. *(Teh-neh-mohs keh eer leh-hohs)*
Are you OK?	¿Está bien? *(Ehs-tah bee-ehn)*
Let me know how you feel.	Dígame cómo se siente. *(Dee-gah-meh koh-moh seh see-ehn-teh)*
I can stop.	Puedo pararme. *(Poo-eh-doh pah-rahr-meh)*
Where are you from?	¿De dónde es usted? *(Deh dohn-deh ehs oos-tehd)*
How did you get here?	¿Cómo llegó aquí? *(Koh-moh yeh-goh ah-kee)*
Is someone with you?	¿Hay alguien con usted? *(Ah-ee ahl-ghee-ehn kohn oos-tehd)*
Do you know how to return?	¿Sabe cómo regresar? *(Sah-beh koh-moh reh-greh-sahr)*

The patient has arrived at a different place. He is not familiar with his surroundings. There are many questions that he can ask. Table 4-4 has other questions that he may ask.

El paciente llegó a un lugar diferente. El no está familiarizado con su alrededor. Hay muchas preguntas que puede hacer. La Tabla 4-4 tiene otras preguntas que él puede hacer.

TABLE 4-4	Other Questions
TABLA 4-4	Otras Preguntas

English	Spanish	Pronunciation
Is it far?	¿Está lejos?	*Ehs-tah leh-hohs*
How far?	¿Qué tan lejos?	*Keh tahn leh-hohs*
Do I have time?	¿Tengo tiempo?	*Tehn-goh tee-ehm-poh*
At what time do they close?	¿A qué hora cierran?	*Ah keh oh-rah see-eh-rahn*
What time is it?	¿Qué hora es?	*Keh oh-rah ehs*
Are there elevators?	¿Hay elevadores?	*Ah-ee eh-leh-bah-doh-rehs*
Are there ramps?	¿Hay rampas?	*Ah-ee ram-pahs*
Where is it?	¿Dónde está?	*Dohn-deh ehs-tah*
Is it the same color?	¿Es del mismo color?	*Ehs dehl mees-moh koh-lohr*
Should I drive?	¿Debo de manejar?	*Deh-boh deh mah-neh-hahr*
Is parking available?	¿Hay estacionamiento?	*Ah-ee ehs-tah-see-oh-nah-mee-ehn-toh*
What is the name of the street?	¿Cuál es el nombre de la calle?	*Koo-ahl ehs ehl nohm-breh deh lah kah-yeh*
Can you go with me?	¿Puede ir conmigo?	*Poo-eh-deh eer kohn-mee-goh*

This is the clinic.
Esta es la clínica.
(*Ehs-tah ehs lah klee-nee-kah*)

Good morning, Miss.
Buenos días, señorita.
(*Boo-eh-nohs dee-ahs, seh-nyoh-ree-tah*)

I was told to come here.
Me dijeron que viniera aquí.
(*Meh dee-heh-rohn keh bee-nee-eh-rah ah-kee*)

I need to see Doctor White.
Necesito ver al doctor White.
(*Neh-seh-see-toh behr ahl dohk-tohr White*)

Have you been here before?
¿Ha estado aquí antes?
(*Ah ehs-tah-doh ah-kee ahn-tehs*)

If you have been here, I need your card.
Si ha estado aquí, necesito su tarjeta.
(*See ah ehs-tah-doh ah-kee, neh-seh-see-toh soo tahr-heh-tah*)

If you haven't, please fill out these papers.

Si no, por favor llene estos papeles.
(See noh, pohr fah-bohr yeh-neh ehs-tohs pah-peh-lehs)

I cannot read English, can you help me?

No puedo leer inglés, ¿puede ayudarme?
(Noh poo-eh-doh leh-ehr een-glehs, poo-eh-deh ah-yoo-dahr-meh)

Yes, please wait.

Sí, espere por favor.
(See, ehs-peh-reh pohr fah-bohr)

This is my first time here.

Esta es mi primera vez aquí.
(Ehs-tah ehs mee pree-meh-rah behs ah-kee)

In that case, tell me your whole name.

En ese caso, dígame su nombre completo.
(Ehn eh-seh kah-soh, dee-gah-meh soo nohm-breh kohm-pleh-toh)

What is your birthdate? year? month? day?

¿Cuál es la fecha de nacimiento? ¿año?/¿mes?/¿día?
(Koo-ahl ehs lah feh-chah deh nah-see-mee-ehn-toh)
(ah-nyoh/mehs/dee-ah)

The computer says that you have an appointment.

La computadora dice que tiene cita.
(Lah kohm-poo-tah-doh-rah dee-seh keh tee-eh-neh see-tah)

You have to go to the floor directly.

Debe ir al piso directamente.
(Deh-beh eer ahl pee-soh dee-rehk-tah-mehn-teh)

The doctor will see you there.

El doctor lo verá ahí.
(Ehl dohk-tohr loh beh-rah ah-ee)

The Surgery floor is in the hospital towers.

El piso de cirugía está en las torres del hospital.
(Ehl pee-soh deh see-roo-hee-ah ehs-tah ehn lahs toh-rehs dehl ohs-pee-tahl)

Ask for unit Six A.

Pregunte por la unidad Seis A.
(Preh-goon-teh pohr lah oo-nee-dahd Seh-ees Ah)

From here, turn to the left, then turn right.

De aquí, dé vuelta a la izquierda, luego voltee a la derecha.
(Deh ah-kee, deh boo-ehl-tah ah lah ees-kee-ehr-dah, loo-eh-goh bohl-teh-eh ah lah deh-reh-chah)

Follow the green line.	Siga la línea verde.
	(See-gah lah lee-nee-ah behr-deh)
The line is on the wall.	La línea está en la pared.
	(Lah lee-nee-ah ehs-tah ehn lah pah-rehd)
Watch for the arrow.	Fíjese en la flecha.
	(Fee-heh-seh ehn lah fleh-chah)
This will take you to the end of the hall.	Esta la llevará al final del pasillo.
	(Ehs-tah lah yeh-bah-rah ahl feen-ahl dehl pah-see-yoh)
There, turn to the left.	Ahí, voltée a la izquierda.
	(Ah-ee, bohl-teh-eh ah lah ees-kee-ehr-dah)
The secretary will help.	La secretaria lo ayudará.
	(Lah seh-kreh-tah-ree-ah loh ah-yoo-dah-rah)
Good luck!	¡Buena suerte!
	(Boo-eh-nah soo-ehr-teh)

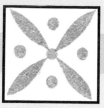

CHAPTER FIVE
Physical Exam

CAPITULO CINCO
Examen Físico

The physical exam is very important. From the moment that we see a person, we start to assess and to note the patient's general well-being. A good review of the body allows us to make a primary diagnosis. With assistance from the laboratory and the x-rays, we are able to make a final diagnosis. The physical exam must be done carefully, since it provides a fundamental base for further decision making. The mental exam is part of the physical exam. It gives us the opportunity to see if the patient is nervous, tense, aggressive, vulnerable, restless, or depressed. We are able to assess whether the patient is oriented to time, person, or place.

El examen físico es muy importante. Desde el momento en que vemos a la persona, podemos darnos cuenta de su estado general. Una buena revisión o exploración del cuerpo nos permitirá hacer un primer diagnóstico. Ayudados por el laboratorio y las radiografías podremos hacer un diagnóstico final. El examen físico debe hacerse con el mayor cuidado posible, ya que es una base fundamental para tomar decisiones posteriores. El examen mental es parte del examen físico; nos permite saber si el paciente está nervioso, tenso, agresivo, vulnerable, inquieto o deprimido. Podremos ver si está orientado en persona, tiempo, lugar, y espacio.

Useful commands and phrases that facilitate the physical exam.

Mandatos y frases útiles que facilitan el examen físico.
(Mahn-dah-tohs ee frah-sehs oo-tee-lehs keh fah-see-lee-tahn ehl ehx-ah-mehn fee-see-koh)

| TABLE 5-1 | Patient's Moods |
| TABLA 5-1 | Actitud del Paciente |

English	Spanish	Pronunciation
nervous	nervioso	*nehr-bee-oh-soh*
tense	tenso	*tehn-soh*
aggressive	agresivo	*ah-greh-see-boh*
irritable	irritable	*ee-ree-tah-bleh*
restless	inquieto	*een-kee-eh-toh*
depressed	deprimido	*deh-pree-mee-doh*
flat	indiferente	*een-dee-feh-rehn-teh*
anxious	ansioso	*ahn-see-oh-soh*
euphoric	eufórico	*eh-oo-foh-ree-koh*

Note that the familiar "tú" is being used.
Note que se está usando la forma familiar "tú".

I am going to examine you.
Voy a examinarte.
(Boh-ee ah ehx-ah-mee-nahr-teh)

Please, sit up in the bed.
Por favor, siéntate en la cama.
(Pohr fah-bohr, see-ehn-tah-teh ehn lah kah-mah)

I am going to check your head:
Voy a revisar tu cabeza:
(Boh-ee ah reh-bee-sahr too kah-beh-sah)

Lift your head.
Levanta la cabeza.
(Leh-bahn-tah lah kah-beh-sah)

Lower your head.
Baja la cabeza.
(Bah-hah lah kah-beh-sah)

Move it side to side.
Muévela de lado a lado.
(Moo-eh-beh-lah deh lah-doh ah lah-doh)

I am going to check your eyes:
Voy a revisar tus ojos:
(Boh-ee ah reh-bee-sahr toos oh-hohs)

Look straight ahead.
Mira hacia adelante.
(Mee-rah ah-see-ah ah-deh-lahn-teh)

Look up.
Mira hacia arriba.
(Mee-rah ah-see-ah ah-ree-bah)

Look down.
Mira hacia abajo.
(Mee-rah ah-see-ah ah-bah-hoh)

Follow my finger.	**Sigue mi dedo.**
	(See-geh mee deh-doh)
Look straight at the light.	**Mira directo a la luz.**
	(Mee-rah dee-rehk-toh ah lah loos)
I am going to check your ears:	**Voy a revisar tus orejas:**
	(Boh-ee ah reh-bee-sahr toohs
	oh-reh-hahs)
Turn your head to the left.	**Voltea la cabeza a la izquierda.**
	(Bohl-teh-ah lah kah-beh-sah ah
	lah ees-kee-ehr-dah)
Turn your head to the right.	**Voltea la cabeza a la derecha.**
	(Bohl-teh-ah lah kah-beh-sah ah
	lah deh-reh-chah)

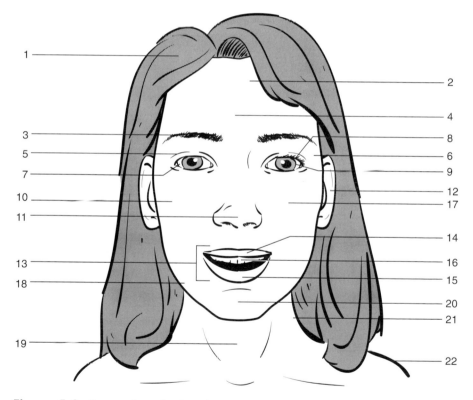

Figure 5-1 Inspecting the Head and Neck. (LA CABEZA Y EL CUELLO).
(1) **El cabello/el pelo** (hair), (2) **el cráneo** (skull), (3) **la ceja** (eyebrow), (4) **la frente** (forehead), (5) **el párpado** (eyelid), (6) **la sién** (temple), (7) **la esclera** (sclera), (8) **la pestaña** (eyelash), (9) **el ojo** (eye), (10) **el pómulo** (cheekbone), (11) **la nariz** (nose), (12) **la oreja/el oído** (ear), (13) **la boca** (mouth), (14) **el labio superior** (upper lip), (15) **el labio inferior** (lower lip), (16) **los dientes** (teeth), (17) **la mejilla** (cheek), (18) **la mandíbula** (mandible), (19) **la manzanilla/la nuez/de adán** (Adam's apple), (20) **la barbilla** (chin), (21) **el cuello** (neck), (22) **la piel** (skin).

I am going to check your nose:	Voy a revisar la nariz: *(Boh-ee ah reh-bee-sahr lah nah-rees)*
Wrinkle your nose.	Arruga la nariz. *(Ah-roo-gah lah nah-rees)*
I am going to check your throat.	Voy a revisar la garganta. *(Boh-ee ah reh-bee-sahr lah gahr-gahn-tah)*
Open your mouth.	Abre la boca. *(Ah-breh lah boh-kah)*
Close your mouth.	Cierra la boca. *(See-eh-rah lah boh-kah)*
Open again.	Abrela otra vez. *(Ah-breh-lah oh-trah behs)*
Say, "ahh."	Di "aaa." *(Dee ah-ah-ah)*
Please, swallow.	Traga, por favor. *(Trah-gah pohr fah-bohr)*
Smile.	Sonríe. *(Sohn-ree-eh)*
I am going to check your mouth.	Voy a revisar tu boca. *(Boh-ee ah reh-bee-sahr tooh boh-kah)*
Your lips should not be dry.	Tus labios no deben estar secos. *(Toohs lah-bee-ohs noh deh-behn ehs-tahr seh-kohs)*
Stick out your tongue.	Saca la lengua. *(Sah-kah lah lehn-goo-ah)*
I am going to check your gums.	Voy a revisar tus encías. *(Boh-ee ah reh-bee-sahr toos ehn-see-ahs)*
I am going to check your teeth.	Voy a revisar tus dientes. *(Boh-ee ah reh-bee-sahr toos dee-ehn-tehs)*
Upper extremities:	Extremidades superiores: *(Ehx-treh-mee-dah-dehs soo-peh-ree-oh-rehs)*
I am going to check the arm.	Voy a revisar tu brazo. *(Boh-ee ah reh-bee-sahr too brah-soh)*
Lift your arm.	Levanta tu brazo. *(Leh-bahn-tah too brah-soh)*
Extend it.	Extiéndelo. *(Ehx-tee-ehn-deh-loh)*
Flex it.	Dóblalo. *(Doh-blah-loh)*

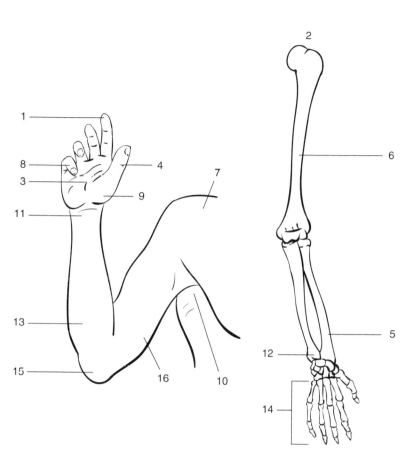

Figure 5-2 Inspecting the Arm and Hand. (BRAZO Y MANO).
(1) **El índice** (index), (2) **los huesos** (bones), (3) **la palma de la mano** (palm of the hand), (4) **el dedo grueso** (thumb), (5) **el radio** (radius), (6) **el húmero** (humerus), (7) **el hombro** (shoulder), (8) **el anular/el chiquito** (little finger), (9) **la mano derecha** (right hand), (10) **la axilla/el sobaco** (armpit/axilla), (11) **la muñeca** (wrist), (12) **la ulna** (ulna), (13) **el antebrazo** (forearm), (14) **los falanges** (phalanges), (15) **el codo** (elbow), (16) **el brazo** (arm).

Rotate it.	**Gíralo./Dale vuelta.** *(Hee-rah-loh/Dah-leh boo-ehl-tah)*
Bend your elbow.	**Dobla el codo.** *(Doh-blah ehl koh-doh)*
I am going to palpate your elbow.	**Voy a palpar tu codo.** *(Boh-ee ah pahl-pahr too koh-doh)*
I am going to palpate your nodes.	**Voy a palpar tus nodos.** *(Boh-ee ah pahl-pahr toos noh-dohs)*
Turn your forearm.	**Voltea el antebrazo.** *(Bohl-teh-ah ehl ahn-teh brah-soh)*

I am going to palpate the shoulder.	**Voy a palpar tu hombro.** *(Boh-ee ah pahl-pahr too ohm-broh)*
Place your arms behind the back.	**Pon los brazos atrás.** *(Pohn lohs brah-sohs ah-trahs)*
Place your hands behind your head.	**Pon tus manos atrás de tu cabeza.** *(Pohn toos mah-nohs ah-trahs deh too kah-beh-sah)*

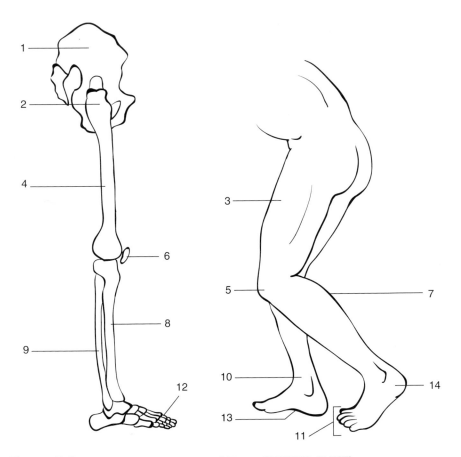

Figure 5-3 Inspecting the Leg and Foot. (PIERNA Y PIE).
(1) **La pelvis** (pelvis), (2) **la cabeza del fémur** (head), (3) **el muslo** (thigh), (4) **el fémur** (femur), (5) **la rodilla** (knee), (6) **la rótula** (knee cap), (7) **la pantorrilla** (calf), (8) **la tibia** (tibia), (9) **la fíbula/el peroné** (fibula), (10) **el tobillo** (ankle), (11) **los dedos** (toes), (12) **los falanges** (phalanges), (13) **la planta** (plantar), (14) **el talón** (heel).

Don't let me extend it.	No me dejes extenderlo. *(Noh meh deh-hehs ehx-tehn-dehr-loh)*
I am going to check your hand.	Voy a revisar tu mano. *(Boh-ee ah reh-bee-sahr too mah-noh)*
I am going to palpate it.	Voy a palparla. *(Boh-ee ah pahl-pahr-lah)*
Open your hand.	Abre tu mano. *(Ah-breh too mah-noh)*
Close it.	Ciérrala. *(See-eh-rah-lah)*
Open the fingers wide.	Separa bien los dedos. *(Seh-pah-rah bee-ehn lohs deh-dohs)*
Don't let me close them.	No me dejes cerrarlos. *(Noh meh deh-hehs seh-rahr-lohs)*
Make a fist.	Haz un puño. *(Ahs oon poo-nyoh)*
Hold my finger.	Agarra mi dedo. *(Ah-gah-rah meeh deh-doh)*
Tighten!	¡Aprieta! *(Ah-pree-eh-tah)*
Lift your hand.	Levanta tu mano. *(Leh-bahn-tah too mah-noh)*
Bend the wrist.	Dobla la muñeca. *(Doh-blah lah moo-nyeh-kah)*
Extend your wrist.	Extiende tu muñeca. *(Ehx-tee-ehn-deh too moo-nyeh-kah)*
I am going to examine your nailbeds.	Voy a examinar la base de tus uñas. *(Boh-ee ah ehx-ah-mee-nahr lah bah-seh deh toos oo-nyahs)*
Lower extremities:	Extremidades inferiores: *(Ehx-treh-mee-dah-dehs een-feh-ree-oh-rehs)*
I am going to examine the leg.	Voy a examinar tu pierna. *(Boh-ee ah ehx-ah-mee-nahr too pee-ehr-nah)*
Lift your leg.	Levanta la pierna. *(Leh-bahn-tah lah pee-ehr-nah)*
Bend it.	Dóblala. *(Doh-blah-lah)*
Bend your hip.	Dobla tu cadera. *(Doh-blah too kah-deh-rah)*
Straighten your knee.	Endereza la rodilla. *(Ehn-deh-reh-sah lah roh-dee-yah)*

Move your leg.	Mueve tu pierna.
	(Moo-eh-beh too pee-ehr-nah)
Forward.	Adelante.
	(Ah-deh-lahn-teh)
Backward.	Atrás.
	(Ah-trahs)
I am going to examine your foot.	Voy a examinar tu pie.
	(Boh-ee ah ehx-ah-mee-nahr too pee-eh)
Turn it to the left.	Voltéalo hacia la izquierda.
	(Bohl-teh-ah-loh ah-see-ah lah ees-kee-ehr-dah)
Turn it to the right.	Voltéalo hacia la derecha.
	(Bohl-teh-ah-loh ah-see-ah lah deh-reh-chah)

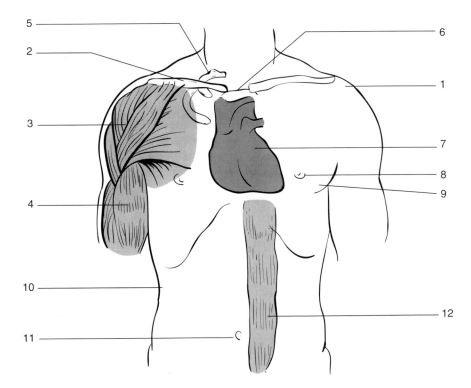

Figure 5-4 Inspecting the chest. (PECHO).
(1) **El hombro** (shoulder), (2) **la clavícula** (clavicle), (3) **el deltoide** (deltoid), (4) **el bíceps** (biceps), (5) **la costilla** (rib), (6) **el esternón** (sternum), (7) **el corazón** (heart), (8) **la areola/el pezón** (areola/nipple), (9) **el pecho/seno/la teta** (chest/breast), (10) **la cintura** (waist), (11) **el ombligo** (umbilicus), (12) **el músculo abdominal** (abdominal muscle).

Push.	**Haz fuerza, empuja.** *(Ahs foo-ehr-sah, ehm-poo-hah)*
Lift your foot.	**Levanta tu pie.** *(Leh-bahn-tah too pee-eh)*
Bend your toes.	**Dobla tus dedos.** *(Doh-blah toos deh-dohs)*
Lower your foot.	**Baja el pie.** *(Bah-hah ehl pee-eh)*
I am going to palpate your feet and ankles.	**Voy a palpar tus pies y tobillos.** *(Boh-ee ah pahl-pahr toos pee-ehs ee toh-bee-yohs)*
Flex the foot upward.	**Dobla el pie hacia arriba.** *(Doh-blah ehl pee-eh ah-see-ah ah-ree-bah)*
Hold it like this.	**Manténlo así.** *(Mahn-tehn-loh ah-see)*
I am going to press on your big toe.	**Voy a apretar tu dedo grueso.** *(Boh-ee ah ah-preh-tahr too deh-doh groo-eh-soh)*
I am going to palpate your knees.	**Voy a palpar tus rodillas.** *(Boh-ee ah pahl-pahr toos roh-dee-yahs)*
Pull your knee to your chest.	**Estira la rodilla hacia el pecho.** *(Ehs-tee-rah lah roh-dee-yah ah-see-ah ehl peh-choh)*
Place your foot on the opposite knee.	**Pon tu pie sobre la rodilla opuesta.** *(Pohn too pee-eh soh-breh lah roh-dee-yah oh-poo-ehs-tah)*
Flex your knee and turn it to the middle.	**Dobla tu rodilla y voltéala hacia adentro.** *(Doh-blah too roh-dee-yah ee bohl-teh-ah-lah ah-see-ah ah-dehn-troh)*
Cross your legs.	**Cruza tus piernas.** *(Kroo-sah toos pee-ehr-nahs)*
Straighten your leg.	**Endereza tu pierna.** *(Ehn-deh-reh-sah too pee-ehr-nah)*
Don't let me bend it.	**No me dejes que la doble.** *(Noh meh deh-hehs keh lah doh-bleh)*
Relax your muscle.	**Relaja tu músculo.** *(Reh-lah-hah too moos-koo-loh)*

Stand up!	¡Levántate!
	(Leh-bahn-tah-teh)
Please, walk.	Camina, por favor.
	(Kah-mee-nah, pohr fah-bohr)
Stop!	¡Para!/¡Detente!
	(Pah-rah/Deh-tehn-teh)
Jump on one foot.	Brinca con un pie.
	(Breen-kah kohn oon pee-eh)
Take your shoes off.	Quítate los zapatos.
	(Kee-tah-teh lohs sah-pah-tohs)
Take your socks off.	Quítate los calcetines.
	(Kee-tah-teh lohs kahl-seh-tee-nehs)
Now, I am going to examine your skin.	Ahora, voy a revisar tu piel.
	(Ah-oh-rah boh-ee ah reh-bee-sahr too pee-ehl)
You have bruises and white spots.	Tiene moretones y manchas blancas.
	(Tee-eh-neh moh-reh-toh-nehs ee mahn-chahs blahn-kahs)
Now, I am going to examine your chest.	Ahora, voy a revisar tu pecho.
	(Ah-oh-rah boy ah reh-bee-sahr too peh-choh)
I am going to listen to your heart.	Voy a escuchar el corazón.
	(Boh-ee ah ehs-koo-chahr ehl koh-rah-sohn)
Don't talk.	No hables.
	(Noh ah-blehs)
Breathe!	¡Respira!
	(Rehs-pee-rah)
Breathe regularly.	Respira regularmente.
	(Rehs-pee-rah reh-goo-lahr-mehn-teh)
Now, take a deep breath.	Ahora, respira hondo.
	(Ah-oh-rah, rehs-pee-rah ohn-doh)
Hold it!	¡Deténlo!
	(Deh-tehn-loh)
Does it hurt to breathe?	¿Te duele al respirar?
	(Teh doo-eh-leh ahl rehs-pee-rahr)
Cough!	¡Tose!
	(Toh-seh)
Cough harder!	¡Tose más fuerte!
	(Toh-seh mahs foo-ehr-teh)

55

Physical Exam

TABLE 5-2	Skin-Related Terms
TABLA 5-2	Terminos Relacionados con la Piel

English	Spanish	Pronunciation
dry	seca	*seh-kah*
bruises/ecchymosis	moretones/equimosis	*moh-reh-toh-nehs/eh-kee-moh-sees*
hematoma	hematoma	*eh-mah-toh-mah*
scratch	raspón	*rahs-pohn*
acne	acné	*ahk-neh*
burns	quemaduras	*keh-mah-doo-rahs*
wound	herida	*eh-ree-dah*
infection	infección	*een-fehk-see-ohn*
inflammation	inflamación	*een-flah-mah-see-ohn*
ulcers	úlceras	*ool-seh-rahs*
fungus	hongos	*ohn-gohs*
red spots/white spots	manchas rojas/manchas blancas	*mahn-chahs roh-hahs/mahn-chahs blahn-kahs*
birthmark	lunar	*loo-nahr*
mole	verruga	*beh-roo-gah*
psoriasis	soriasis	*soh-ree-ah-sees*
eczema	eczema	*ehk-seh-mah*
freckles	pecas	*peh-kahs*

I am going to palpate your chest.	Voy a palpar el pecho. *(Boh-ee ah pahl-pahr ehl peh-choh)*
Relax.	Descansa. *(Dehs-kahn-sah)*
Sit upright!	¡Siéntate derecho! *(See-ehn-tah-teh deh-reh-choh)*
Please, lie down.	Acuéstate, por favor. *(Ah-koo-ehs-tah-teh pohr fah-bohr)*
I am going to palpate the breast.	Voy a palpar el seno. *(Boh-ee ah pahl-pahr ehl seh-noh)*
I am going to palpate the axillary nodes.	Voy a palpar los nodos de la axila. *(Boh-ee ah pahl-pahr lohs noh-dohs deh lah ahx-ee-lah)*
I am going to tap.	Voy a percutir/golpear. *(Boh-ee ah pehr-koo-teer/gohl-peh-ahr)*

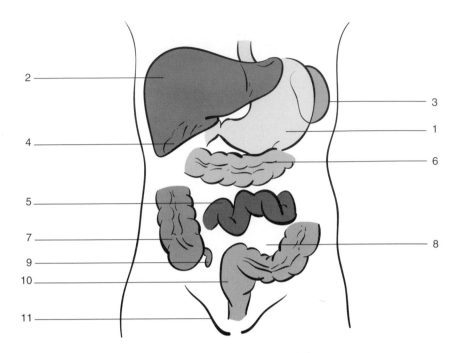

Figure 5-5 Inspecting the abdomen. (ABDOMEN).
(1) **el estómago** (stomach), (2) **el hígado** (liver), (3) **el bazo** (spleen), (4) **la vesícula biliar/la hiel** (gallbladder), (5) **el intestino chico/delgado** (small intestine), (6) **el intestino transverso** (transverse intestine), (7) **el asendiente grueso** (ascending colon), (8) **el vientre/área pélvica** (lower pelvic area), (9) **la apéndice** (appendix), (10) **el recto** (rectum), (11) **la ingle** (groin).

I am going to auscultate.	Voy a auscultar/escuchar. *(Boh-ee ah ah-oos-kool-tahr/ehs-koo-chahr)*
I am going to listen to your heartbeat.	Voy a oír tu pulso apical/los latidos del corazón. *(Boh-ee ah oh-eer too pool-soh ah-pee-kahl/lohs lah-tee-dohs dehl koh-rah-sohn)*
I am going to palpate your carotid pulse.	Voy a palpar tu pulso en la carótida/en el cuello. *(Boh-ee ah pahl-pahr too pool-soh ehn lah kah-roh-tee-dah/ehn ehl koo-eh-yoh)*
I am going to take the radial pulse.	Voy a tomar tu pulso radial. *(Boh-ee ah toh-mahr too pool-soh rah-dee-ahl)*

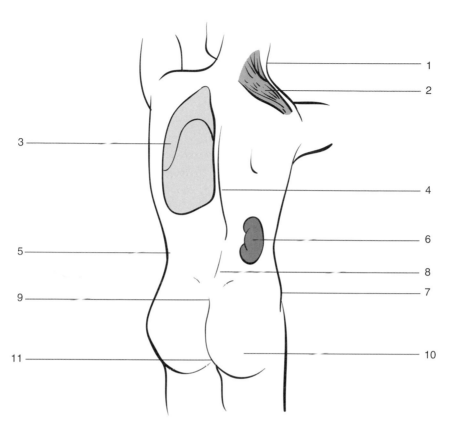

Figure 5-6 Inspecting the Back. (LA ESPALDA).
(1) **La nuca** (nape),(2) **el trapezolde** (trapezius), (3) **el pulmón** (lung), (4) **la vér-tebra** (spine), (5) **la cintura** (waist), (6) **el riñón** (kidney), (7) **la cadera** (hip), (8) **el lumbar** (lumbar), (9) **el sacro** (sacrum), (10) **la nalga** (buttock), (11) **el ano/la cola** (anus).

I am going to observe the jugular vein.	**Voy a observar tu vena yugular.** *(Boh-ee ah ohb-sehr-bahr too beh-nah yoo-goo-lahr)*
Now, I am going to examine your abdomen.	**Ahora, voy a revisar tu abdomen/vientre.** *(Ah-oh-rah boh-ee ah reh-bee-sahr too ahb-doh-mehn/bee-ehn-treh)*
I am going to check your liver.	**Voy a revisar tu hígado.** *(Boh-ee ah reh-bee-sahr too ee-gah-doh)*

I am going to palpate lightly.	Voy a palpar/tocar ligero. *(Boh-ee ah pahl-pahr/toh-kahr lee-heh-roh)*
I am going to palpate deeply.	Voy a palpar hondo. *(Boh-ee ah pahl-pahr ohn-doh)*
Tell me if it hurts.	Dime si duele. *(Dee-meh see doo-eh-leh)*
Does it hurt when I press?	¿Duele cuando presiono? *(Doo-eh-leh koo-ahn-doh preh- see-oh-noh)*
Does it hurt when I let go?	¿Duele cuando retiro la mano? *(Doo-eh-leh koo-ahn-doh reh- tee-roh lah mah-noh)*
I am going to palpate with both hands.	Voy a palpar/tocar con las dos manos. *(Boh-ee ah pahl-pahr/toh-kahr kohn lahs dohs mah-nohs)*
Raise your head.	Levanta tu cabeza. *(Leh-bahn-tah too kah-beh-sah)*
I am going to check how strong your abdominal muscle is.	Voy a ver la fuerza del músculo abdominal. *(Boh-ee ah behr lah foo-ehr-sah dehl moos-koo-loh ahb-doh-mee- nahl)*
Turn onto your side.	Voltéate de lado. *(Bohl-teh-ah-teh deh lah-doh)*
Left . . .	Izquierdo. . . . *(Ees-kee-ehr-doh)*
Right . . .	Derecho . . . *(Deh-reh-choh)*
Take a deep breath.	Respira hondo. *(Rehs-pee-rah ohn-doh)*
Let it out.	Exhala. *(Ehx-ah-lah)*
I am going to palpate the groin.	Voy a palpar las ingles. *(Boh-ee ah pahl-pahr lahs een-glehs)*
Push down.	Empuja. *(Ehm-poo-hah)*
I am going to examine the rectum.	Voy a examinar el recto. *(Boh-ee ah ehx-ah-mee-nahr ehl rehk-toh)*
I am going to collect a stool sample.	Voy a recoger una muestra de excremento. *(Boh-ee ah reh-koh-hehr oo-nah moo-ehs-trah deh ehx-kreh-mehn- toh)*

I am going to examine the genitalia.	Voy a examinar los genitales. *(Boh-ee ah ehx-ah-mee-nahr lohs heh-nee-tah-lehs)*
I am going to examine your back.	Voy a examinar tu espalda. *(Boh-ee ah ehx-ah-mee-nahr too ehs-pahl-dah)*
I am going to listen to the lungs.	Voy a oír los pulmones. *(Boh-ee ah oh-eer lohs pool-moh-nehs)*
Breathe through the mouth.	Respira con la boca abierta. *(Rehs-pee-rah kohn lah boh-kah ah-bee-ehr-tah)*
Again.	Otra vez. *(Oh-trah behs)*
Repeat one, two, three.	Repite uno, dos, tres. *(Reh-pee-teh oo-noh, dohs, trehs)*
Now, stand up.	Ahora, levántate. *(Ah-oh-rah, leh-bahn-tah-teh)*
Now, bend over.	Ahora, agáchate. *(Ah-oh-rah, ah-gah-chah-teh)*
Cross your arms.	Cruza tus brazos. *(Kroo-sah toos brah-sohs)*
Twist your waist.	Tuerce la cintura. *(Too-ehr-seh lah seen-too-rah)*
Repeat the word "99."	Repite las palabras "noventa y nueve". *(Reh-pee-teh lahs pah-lah-brahs "noh-behn-tah ee noo-eh-beh")*
Say your name.	Di tu nombre. *(Dee too nohm-breh)*
Bend your shoulder.	Dobla tu hombro. *(Doh-blah too ohm-broh)*
I have finished the exam.	Terminé de revisarte. *(Tehr-mee-neh deh reh-bee-sahr-teh)*
Any questions?	¿Alguna pregunta? *(Ahl-goo-nah preh-goon-tah)*

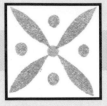

CHAPTER SIX
Admitting A Patient

CAPITULO SEIS
Admitiendo al Paciente

M any Hispanic patients take someone with them to the hospital. This person is able to translate for the patient. However, there's nothing like being able to greet the patient in his language and be able to elicit first-hand information. Do not be annoyed if the patient brings with him several members of his family. Hispanics tend to be supportive of each other and feel better when family is around. Be patient. Alert the patient that you will be asking many questions.

Muchos pacientes hispanos llevan a una persona con ellos al hospital. Esta persona sirve de intérprete. Pero, no hay comparación, como el poder saludar al paciente en su lengua y tomar información de primera. No se moleste si el paciente va acompañado por varios miembros de su familia. Los hispanos tienden a apoyarse uno al otro y se sienten mejor cuando hay familiares alrededor. Tenga paciencia. Avísele al paciente que va a hacerle muchas preguntas.

What can I help you with?	¿En que puedo ayudarlo? *(Ehn keh poo-eh-doh ah-yoo-dahr-loh)*
Tell me why you are here.	Dígame por qué está aquí. *(Dee-gah-meh pohr keh ehs-tah ah-kee)*
What's happening?	¿Qué le pasa? *(Keh leh pah-sah)*
How did you get here?	¿Cómo llegó aquí? *(koh-moh yeh-goh ah-kee)*

Did you come by car?	¿Vino en carro? *(Bee-noh ehn kah-roh)*
Did you arrive in a wheelchair?	¿Llegó en silla de ruedas? *(Yeh-goh ehn see-yah deh roo-eh-dahs)*
Did you walk?	¿Caminó? *(Kah-mee-noh)*
You have to give permission for treatment.	Tiene que dar permiso para el tratamiento. *(Tee-eh-neh keh dahr pehr-mee-soh pah-rah ehl trah-tah-mee-ehn-toh)*
Can you write?	¿Puede escribir? *(Poo-eh-deh ehs-kree-beer)*
Please, sign here.	Por favor, firme aquí. *(Pohr fah-bohr, feer-meh ah-kee)*
What brought you to the hospital?	¿Qué lo trajo al hospital? *(Keh loh trah-hoh ahl ohs-pee-tahl)*
What problem do you have?	¿Qué problema tiene? *(Keh proh-bleh-mah tee-eh-neh)*
Do you have high blood pressure?	¿Tiene la presión alta? *(Tee-eh-neh lah preh-see-ohn ahl-tah)*
Are you dizzy?	¿Tiene mareos? *(Tee-eh-neh mah-reh-ohs)*
Do you get headaches?	¿Tiene dolor de cabeza? *(Tee-eh-neh doh-lohr deh kah-beh-sah)*

See Table 6-1 for similar medical terms.
Vea la Tabla 6-1 con términos médicos similares.

I am going to ask many questions!	¡Voy a hacerle muchas preguntas! *(Boh-ee ah ah-sehr-leh moo-chahs preh-goon-tahs)*
Do you speak English?	¿Habla inglés? *(Ah-blah een-glehs)*
Can you read?	¿Puede leer? *(Poo-eh-deh leh-ehr)*
Where do you work?	¿Dónde trabaja? *(Dohn-deh trah-bah-hah)*
What is your occupation?	¿Qué clase de trabajo tiene? *(Keh klah-seh deh trah-bah-hoh tee-eh-neh)*

TABLE 6-1	Similar Medical Terms
TABLA 6-1	Terminos Médicos Similares

English	Spanish	Pronunciation
anemia	anemia	*ah-neh-mee-ah*
cardiac	cardíaco	*kahr-dee-ah-koh*
dehydrated	deshidratado	*deh-see-drah-tah-doh*
epilepsy	epilepsia	*eh-pee-lehp-see-ah*
inflammation	inflamación	*een-flah-mah-see-ohn*
neurotic	neurótico	*neh-oo-roh-tee-koh*
organ	órgano	*ohr-gah-noh*
pancreas	páncreas	*pahn-kreh-ahs*
rheumatic	reumático	*reh-oo-mah-tee-koh*
valve	válvula	*bahl-boo-lah*
vision	visión	*bee-see-ohn*
vomit	vómito	*boh-mee-toh*

How many years did you go to school?
¿Cuántos años fué a la escuela?
(Koo-ahn-tohs ah-nyohs foo-eh ah lah ehs-koo-eh-lah)

What is your religion?
¿Cuál es su religión?
(Koo-ahl ehs soo reh-lee-hee-ohn)

Who takes care of you at home?
¿Quién lo cuida en casa?
(Kee-ehn loh koo-ee-dah ehn kah-sah)

Table 6-2 will help you with pronunciation of commonly used words.
La Tabla 6-2 le ayudará con la pronunciación de palabras comúnes.

Husband? Wife? Children?
¿Esposo? ¿Esposa? ¿Hijos?
(Ehs-poh-soh Ehs-poh-sah Ee-hohs)

Do you have a family doctor?
¿Tiene un doctor familiar?
(Tee-eh-neh oon dohk-tohr fah-mee-lee-ahr)

Do you have allergies?
¿Tiene alergias?
(Tee-eh-neh ah-lehr-hee-ahs)

Are you allergic to foods?
¿Es alérgico a comidas?
(Ehs ah-lehr-hee-koh ah koh-mee-dahs)

English	Spanish	Pronunciation

TABLE 6-2 **Pronunciation Of Selected Words**
TABLA 6-2 Pronunciación de Palabras Selectas

English	Spanish	Pronunciation
help	ayuda	*ah-yoo-dah*
work	trabajo	*trah-bah-hoh*
hospital	hospital	*ohs-pee-tahl*
chest	pecho	*peh-choh*
reason	razón	*rah-sohn*
ask	preguntar	*preh-goon-tahr*
speak	hablar	*ah-blahr*
read	leer	*leh-ehr*
allergies	alergias	*ah-lehr-hee-ahs*
smoke	fumar	*fooh-mahr*
alcohol	alcohol	*ahl-kohl*
visit	visita	*bee-see-tah*
permission	permiso	*pehr-mee-soh*
last	última	*ool-tee-mah*

To drugs? To plants?	¿A medicamentos? ¿A plantas? *(Ah meh-dee-kah-mehn-tohs Ah plahn-tahs)*
Do you smoke?	¿Fuma usted? *(Foo-mah oos-tehd)*
How many cigarettes per day?	¿Cuántos cigarrillos por día? *(Koo-ahn-tohs see-gah-ree-yohs pohr dee-ah)*
Do you drink alcohol?	¿Toma bebidas alcohólicas? *(Toh-mah beh-bee-dahs ahl-koh-lee-kahs)*
What kind of drinks?	¿Qué clase de bebidas? *(Keh klah-seh deh beh-bee-dahs)*
How much do you drink per day?	¿Cuánto alcohol toma por día? *(Koo-ahn-toh ahl-kohl toh-mah pohr dee-ah)*
Do you use drugs/medicine?	¿Usa drogas/medicamento? *(Oo-sah droh-gahs/meh-dee-kah-mehn-toh)*
What drugs/medicine do you use?	¿Qué drogas/medicamento usa? *(Keh droh-gahs/meh-dee-kah-mehn-toh oo-sah)*

Have you had blood transfusions?	¿Ha tenido transfusiones de sangre? *(Ah teh-nee-doh trahns-foo-see-oh-nehs deh sahn-greh)*
Reaction to transfusions?	¿Reacción a transfusiones? *(Reh-ahk-see-ohn ah tranhs-foo-see-oh-nehs)*
What medicines do you take?	¿Qué medicinas toma? *(Keh meh-dee-see-nahs toh-mah)*
When was the last time that you took medicine?	¿Cuándo fue la última vez que tomó medicina? *(Koo-ahn-doh foo-eh lah ool-tee-mah behs keh toh-moh meh-dee-see-nah)*
Have you had surgeries?	¿Ha tenido operaciones? *(Ah teh-nee-doh oh-peh-rah-see-oh-nehs)*
What kind of surgery?	¿Qué clase de operaciones? *(Keh klah-seh deh oh-peh-rah-see-oh-nehs)*
Have you had broken bones?	¿Ha tenido huesos rotos/fracturados? *(Ah teh-nee-doh oo-eh-sohs roh-tohs/frahk-too-rah-dohs)*
Car accidents?	¿Accidentes de auto? *(Ahk-see-dehn-tehs deh ah-oo-toh)*
Did you bring valuables?	¿Trajo algo de valor? *(Trah-hoh ahl-goh deh bah-lohr)*
Glasses?	¿Anteojos/lentes? *(Ahn-teh-oh-hohs/lehn-tehs)*
Jewelry? Cash?	¿Joyas? ¿Dinero? *(Hoh-yahs Dee-neh-roh)*
Artificial eye?	¿Ojo artificial? *(Oh-hoh ahr-tee-fee-see-ahl)*
Hearing aid?	¿Aparato para oír? *(Ah-pah-rah-toh pah-rah oh-eer)*
Dentures?	¿Dentadura postiza? *(Dehn-tah-doo-rah pohs-tee-sah)*
The hospital is not responsible.	El hospital no se hace responsable. *(Ehl ohs-pee-tahl noh seh ah-seh rehs-pohn-sah-bleh)*
Do you have special problems?	¿Tiene problemas especiales? *(Tee-eh-neh proh-bleh-mahs ehs-peh-see-ah-lehs)*

Do you take a special diet?	¿Toma dieta especial? *(Toh-mah dee-eh-tah ehs-peh-see-ahl)*
What foods do you like?	¿Qué alimentos le gustan? *(Keh ah-lee-mehn-tohs leh goos-tahn)*
What foods do you dislike?	¿Qué alimentos le disgustan? *(Keh ah-lee-mehn-tohs leh dees-goos-tahn)*
Do you need to see a dietitian?	¿Necesita ver a la dietista? *(Neh-seh-see-tah behr ah lah dee-eh-tees-tah)*

Table 6-3 gives a list of special diets.
La Tabla 6-3 le da una lista de dietas especiales.

Do you have tuberculosis?	¿Tiene tuberculosis? *(Tee-eh-neh too-behr-koo-loh-sees)*
Chest pain?	¿Dolor en el pecho? *(Doh-lohr ehn ehl peh-choh)*
Diabetes?	¿Diabetes? *(Dee-ah-beh-tehs)*
Cancer?	¿Cáncer? *(Kahn-sehr)*
How many persons in your family?	¿Cuántas personas forman su familia? *(Koo-ahn-tahs pehr-soh-nahs fohr-mahn soo fah-mee-lee-ah)*
Do you live by yourself?	¿Vive solo? *(Bee-beh soh-loh)*

TABLE 6-3 Types of Diets
TABLA 6-3 Tipos de Dietas

English	Spanish	Pronunciation
regular	regular	*reh-goo-lahr*
liquid	líquida	*lee-kee-dah*
low sodium	baja en sal/poca sal	*bah-hah ehn sahl/poh-kah sahl*
diabetic	diabética	*dee-ah-beh-tee-kah*
low cholesterol	poco colesterol	*poh-koh koh-lehs-teh-rohl*
low fat	poca grasa	*poh-kah grah-sah*
pureed	puré	*poo-reh*

How do you spend the day?	¿Cómo pasa el día?
	(Koh-moh pah-sah ehl dee-ah)
At what time do you get up?	¿A qué hora se levanta?
	(Ah keh oh-rah seh leh-bahn-tah)
At what time do you go to bed?	¿A qué hora se acuesta?
	(Ah keh oh-rah seh ah-koo-ehs-tah)
How many hours do you sleep?	¿Cuántas horas duerme?
	(Koo-ahn-tahs oh-rahs doo-ehr-meh)
Do you sleep during the day?	¿Duerme durante el día?
	(Doo-ehr-meh doo-rahn-teh ehl dee-ah)
How long?	¿Cuánto tiempo?
	(Koo-ahn-toh tee-ehm-poh)
Who helps you at home?	¿Quién le ayuda en casa?
	(Kee-ehn leh ah-yoo-dah ehn kah-sah)
Can you do house chores?	¿Puede hacer quehacers?
	(Poo-eh-deh ah-sehr keh-ah-seh-rehs)
Do you get tired easily?	¿Se cansa con facilidad?
	(Seh kahn-sah kohn fah-see-lee-dahd)
Do you need to see a social worker?	¿Necesita ver a la trabajadora social?
	(Neh-seh-see-tah behr ah lah trah-bah-hah-doh-rah soh-see-ahl)
Do you want to see a priest?	¿Necesita ver al sacerdote?
	(Neh-seh-see-tah behr ahl sah-sehr-doh-teh)

See Table 6-4 for more helpful words and phrases.
Vea la Tabla 6-4 para más palabras y frases útiles.

TABLE 6-4	Helpful Words and Phrases
TABLA 6-4	Palabras y Frases Útiles

English	Spanish	Pronunciation
hospital policy	reglas del hospital	*reh-glahs dehl ohs-pee-tahl*
routine	la rutina	*lah roo-tee-nah*
no smoking	no se permite fumar	*noh seh pehr-mee-teh foo-mahr*
instructions	instrucciones	*eens-trook-see-ohn-ehs*
chaplain/	capellán/	*kah-peh-yahn/*
priest	sacerdote/cura	*sah-sehr-doh-teh/koo-rah*
visiting hours	horas de visita	*oh-rahs deh bee-see-tah*

I will show you your room.	Le mostraré su cuarto. *(Leh mohs-trah-reh soo koo-ahr-toh)*
You cannot smoke here.	No puede fumar aquí. *(Noh poo-eh-deh foo-mahr ah-kee)*
This is the call bell.	Este es el timbre. *(Ehs-teh ehs ehl teem-breh)*
The meals are served at seven AM.	Los alimentos se sirven a las siete de la mañana. *(Lohs ah-lee-mehn-tohs seh seer-behn ah lahs see-eh-teh deh lah mah-nyah-nah)*
At eleven thirty.	A las once y media. *(Ah lahs ohn-seh ee meh-dee-ah)*
At five PM.	A las cinco de la tarde. *(Ah lahs seen-koh deh lah tahr-deh)*
Phone for local calls.	Teléfono para llamadas locales. *(Teh-leh-foh-noh pah-rah yah-mah-dahs loh-kah-lehs)*
This is the radio.	Este es el radio. *(Ehs-teh ehs ehl rah-dee-oh)*
The television has four channels.	El televisor tiene cuatro canales. *(Ehl teh-leh-bee-sohr tee-eh-neh koo-ah-troh kah-nah-lehs)*
There is an educational channel.	Hay un canal educativo. *(Ah-ee oon kah-nahl eh-doo-kah-tee-boh)*
These buttons move the bed up/down.	Estos botones mueven la cama arriba/abajo. *(Ehs-tohs boh-toh-nehs moo-eh-behn lah kah-mah ah-ree-bah/ah-bah-hoh)*
You can raise the head.	Puede levantar la cabeza. *(Poo-eh-deh leh-bahn-tahr lah kah-beh-sah)*
You can raise the feet.	Puede levantar los pies. *(Poo-eh-deh leh-bahn-tahr lohs pee-ehs)*
The rails lower down.	El barandal se baja. *(Ehl bah-rahn-dahl seh bah-hah)*
Visits are from two to eight PM.	Las visitas son de las dos a las ocho de la noche. *(Lahs bee-see-tahs sohn deh lahs dohs ah lahs oh-choh deh lah noh-cheh)*

Wear this bracelet all the time.	Use esta pulsera todo el tiempo.
	(Oo-seh ehs-tah pool-seh-rah toh-doh ehl tee-ehm-poh)
Your towels are in the bathroom.	Sus toallas están en el baño.
	(Soos too-ah-yahs ehs-tahn ehn ehl bah-nyoh)
There is an emergency light.	Hay una luz para emergencias.
	(Ah-ee oo-nah loos pah-rah eh-mehr-hehn-see-ahs)
Pull the cord in the bathroom.	Jale el cordón en el baño.
	(Hah-leh ehl kohr-dohn ehn ehl bah-nyoh)
The bell will sound.	La campana sonará.
	(Lah kahm-pah-nah soh-nah-rah)
Your family will bring you clothes.	Su familia le traerá ropa.
	(Soo fah-mee-lee-ah leh trah-eh-rah roh-pah)
Change into this gown.	Póngase esta bata.
	(Pohn-gah-seh ehs-tah bah-tah)
Rest now.	Descanse ahora.
	(Dehs-kahn-seh ah-oh-rah)
Do you have questions?	¿Tiene dudas?
	(Tee-eh-neh doo-dahs)
I will return to ask you more questions.	Regresaré para hacerle más preguntas.
	(Reh-greh-sah-reh pah-rah ah-sehr-leh mahs preh-goon-tahs)

Table 6-5 will help you review common questions.
La tabla 6-5 le ayudará a repasar preguntas comunes.

TABLE 6-5	Common Questions
TABLA 6-5	Preguntas Comúnes

English	Spanish	Pronunciation
Do you have . . . ?	¿Tiene . . . ?	*Tee-eh-neh*
How did you . . . ?	¿Cómo hizo . . . ?	*Koh-moh ee-soh*
What kind?	¿Qué clase?	*Keh klah-seh*
What's the matter?	¿Qué pasa?	*Keh pah-sah*
How many?	¿Cuántos?	*Koo-ahn-tohs*
Have you had . . . ?	¿Ha tenido . . . ?	*Ah teh-nee-doh*
What is . . . ?	¿Qué es . . . ?	*Keh ehs*
Can you . . . ?	¿Puede usted . . . ?	*Poo-eh-deh oos-tehd*

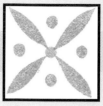

CHAPTER SEVEN
Consent to Procedures/Treatment

CAPITULO SIETE
Consentimiento a Procedimientos/Cirugía

Asking a patient's consent for procedures and surgery is an extremely important activity, especially when the patient does not understand English. As a health care provider, you are charged with explaining the procedure, the benefits, and the risks that the patient is exposed to when he agrees to have a procedure or surgery performed.

El pedir al paciente el consentimiento para procedimientos y cirugía es una actividad muy importante, especialmente cuando el paciente no entiende el inglés. Siendo un proveedor de cuidados de salud, usted está encargado de explicar el procedimiento, los beneficios y los riesgos al cuales se expone cuando él está de acuerdo en tener un procedimiento o una cirugía.

In general, the consent has to be signed by the patient. Sometimes, when the patient is unable to sign, a relative signs it. We sometimes ask the patient to sign a power of attorney so that a relative or friend is able to give permission for treatment.

En general, el consentimiento debe ser firmado por el paciente. Algunas veces, cuando el paciente no puede firmar, un pariente lo firma. A veces, nosotros le pedimos al paciente que firme un documento dando poder a un pariente o un amigo para que pueda dar permiso para el tratamiento.

Good morning Mrs. Chapa!

¡Buenos días Señora Chapa!
(*Boo-eh-nohs dee-ahs Seh-nyoh-rah Chah-pah!*)

Tomorrow you are going to have your surgery.

Mañana le van a hacer la cirugía.
(*Mah-nyah-nah leh bahn ah ah-sehr lah see-roo-hee-ah.*)

Did the doctor explain the procedure to you?

¡Le explicó él médico el procedimiento?
(*Leh ehx-plee-koh ehl meh-dee-koh ehl proh-seh-dee-mee-ehn-toh?*)

Yes, my doctor told me about the benefits and the risks.

Sí, mi doctor me dijo los beneficios y los riesgos.
(*See, mee dohk-tohr meh dee-hoh lohs beh-neh-fee-see-ohs ee lohs ree-ehs-gohs*)

The anesthesiologist will visit you in the afternoon.

El anestesiólogo la visitará en la tarde.
(*Ehl ah-nehs-teh-see-oh-loh-goh lah bee-see-tah-rah ehn lah tahr-deh*)

If you have questions, please let me know.

Si tiene preguntas, por favor avíseme.
(*See tee-eh-neh preh-goon-tahs, pohr fah-bohr ah-bee-seh-meh*)

Does this surgery require a blood transfusion?

¿Esta cirugía requiere transfusión de sangre?
(*Ehs-tah see-roo-hee-ah reh-kee-eh-reh trahns-foo-see-ohn deh sahn-greh*)

No, it does not require it.

No, no lo requiere.
(*Noh, noh loh reh-kee-eh-reh*)

Will your husband be here?

¿Estará aquí su esposo?
(*Ehs-tah-rah ah-kee soo ehs-poh-soh*)

No, he is working out of state.

No, él trabaja fuera del estado.
(*Noh, ehl trah-bah-hah foo-eh-rah dehl ehs-tah-doh*)

My daughter will be here.

Mi hija estará aquí.
(*Mee ee-hah ehs-tah-rah ah-kee*)

Let's go over the consent form.

Vamos a ver la forma de consentimiento.
(*Bah-mohs ah behr lah fohr-mah deh kohn-sehn-tee-mee-ehn-toh*)

CONSENT FOR TREATMENT

Date: _____   Time: _____

I hereby give my permission for the following treatment: _____

To be performed by Dr. _____

and his assistants.

I consent to the treatment in addition to or different from those now being planned.

I hereby certify that I have been informed of the treatment and have been told of the benefits and risks.

_____
Witness

Name: _____

_____
Address: ____ _____

_____
Signature of Patient

_____ _____
Signature of person authorized to consent for patient

_____
Relationship to Patient

A

CONSENTIMIENTO PARA TRATAMIENTO

Fecha: _____   Hora: _____

Doy permiso para el siguiente tratamiento: _____

Llevado a cabo por el doctor: _____ _____

y sus asistentes.

Doy permiso para el tratamiento en adición o diferente del tratamiento planeado.

Yo certifico que me han informado acerca del tratamiento y me han dicho sus beneficios y riesgos.

_____
Testigo

Nombre: _____

_____
Dirección: _____

_____
Firma del Paciente

_____
Firma de la persona autorizada para dar consentimiento

_____ _____
Relación al Paciente

B

Figure 7-1 **A,** Consent for treatment. **B, Consentimiento para tratamiento.**

OUR LADY OF THE LAKE REGIONAL MEDICAL CENTER
BATON ROUGE, LA

CONSENT FOR OPERATION OR OTHER PROCEDURE

DATE _____, 20 _____   TIME _____ AM ____ PM ____

I hereby give Doctor _____ and/or any assistant engaged by him
Physician's Name

Permission to perform

_____
Name of Procedure

On _____, under such anesthetics, with the exception of
_____, as he or the anesthesiologist in their discretion deem
necessary or desirable. I also authorize the above named physician engaged or
designated by him to perform any procedure different from those listed above if during
the course of the operation or procedure of thereafter any conditions occur or are
encountered which in his judgement make such different procedure necessary or
desirable.

I UNDERSTAND AND ACKNOWLEDGE THAT THE FOLLOWING KNOWN RISKS
MAY BE ASSOCIATED WITH THIS PROCEDURE INCLUDING ANESTHESIA:
DEATH, BRAIN DAMAGE, QUADRIPLEGIA (Paralysis of all arms and legs),
PARAPLEGIA (paralysis of both legs), LOSS OR LOSS OF FUNCTION OF ANY
ORGAN OR LIMB, DISFIGURING SCARS.

I FURTHER ACKNOWLEDGE THAT ALL QUESTIONS I HAVE ASKED ABOUT THE
PROCEDURE HAVE BEEN ANSWERED IN A SATISFACTORY MANNER BY MY
PHYSICIAN.

The nature and purposes of the operation, possible alternative methods of treatment,
the risks involved, and the possibility of complications have been fully explained to me
by my physician. No guarantee or assurance has been given by anyone as to the
results that may be obtained.

I further authorize Our Lady of the Lake Regional Medical Center to retain, preserve,
and use for scientific, diagnostic, therapeutic, or educational purposes or disposal at
their convenience any specimens or tissue from me during my hospitalization.

I HAVE READ AND UNDERSTAND THE ABOVE FORM WHICH WAS COMPLETED
PRIOR TO MY SIGNING.

_____   _____
Witness   Signature of Patient

_____   _____
Witness*   Signature of Other Than Patient**

                                 _____
                                 Relationship to the Patient

* Two witnesses are required if consent is via telephone or if patient cannot sign his
name and only makes a mark.
** To be signed by personnel legally authorized to consent for the patient.

A

Figure 7-2 A, Consent for operation or other procedure.   *Continued*

OUR LADY OF THE LAKE REGIONAL MEDICAL CENTER
BATON ROUGE, LA

CONSENTIMIENTO PARA OPERACIÓN U OTRO PROCEDIMIENTO

FECHA _____, 20 ____   HORA _____ AM ____ PM ____

Por la presente doy permiso al Doctor _____ y/o cualquier asistente en su servicio

Permiso para llevar a cabo

_____

Nombre del Procedimiento

En _____, bajo anestesia, con la excepción de _____, con la discreción
necesaria de él o el anestesiólogo. También autorizo al doctor mencionado arriba o a
quien designe para que lleve a cabo cualquier procedimiento diferente a los que
están en la lista si durante el curso de la operación o del procedimiento o de alguna
otra condición que ocurra o en las cuales en su juicio hacen esos procedimientos
diferentes que sean necesarios o deseados.

YO ENTIENDO Y CONFIRMO QUE LOS SIGUIENTES RIESGOS PUEDEN ESTAR
ASOCIADOS CON ESTE PROCEDIMIENTO QUE INCLUYE ANESTESIA, MUERTE,
DAÑO AL CEREBRO, CUADRIPLÉJIA (PARÁLISIS DE LOS BRAZOS Y PIERNAS),
PARAPLÉJÍA (PARÁLISIS DE AMBAS PIERNAS), PÉRDIDA O PÉRDIDA DE LA
FUNCIÓN DE CUALQUIER ORGANO O MIEMBRO, CICATRICES
DISFIGURANTES.

YO CONFIRMO QUE TODAS LAS PREGUNTAS QUE HE HECHO SOBRE EL
PROCEDIMEIENTO SE HAN CONTESTADO DE UNA MANERA SATISFACTORIA
POR MI MÉDICO.

La naturaleza y la intención de la operación, los métodos alternativos al tratamiento,
los riesgos involucrados, y la posibilidad de complicaciones me los explicó bien mi
médico. Nadie me a garantizado o asegurado los resultados que se obtengan.

Además yo autorizo al Centro Médico de Nuestra Señora Del Lago a retener,
preservar, y usar para acciones científicas, de diagnóstico, de terápia, u objetivos
educacionales o disponer a su conveniencia cualquier muestra o tejidos que me
hayan substraído durante mi hospitalización.

HE LEÍDO Y ENTIENDO LA FORMA QUE SE COMPLETÓ ANTES DE QUE YO
FIRMARA.

_____   _____
Testigo   Firma del Paciente

_____   _____
Testigo*   Firma de otra persona**

                                           _____
                                           Relación al Paciente

* Dos testigos se requieren si el consentimiento se dá por teléfono o si el paciente no
puede firmar su nombre y solo hace una marca.
** Se firma por una persona autorizada legalmente para dar consentimiento por el
paciente.

B

Figure 7-2, cont'd. B, Consentimiento para operación u otro procedimiento.
(Courtesy Our Lady of the Lake Regional Medical Center, Baton Rouge, Louisiana.)

1. Legal Relationship Between Hospital and Physician

I understand that, unless I am specifically otherwise informed, in writing, all physicians furnishing services to me, including the pathologist, anesthesiologist, emergency room physician, and the like, are independent contractors and are not employees or agents of the Hospital. I am under the care and supervision of my attending physician and it is the responsibility of the Hospital and its staff to carry out the instructions of my physician. It is my physician's responsibility to obtain my informed consent, when required, for medical or surgical treatment, special diagnostic or therapeutic procedures, or hospital services rendered to me under general and special instructions of my physician.

I understand that there will be a separate charge for professional services, such as physician services. I understand that the Hospital does bill for some professional fees; otherwise, the professional fees are not included in the Hospital's bill.

2. Assignment of Benefits

This assignment of benefits allows the Hospital and/or hospital based physicians to be paid directly by my health insurance carrier or other health benefit plan for the services the Hospital and/or hospital based physicians provides to me, my minor child, or other person entitled to health care benefits for this admission. In return for the services rendered and to be rendered by the Hospital and/or hospital based physicians. I hereby irrevocably assign and transfer to the Hospital and/or hospital based physicians all right, title, and interest in all benefits payable for the health care rendered, which are provided in any and all insurance policies and health benefit plans from which my dependents or I am entitled to recover. This assignment and transfer shall be for the purpose of granting the Hospital and/or hospital based physicians an independent right of recovery against my insurer or health benefit plan, but shall not be construed as an obligation of the Hospital and/or hospital based physicians to pursue any such right of recovery. In no event will the Hospital and/or hospital based physicians retain benefits in excess of the amount owed to the Hospital and/or hospital based physicians for the care and treatment rendered during this admission. I have read and been given the opportunity to ask questions about this assignment of benefits, and I have signed this document freely and without inducement, other than the rendition of services by the Hospital and/or hospital based physicians.

3. Medicare Patient Certification

I certify that the information given by me in applying for payment under Title XVIII or Title XIX of the Social Security Act is correct. I authorize any holder or medical or other information about me to release to the Social Security

5. Organ Donation

I understand that I have the right to donate any of my organs or tissues for transplantation and that I may do so by completing an anatomical gift form.

Please initial if applicable: I Have signed an organ donor card and have been requested to supply a copy to the Hospital. _____

6. Patient Self-Determination Act

I acknowledge that I have been given information regarding this state's law on living wills and advance directives. Advance directives are documents such as living wills, durable powers of attorney, or health care surrogate appointments.

Please Initial the Following Applicable Statements:

I have executed an Advance Directive and have been requested to supply a copy to the Hospital. _____

I have reviewed the Advance Directive on file at the Hospital and it is my current Advance Directive. _____

I have not executed an Advance Directive. _____

I have received information about Advance Directives as required by federal law. _____

Do you wish to execute an Advance Directive at this time?

☐ Yes ☐ No

7. Patient Rights

I acknowledge that I have been given information and instructions regarding my Patient Rights. My Patient Rights include, but are not limited to, the right to make medical decisions, including the right to accept or refuse medical treatment, participate in my plan of care and receive care in a safe setting, free from verbal or physical abuse or harassment. I acknowledge that I have also received information about the Hospital's grievance process.

Please Initial: Agree _____ **Disagree** _____

8. Personal Valuables

I understand that the Hospital maintains a safe for the safekeeping of money and valuables, and the Hospital shall not be liable for the loss or damage to any money, jewelry, documents, furs, fur coats and fur garments or other articles of unusual value and small size, unless placed therein, and shall not be liable for loss or damage to any other personal property, unless deposited with the Hospital for safekeeping.

Administration or its intermediaries or carriers any information need for this or a related Medicare claim. I permit a copy of the authorization to be used in place of the original and request payment of authorized benefits be make on my behalf.

4. Consent to Medical and Surgical Procedures

I, the undersigned, consent to the procedures which may be performed during this hospitalization or on an outpatient basis, including emergency treatment or services, and which may include but are not limited to laboratory procedures, x-ray examination, diagnostic procedures, medical, nursing or surgical treatment or procedures, anesthesia, or hospital services rendered to me under the general and special instructions of my physician.

This course includes testing for blood-borne infectious diseases, Including but not limited to hepatitis, Acquired Immune Deficiency Syndrome (AIDS), and Human Immunodeficiency Virus (HIV), if a Physician orders such test(s) for diagnostic purposes.

Please Initial: Agree _____ Disagree _____

9. Weapons/Explosive/Drugs

I understand and agree that if the Hospital at any time believes there may be a weapon, explosive devices, illegal substances or drug, or any alcoholic beverage in my room or with my belongings, the Hospital may search my room and my belongings, confiscate any of the above items that are found, and dispose of them as appropriate including delivery of any item to law enforcement authorities.

10. Private Room

I understand and agree that if I request a private room for myself or the patient, I am responsible for any additional charges associated with that request.

11. Financial Agreement

I, the undersigned, agree whether I sign as parent, guardian, spouse, agent, guarantor, or as patient, that in consideration of the services to be rendered to the patient, I hereby individually obligate myself to pay the account of the Hospital in accordance with the regular rates and terms of the Hospital. Should the account be referred to an attorney or collection agency for collection, I shall pay attorney's fees and collection expenses.

Date	I hereby certify and state that I have read, and that I fully and completely understand this Condition of Admission and Authorization for Medical Treatment, and that I have signed this Conditions of Admission and Authorization for Medical Treatment knowingly, freely, and voluntarily. Moreover, I certify and state that I have received no promises, assurances, or guarantees from anyone as to the results that may be obtained by any medical treatment or services.
Time ☐ A.M. ☐ P.M.	

Patient Identification

Patient/Parent/Guardian/Conservator
X

Spouse (if married/available)
X

Witness (to Signature only)
X

East Houston Regional Medical Center
Conditions of Admission and
Authorization for Medical Treatment
A

Figure 7-3 A, Conditions of admission and authorization for medical treatmenet.

Continued

1. **Relación legal entre el hospital y el médico**
Entiendo que, a menos que se me informe por escrito, todos los médicos que me presten sevicios, incluyendo el patólogo, anetesiólogo, o médico del departamento de urgencias, son empleados bajo contrato y no empleados o agentes del hospital. Yo estoy bajo el cuidado y supervisión de mi médico y es la responsabilidad del hospital y sus empleados el seguir sus instrucciones. Es la responsabilidad de mi médico el obtener mi consentimiento para tratamiento médico o quirúrgico, procedimientos especiales de diagnóstico o terapeúticos, o servicios hospitalarios que se me presten bajo instrucciones generales y especiales de mi médico.
Entiendo que habrá gastos en separado por servicios profesionales tales como servicios médicos. Entiendo que el hospital cobra por servicios profesionales que no estan incluidos en la cuenta del hopsital.

2. **Asignación de Beneficios**
Esta asignación de beneficios permite que le page al hospital o a los médicos directamente, por medio de mi seguro de salud u otros planes de beneficios, por los servicios que el hospital o los médicos en el hospital me porveen a mí, a mis hijos, u otras personas que merezcan estos beneficios de salud por este ingreso. En cambio por los servicios que me proveen en el hospital, yo asigno y traspaso al hospital y a los médicos todos los derechos, e interés en todos los beneficios pagados por el cuidado de salud, que se proveen por las pólizas de seguro y los planes de cuideado de salud a los cuales mis dependientes y yo estamos autorizados a recupar. Esta asignación y traspaso se hace con la intensión de dar al hospital y a los médicos el derecho independiente a cobrar a la compañía de seguro o a cualquier otro plan de beneficios, pero no tener obligación de proseguir con dichos derechos. En todo caso, el hospital o los médicos no se quedarán con el exceso del pago que se les debe por el cuidado y tratamiento durante este ingreso al hospital. He leído y se me ha dado la oportunidad de hacer preguntas sobre la asignación de beneficios, y he firmado este documento libremente y sin persuación a parte de los servicios prestados por el hospital o los médicos.

3. **Certificación de Paciente de Medicare**
Yo certifico que la información que se me ha dado sobre el pago bajo el titulo XVIII o Titulo XIX del Acto del Seguro Social es correcta. Yo autorizo a cualquier agente relacionado con este reclamo de Medicare a dar información médica necesaria a la Administración del Seguro Social o a sus intermediarios. Yo doy permiso para que una copia de la autorización se use en lugar de la original y que se solicite pago de beneficios autorizados en mi nombre.

Por favor encriba si es aplicable: He firmado una tarjeta de donación y se me a pedido que dé una copia al hospital. _____

6. **Acto de Auto-Determinación del Paciente**
Confirmo que se me ha dado información sobre las leyes de este estado relacionadas con testamentos actuales y directivas avanzadas. Los testamentos actuales son documentos tales como testamentos vivos, poderes de derechos, o asignaciones de cuidados.

Por favor inscriba las iniciales en las declaraciones que sean aplicables:

He ejecutado las Directivas Avanzadas y se me a pedido que de una copia al Hospital. _____

He repasado la Directiva Avanzada en el archivo del Hospital y está al corriente. _____

No he ejecutado una Directiva Avanzada. _____

He recivido información sobre las Directivas Avanzadas como requiere la ley. _____

Desea ejecutar una Directiva Avanzada ahora?

____ Si   ____ No

7. **Derechos del Paciente**
Confirmo que se me ha dado información e instrucciones relacionadas con derechos de Paciente. Mis derechos incluyen, pero no se limitan, al derecho de hacer decisiones medicas, incluyendo el derecho a aceptar o rehusar tratamiento médico, participar en el cuidado de mi salud y recivir cuidado en ambiente sano, libre de abuso fisico o verbal. Confirmo que he recivido información acerca del proceso de quejas del Hospital.

Por favor inscribe: Estoy de acuerdo
No estoy de acuerdo _____

8. **Valores Personales (objetos de Valor)**
Entiendo que el Hospital provee una caja fuerte para guardar dinero y objetos de valor, que el Hosptial no es responsable por la pérdida o daño de dinero, joyeria, documentos, pieles, abrigo de pieles y artículos de piel u otros artículos de valor extraordinario y tamaño pequeño, a menos que esten identificados, y no se hace responsable por perdida o daño a cualquier propiedad pesonal, a menos que esté depositada en la caja fuete del Hospital.

4. Consentimiento a Procedimientos Médicos o Quirúrgicos
Yo, el abajo informante, estoy de acuerdo con los procedimientos que se lleven a cabo durante esta hospitalización o en consultas externas, incluyendo tratamiento de urgencia o servicios que incluyen, pero no se limitan a procedimientos de laboratorio, rayos X, anestesia, o servicios hospitalarios que me presten bajo las instrucciones generales o especiales de mi médico.

Este consentimiento incluye examen sobre enfermedades infecciosas, incluyendo pero no limitadas a hepatitis, SIDA, y el virus de Immunodeficiencia (VIH), si el médico ordena tales examenes con próposito de diagnosticar.

Por Favor Escriba sus Iniciales: **apruebo** _____
No apruebo _____

5. Donación de Organos
Entiendo que tengo derecho de donar cualquiera de mis organos o tejidos para transplante y que puedo hacer este al completar la forma de regalo anatómico.

9. Armas/Explosivos/Drogas
Entiendo y estoy de acuerdo que si el Hospital en cualquier tiempo piensa que haya una arma, explosivos, drogas o substancias ilegales, o bebidas alcóholicas en mi cuarto o en mis pertenencias personales, el Hospital puede investigar mi cuarto y mis pertenencias, confiscar los atículos que se encuentren, y disponer de ellos apropiadamente, incluyendo la entrega de cualquier artículo a las autoridades jurídicas.

10. Cuarto Privado
Entiendo y certifico que si yo pido un cuarto privado para mí o para el paciente, yo soy responsable por gastos adicionales.

11. Consentimiento Financiero
Yo, el abajo firmante, consiento, si firmo como padre, tutor, esposo, agente, gerente, o paciente, que, en consideración de los servicios prestados al paciente, yo me obligo individualmente a pagar la cuenta del Hospital de acuerdo con los términos y cargos del Hospital. En caso de que la cuenta se lleve a un abogado o a la agencia de cobros para su cobro, yo pagaré los honorarios del doctor y los gastos de cobro.

Yo certifico que he leído y entiendo por completo esta Condición de Admisión y Autorización para Tratamiento Médico, y que he firmado esta forma, libre y voluntariamente. Además, yo certifico que no he recivido promesas, aseguranzas, o garantías de nadie sobre los resultados por cualquier tratamiento medico o servicios obtenidos.

Patient Identification

Fecha _____ ☐ A.M.
Hora _____ ☐ P.M.

Paciente/Padre/Guardian/Conservador
X

Cónyuge (si casado/disponible)
X

Testigo (solo para la firma)
X

**East Houston Regional Medical Center
Condición de Admisión y**
Autorización para Tratamiento Medico

B

Figure 7-3, cont'd. **B,** Condiciones de admisión y autorización para tratamiento médico. (Courtesy East Houston Regional Medical Center.)

CONSENT FOR ANESTHESIA

Date: _____   Time: _____

- I _____, hereby request that Dr. _____, anesthesiologist, or any other anesthesiologist, designated by the hospital, administer anesthesia and provide the care necessary for me. I understand that the use of anesthetics be supervised by the anesthesiologist or his designee. I authorize the anesthesiologist to obtain assistance of other physicians, residents, interns, nurse anesthetists or others as considered advisable.
- The anesthesiologist or his designee has explained to me the type of anesthetic to be used and the risks. I have been informed of alternative methods of anesthesia and the risks involved in the use of alternative anesthetics. I can refuse the anesthetic. I have discussed the above with the anesthesiologist, or his designee, and had received satisfactory answers.

_____   _____
Signature of Patient   Date and Time

Reason patient did not sign consent

_____
_____
_____

A

CONSENTIMIENTO PARA ANESTESIA

Fecha: _____   Hora: _____

- Yo _____, por este medio, pido que el Dr. _____, anestesiólogo, o cualquier otro anestesiólogo, designado por el hospital, me administre anestesia y cuidado necesario. Yo entiendo que el uso de anestético será supervisado por el anestesiólogo o una persona designada. Yo autorizo al anestesiólogo para que obtenga asistencia de otros doctores, residentes, internos, enfermera anestesióloga u otros como lo considere prudente.
- El anestesiólogo o la persona designada me ha explicado el tipo de anestesia que se usará y los riesgos. Se me ha informado sobre métodos alternativos de anestesia y los riesgos involucrados en el uso de anestesia alternativa. Yo puedo rehusar la anestesia. He discutido lo mencionado arriba con el anestesiólogo, o la persona designada, y estoy satisfecho con las respuestas.

_____   _____
Firma del Paciente   Fecha y Hora

Razón por la cual el paciente no firmó el consentimiento

_____
_____
_____

B

Figure 7-4 **A,** Consent for anesthesia. **B, Consentimiento para anestesia.**

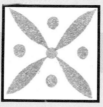

CHAPTER EIGHT
Discharging a Patient

CAPITULO OCHO
Dando de Alta al Paciente

A discharge planner is an advocate for the patient and the hospital. He is expected to devise a treatment plan for the patient. He has an important role in the prevention of illness, facilitates patient education, and alerts the patient and his family of health hazards.

La persona encargada de dar de alta al paciente es un intermediario entre el paciente y el hospital. Se espera que él diseñe un plan de cuidado para el paciente. El desempeña un papel muy importante en la prevención de enfermedades, facilita la educación del paciente y aconseja a él y a su familia sobre los peligros contra la salud.

The discharge planner identifies the patient, reads the hospital chart, and consults with the doctors, nurses, and social services. He interviews the patient within two working days of admission. He documents the intervention and sets health care goals for the patient.

La persona encargada de dar de alta al paciente, lo identifica, lee los archivos médicos, y consulta a los doctores, enfermeras, y trabajadores sociales. El entrevista al paciente a los dos dias de ingreso al hospital. El documenta la intervención y determina las metas del cuidado para el paciente.

Some of the tools that the discharge planner needs include: a list of community resources, a patient profile, the patient's discharge plan form, and a checklist to assure that he has addressed all the patient's needs.

Algunos instrumentos que la persona necesita incluyen: una lista de los recursos comunitarios, la forma para el plan de dar de alta, una lista para checar todas las necesidades del paciente.

TABLE 8-1	Key Words
TABLA 8-1	Palabras Clave

English	Spanish	Pronunciation
check	revise	*reh-bee-seh*
crutches	muletas	*moo-leh-tahs*
elder	anciana (feminine)	*ahn-see-ah-nah*
hazard	peligro	*peh-lee-groh*
ice	hielo	*ee-eh-loh*
in charge	encargado	*ehn-kahr-gah-doh*
medical file	archivo médico	*ahr-chee-boh meh-dee-koh*
numb	adormecido	*ah-dohr-meh-see-doh*
prevention	prevención	*preh-behn-see-ohn*
resources	recursos	*reh-koor-sohs*
sensation	sensación	*sehn-sah-see-ohn*
tight	apretado	*ah-preh-tah-doh*

Mr. Smith has a broken leg with waist-to-ankle cast. His elderly mother takes him home.

El señor Smith tiene una pierna rota y yeso de la cintura al tobillo. Su madre anciana lo lleva a casa.
(Ehl seh-nyohr Smith tee-eh-neh oo-nah pee-ehr-nah roh-tah ee yeh-soh deh lah seen-too-rah ahl toh-bee-yoh. Soo mah-dreh ahn-see-ah-nah loh yeh-bah ah kah-sah)

Mr. Smith, I need to talk to you about your care at home.

Señor Smith, necesito hablarle acerca del cuidado en casa.
(Seh-nyohr Smith, neh-seh-see-toh ah-blahr-leh ah-sehr-kah dehl koo-ee-dah-doh ehn kah-sah)

About your medical needs:

Sobre sus necesidades médicas:
(Soh-breh soos neh-seh-see-dah-dehs meh-dee-kahs):

Care of the cast

Cuidado del yeso
(Koo-ee-dah-doh dehl yeh-soh)

Check your foot at least every hour for twenty-four hours.

Revise su pie al menos cada hora por veinticuatro horas.
(Reh-bee-seh soo pee-eh ahl meh-nohs kah-dah oh-rah pohr veh-een-tee-koo-ah-troh oh-rahs)

If you notice an abnormal color or loss of sensation, call the doctor.

Si nota un color anormal o falta de sensación, llame al doctor.
(See noh-tah oon koh-lohr ah-nohr-mahl oh fahl-tah deh sehn-sah-see-ohn, yah-meh ahl dohk-tohr.

Have your mother do the checks if you are asleep.

Su madre puede checarlo si usted está dormido.
(Soo mah-dreh poo-eh-deh cheh-kahr-loh see oos-tehd ehs-lah dohr-mee-doh)

Use crutches to avoid weight-bearing.

Use las muletas para no poner peso en la pierna.
(Oo-seh lahs moo-leh-tahs pah-rah noh poh-nehr peh-soh ehn lah pee-ehr-nah)

Elevate the leg above heart level.

Eleve la pierna arriba del nivel del corazón.
(Eh-leh-beh lah pee-ehr-nah ah-ree-bah dehl nee-behl dehl koh-rah-sohn)

You can take pain pills.

Puede tomar pastillas para el dolor.
(Poo-eh-deh toh-mahr pahs-tee-yahs pah-rah ehl doh-lohr)

Call your doctor immediately if:

Llame a su doctor inmediatamente si:
(Yah-meh ah soo dohk-tohr een-meh-dee-ah-tah-mehn-teh see)

Your cast feels tight.

El yeso se siente apretado.
(Ehl yeh-soh seh see-ehn-teh ah-preh-tah-doh)

You have burning pain.

Tiene ardor.
(Tee-eh-neh ahr-dohr)

Your toes are discolored or numb.

Si los dedos están descoloridos o adormecidos.
(See lohs deh-dohs ehs-tahn dehs-koh-loh-ree-dohs oh ah-dohr-meh-see-dohs)

If you have a wheelchair, use it.

Si tiene una silla de ruedas, úsela.
(See tee-eh-neh oo-nah see-yah deh roo-eh-dahs, oo-seh-lah)

Avoid the following:

Evite lo siguiente:
(Eh-bee-teh loh see-gee-ehn-teh)

Getting the cast wet.

Mojar el yeso.
(Moh-hahr ehl yeh-soh)

Wrapping tape on the cast.

Enredar cinta alrededor del yeso.
(Ehn-reh-dahr seen-tah ahl-reh-
deh-dohr dehl yeh-soh)

Sticking objects inside the cast.

Meter objetos dentro del yeso.
(Meh-tehr ohb-heh-tohs dehn-troh
dehl yeh-soh)

Return for follow-up in one to
three days.

Regrese para un seguimiento de
uno a tres días.
(Reh-greh-seh pah-rah oon seh-ghee-
mee-ehn-toh deh oo-noh ah trehs
dee-ahs)

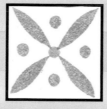

CHAPTER NINE
The Clerical Staff

CAPITULO NUEVE
Las Secretarias

The clerical staff is very important. They are the ones that first greet the patient. Their ability to be pleasant and courteous and to give the appropriate information will speed up the process of admitting the patient to the hospital or referring him to another department.

Las secretarias son muy importantes. Ellas son las primeras personas que saludan al paciente. La habilidad de ser amables y atentas y de dar información apropiada asegura que el proceso de admitir al paciente al hospital o de mandarlo a otro departamento sea mas rápido.

Good afternoon!	¡Buenas tardes! *(Boo-eh-nahs tahr-dehs)*
Are you the patient?	¿Es usted el/la paciente? *(Ehs oos-tehd ehl/lah pah-see-ehn-teh)*
Do you speak English?	¿Habla usted inglés? *(Ah-blah oos-tehd een-glehs)*
Is he/she with you?	¿El/Ella viene con usted? *(Ehl/Eh-yah bee-eh-neh kohn oos-tehd)*
Does he/she speak English?	¿El/Ella habla inglés? *(Ehl/Eh-yah ah-blah een-glehs)*
How may I help you?	¿En qué puedo servirle? *(Ehn keh poo-eh-doh sehr-beer-leh)*
What happened to you?	¿Qué le pasó? *(Keh leh pah-soh)*

Please sit down.	Por favor, siéntese.
	(Pohr fah-bohr, see-ehn-teh-seh)
I need to ask you some questions.	Necesito hacerle unas preguntas.
	(Neh-seh-see-toh ah-sehr-leh oo-nahs preh-goon-tahs)
I have to enter the information in the computer.	Tengo que poner la información en la computadora.
	(Tehn-goh keh poh-nehr lah een-fohr-mah-see-ohn ehn lah kohm-poo-tah-doh-rah)
What is your name?	¿Cómo se llama usted?
	(Koh-moh seh yah-mah oos-tehd)
What is your last name?	¿Cómo se apellida?
	(Koh-moh seh ah-peh-yee-dah)
Have you been in this hospital?	¿Ha estado en este hospital?
	(Ah ehs-tah-doh ehn ehs-teh ohs-pee-tahl)
Have you been to the emergency room?	¿Ha estado en el cuarto de emergencia/urgencias?
	(Ah ehs-tah-doh ehn ehl koo-ahr-toh deh eh-mehr-hehn-see-ah/oor-hehn-see-ahs)
When was the last time you were here?	¿Cuándo fue la última vez que estuvo aquí?
	(Koo-ahn-doh foo-eh lah ool-tee-mah behs keh ehs-too-boh ah-kee)
Is this your first time in the hospital?	¿Es su primera vez en el hospital?
	(Ehs soo pree-meh-rah behs ehn ehl ohs-pee-tahl)
Do you have a hospital card?	¿Tiene usted tarjeta de hospital?
	(Tee-eh-neh oos-tehd tahr-heh-tah deh ohs-pee-tahl)
What is your Social Security number?	¿Cuál es su número de Seguro Social?
	(Koo-ahl ehs soo noo-meh-roh deh Seh-goo-roh Soh-see-ahl)
Please repeat slowly.	Por favor, repita despacio.
	(Pohr fah-bohr, reh-pee-tah dehs-pah-see-oh)
Date of birth?	¿Fecha de nacimiento?
	(Feh-chah deh nah-see-mee-ehn-toh)
When (in what year) were you born?	¿En qué año nació?
	(Ehn keh ah-nyoh nah-see-oh)

How old are you?	¿Cuántos años tiene?
	(Koo-ahn-tohs ah-nyohs tee-eh-neh)
Do you have health insurance?	¿Tiene seguro de salud?
	(Tee-eh-neh seh-goo-roh deh sah-lood)
What is the name of the insurance?	¿Cuál es el nombre del seguro?
	(Koo-ahl ehs ehl nohm-breh dehl seh-goo-roh)
Will it pay for the hospital?	¿Paga por la hospitalización?
	(Pah-gah pohr lah ohs-pee-tah-lee-sah-see-ohn)
Who is going to pay the hospital?	¿Quién va a pagar el hospital?
	(Kee-ehn bah ah pah-gahr ehl ohs-pee-tahl)
Do you have Medicare?	¿Tiene Medicare?
	(Tee-eh-neh Meh-dee-kehr)
Do you have your Medicare card?	¿Tiene su tarjeta de Medicare?
	(Tee-eh-neh soo tahr-heh-tah deh Meh-dee-kehr)
Do you have a driver's license?	¿Tiene licencia para manejar?
	(Tee-eh-neh lee-sehn-see-ah pah-rah mah-neh-hahr)
What is your address?	¿Cuál es su dirección?
	(Koo-ahl ehs soo dee-rehk-see-ohn)
Where do you live?	¿Dónde vive usted?
	(Dohn-deh bee-beh oos-tehd)
What is the street name?	¿Cuál es el nombre de la calle?
	(Koo-ahl ehs ehl nohm-breh deh lah kah-yeh)
Is that an apartment?	¿Es apartamento?
	(Ehs ah-pahr-tah-mehn-toh)
Is it a house?	¿Es una casa?
	(Ehs oo-nah kah-sah)
What is the zip code?	¿Cuál es el código postal?
	(Koo-ahl ehs ehl koh-dee-goh pohs-tahl)
What is your phone number?	¿Cuál es su número de teléfono?
	(Koo-ahl ehs soo noo-meh-roh deh teh-leh-foh-noh)
Do you work?	¿Trabaja usted?
	(Trah-bah-hah oos-tehd)
Where do you work?	¿Dónde trabaja usted?
	(Dohn-deh trah-bah-hah oos-tehd)

What is the address?	¿Cuál es la dirección? *(Koo-ahl ehs lah dee-rehk-see-ohn)*
Is it here in town?	¿Está en esta ciudad? *(Ehs-tah ehn ehs-tah see-oo-dahd)*
What work do you do?	¿Qué trabajo hace usted? *(Keh trah-bah-hoh ah-seh oos-tehd)*
Where were you born?	¿Dónde nació usted? *(Dohn-deh nah-see-oh oos-tehd)*
Are you single?	¿Es usted soltero/soltera? *(Ehs oos-tehd sohl-teh roh/sohl-teh-rah)*
Are you married?	¿Es usted casado(a)? *(Ehs oos-tehd kah-sah-doh/kah- sah-dah)*
Are you divorced?	¿Es usted divorciado(a)? *(Ehs oos-tehd dee-bohr-see-ah- doh/dee-bohr-see-ah-dah)*
Are you a widow/widower?	¿Es usted viudo(a)? *(Ehs oos-tehd bee-oo-doh/bee- oo-dah)*
Common-law wife/husband?	¿Unión libre? *(Oo-nee-ohn lee-breh)*
What is your religion?	¿Cuál es su religión? *(Koo-ahl ehs soo reh-lee-heh-ohn)*
Who can we call in case of an emergency?	¿A quién le llamamos en caso de emergencia? *(Ah kee-ehn leh yah-mah-mohs ehn kah-soh deh eh-mehr-hehn- see-ah)*
Do you have a family doctor?	¿Tiene usted doctor familiar? *(Tee-eh-neh oos-tehd dohk-tohr fah-mee-lee-ahr)*
Do you want to see our doctor?	¿Quiere ver a nuestro doctor? *(Kee-eh-reh behr ah noo-ehs- troh dohk-tohr)*
Do you prefer to call your doctor?	¿Prefiere llamar a su doctor? *(Preh-fee-eh-reh yah-mahr ah soo dohk-tohr)*
You must pay a deposit.	Debe pagar un depósito. *(Deh-beh pah-gahr oon deh-poh- see-toh)*
You don't have to pay in full/cash.	No tiene que pagar en efectivo/al contado. *(Noh tee-eh-neh keh pah-gahr ehn eh-fehk-tee-boh/ahl kohn- tah-doh)*

You can pay on terms.	**Puede pagar a plazos.** *(Poo-eh-deh pah-gahr ah plah-sohs)*
You need to sign this form.	**Debe firmar esta forma.** *(Deh-beh feer-mahr ehs-tah fohr-mah)*
You are giving us permission to treat you here.	**Nos da permiso de tratarlo aquí.** *(Nohs dah pehr-mee-soh deh trah-tahr-loh ah-kee)*
Please sign here.	**Por favor, firme aquí.** *(Pohr fah-bohr, feer-meh ah-kee)*
Can you write?	**¿Puede escribir?** *(Poo-eh-deh ehs-kree-beer)*
You can write an "X."	**Puede escribir una "X".** *(Poo-eh-deh ehs-kree-beer oo-nah eh-kees)*
How long have you been sick?	**¿Desde cuándo está enfermo/enferma?** *(Dehs-deh koo-ahn-doh ehs-tah ehn-fehr-moh/ehn-fehr-mah)*
Days? Months?	**¿Días? ¿Meses?** *(Dee-ahs Meh-sehs)*
Why are you here?	**¿Por qué está aquí?** *(Pohr keh ehs-tah ah-kee)*
What is the worst problem?	**¿Cuál es su peor problema?** *(Koo-ahl ehs soo peh-ohr proh-bleh-mah)*
What is hurting you?	**¿Qué le duele?** *(Keh leh doo-eh-leh)*
Start at the beginning.	**Comience desde el principio.** *(Koh-mee-ehn-seh dehs-deh ehl preen-see-pee-oh)*
When did this happen?	**¿Cuándo le pasó esto?** *(Koo-ahn-doh leh pah-soh ehs-toh)*
Do you have relatives/friends?	**¿Tiene parientes/amigos?** *(Tee-eh-neh pah-ree-ehn-tehs/ah-mee-gohs)*
Where are they?	**¿Dónde están?** *(Dohn-deh ehs-tahn)*
What is your brother's/sister's name?	**¿Cómo se llama su hermano/hermana?** *(Koh-moh seh yah-mah soo ehr-mah-noh/ehr-mah-nah)*
What is your husband's/wife's name?	**¿Cómo se llama su esposo/esposa?** *(Koh-moh seh yah-mah soo ehs-poh-soh/ehs-poh-sah)*

Thank you for the information.

Gracias por la información.
(*Grah-see-ahs pohr lah een-fohr-mah-see-ohn*)

Please, sit down in the waiting room.

Por favor, siéntese en la sala de espera.
(*Pohr fah-bohr, see-ehn-teh-seh ehn lah sah-lah deh ehs-peh-rah*)

There are a lot of patients.

Hay muchos pacientes.
(*Ah-ee moo-chohs pah-see-ehn-tehs*)

You will have to wait.

Tendrá que esperar usted.
(*Tehn-drah keh ehs-peh-rahr oos-tehd*)

Wait 30 minutes.

Espere treinta minutos.
(*Ehs-peh-reh treh-een-tah mee-noo-tohs*)

You may be here about four hours.

Estará aquí cerca de cuatro horas.
(*Ehs-tah-rah ah-kee sehr-kah deh koo-ah-troh oh-rahs*)

A nurse will see you.

Una enfermera la atenderá.
(*Ooh-nah ehn-fehr-meh-rah lah ah-tehn-deh-rah*)

Do you need to call a taxi?

¿Necesita llamar un taxi/ carro de sitio?
(*Neh-seh-see-tah yah-mahr oon tahx-ee/kah-roh deh see-tee-oh*)

Do you want to go home?

¿Quiere ir a su casa?
(*Kee-eh-reh eer ah soo kah-sah*)

You need to be admitted.

Necesita internarse.
(*Neh-seh-see-tah een-tehr-nahr-seh*)

Please wait a few minutes.

Por favor, espere unos minutos.
(*Poh fah-bohr, ehs-peh-reh oo-nohs mee-noo-tohs*)

I will call transportation.

Llamaré al transporte.
(*Yah-mah-reh ahl trahns-pohr-teh*)

Someone will take you to your room.

Alguien lo llevará a su cuarto.

(*Ahl-ghee-ehn loh yeh-bah-rah ah soo koo-ahr-toh*)

You will be all right!

¡Va a estar bien!
(*Bah ah ehs-tahr bee-ehn*)

Don't worry!

¡No se preocupe!
(*Noh seh preh-oh-koo-peh*)

Unit 2

Home Situations

UNIDAD 2

Situaciones en el Hogar

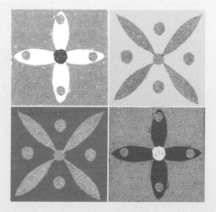

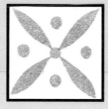

CHAPTER TEN
A Home Visit

CAPITULO DIEZ
Una Visita al Hogar

A home visit gives you the opportunity to assess several members of the family. It is also a convenient time to assess the home environment and to determine how the family members are coping with their needs. The community worker approaches Mr. Ríos, the grandfather. Mr. Ríos suffered a stroke 5 months ago and is recuperating.

Una visita al hogar proporciona la oportunidad de asesorar a varios miembros de la familia. También es una ocasión conveniente para evaluar el ambiente familiar y determinar cómo se están dando abasto con sus necesidades. El trabajador comunitario se dirige al señor Ríos, el abuelo. El señor Ríos sufrió un ataque de apoplejía (derrame cerebral) hace cinco meses y se está recuperando.

Mr. Ríos, how are you?	Señor Ríos, ¿cómo está? *(Seh-nyohr Ree-ohs, koh-moh ehs-tah)*
Good afternoon!	¡Buenas tardes! *(Boo-eh-nahs tahr-dehs)*
Do you remember me?	¿Se acuerda de mí? *(Seh ah-koo-ehr-dah deh mee)*
I am the medical student.	Yo soy el/la estudiante de medicina. *(Yo soh-ee: ehl/lah ehs-too-dee-ahn-teh deh meh-dee-see-nah)*
The nurse.	El/la enfermero(a). *(Ehl/lah ehn-fehr-meh-roh[ah])*

Therapist.	El/la terapista. *(Ehl/lah teh-rah-pees-tah)*
I want to talk to you.	Quiero hablar con usted. *(Kee-eh-roh ah-blahr kohn oos-tehd)*
Can you get out of bed?	¿Puede salir de la cama? *(Poo-eh-deh sah-leer deh lah kah-mah)*
Please, raise this arm.	Por favor, levante este brazo. *(Pohr fah-bohr, leh-bahn-teh ehs-teh brah-soh)*
Now raise the left arm.	Ahora levante el brazo izquierdo. *(Ah-oh-rah leh-bahn-teh ehl brah-soh ees-kee-ehr-doh)*
I will help you sit.	Le ayudaré a sentarse. *(Leh ah-yoo-dah-reh ah sehn-tahr-seh)*
Stay sitting.	Quédese sentado. *(Keh-deh-seh sehn-tah-doh)*
I have some paper.	Tengo papel. *(Tehn-goh pah-pehl)*
I want you to write your name and today's date.	Quiero que escriba su nombre y la fecha de hoy. *(Kee-eh-roh keh ehs-kree-bah soo nohm-breh ee lah feh-chah deh oh-ee)*
Now, stand up and walk.	Ahora, levántese y camine. *(Ah-oh-rah, leh-bahn-teh-seh ee kah-mee-neh)*
Walk six paces.	Camine seis pasos. *(Kah-mee-neh seh-ees pah-sohs)*
Do not hold on to the wall.	No se agarre de la pared. *(Noh seh ah-gah-reh deh lah pah-rehd)*
Sit in the chair.	Siéntese en la silla. *(See-ehn-teh-seh ehn lah see-yah)*
Please cross your leg.	Por favor, cruce la pierna. *(Pohr fah-bohr, kroo-seh lah pee-ehr-nah)*
Lift your right foot.	Levante el pie derecho. *(Leh-bahn-teh ehl pee-eh deh-reh-choh)*
Have you had swelling:	¿Ha tenido hinchazón:? *(Ah teh-nee-doh een-chah-sohn)*

On your feet?	¿En los pies?
	(Ehn lohs pee-ehs)
Ankles?	¿Tobillos?
	(Toh-bee-yohs)
Eyelids?	¿Párpados?
	(Pahr-pah-dohs)
Are you taking your medicines?	¿Está tomando sus medicinas?
	(Ehs-tah toh-mahn-doh soos meh-dee-see-nahs)
How many times a day?	¿Cuántas veces al día?
	(Koo-ahn-tahs beh-sehs ahl dee-ah)
Do you sleep during the day?	¿Duerme durante el día?
	(Doo-ehr-meh doo-rahn-teh ehl dee-ah)
At what time do you go to sleep?	¿A qué hora se acuesta a dormir?
	(Ah keh oh-rah seh ah-koo-ehs-tah ah dohr-meer)
At what time do you get up?	¿A qué hora se levanta?
	(Ah keh oh-rah seh leh-bahn-tah)
Do you wake up at night?	¿Se despierta en la noche?
	(Seh dehs-pee-ehr-tah ehn lah noh-cheh)
Your appetite is good?	¿Tiene buen apetito?
	(Tee-eh-neh boo-ehn ah-peh-tee-toh)
Is your appetite bad?	¿Tiene mal apetito?
	(Tee-eh-neh mahl ah-peh-tee-toh)
How many times do you eat per day?	¿Cuántas veces come por día?
	(Koo-ahn-tahs beh-sehs koh-meh pohr dee-ah)
What did you eat for breakfast?	¿Qué comió en el desayuno?
	(Keh koh-mee-oh ehn ehl deh-sah-yoo-noh)
Tell me what foods.	Dígame qué alimentos.
	(Dee-gah-meh keh ah-lee-mehn-tohs)
Do you drink coffee?	¿Toma café?
	(Toh-mah kah-feh)
How many cups per day?	¿Cuántas tazas diarias?
	(Koo-ahn-tahs tah-sahs dee-ah-ree-ahs)

How many glasses of water do you drink?	¿Cuántos vasos de agua toma? *(Koo-ahn-tohs bah-sohs deh ah-goo-ah toh-mah)*
When was the last time you used the toilet?	¿Cuándo fue la última vez que hizo del baño/que obró? *(Koo-ahn-doh foo-eh lah ool-tee-mah behs keh ee-soh dehl bah-nyoh/keh oh-broh)*
Are you constipated?	¿Está estreñido? *(Ehs-tah ehs-treh-nyee-doh)*
Do you have diarrhea?	¿Tiene diarrea? *(Tee-eh-neh dee-ah-reh-ah)*
How often do you urinate?	¿Cuántas veces orina? *(Koo-ahn-tahs beh-sehs oh-ree-nah)*
What was the color of the urine?	¿Cuál era el color de la orina? *(Koo-ahl eh-rah ehl koh-lohr deh lah oh-ree-nah)*
Did you see blood in the urine?	¿Vio sangre en la orina? *(Bee-oh sahn-greh ehn lah oh-ree-nah)*
Do you dribble?	¿Se orina sin sentir? *(Seh oh-ree-nah seen sehn-teer)*
Do you have problems with starting to urinate?	¿Tiene dificultad para empezar a orinar? *(Tee-eh-neh dee-fee-kool-tahd pah-rah ehm-peh-sahr ah oh-ree-nahr)*

TABLE 10-1   Personal Pronouns
TABLA 10-1   Pronombres Personales

English	Spanish	Pronunciation
I	Yo	*Yoh*
You (familiar)	Tú	*Too*
You (formal)	Usted	*Oos-tehd*
He	Él	*Ehl*
She	Ella	*Eh-yah*
We (masculine)	Nosotros	*Noh-soh-trohs*
We (feminine)	Nosotras	*Noh-soh-trahs*
They (masculine)	Ellos	*Eh-yohs*
They (feminine)	Ellas	*Eh-yahs*

Do you have hesitancy?	¿Se corta el chorro de la orina? *(Seh kohr-tah ehl choh-roh deh lah oh-ree-nah)*
Do you have questions?	¿Tiene preguntas? *(Tee-eh-neh preh-goon-tahs)*
Thank you for the information.	Gracias por la información. *(Grah-see-ahs pohr lah een-fohr-mah-see-ohn)*

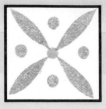

CHAPTER ELEVEN
Home Health/Hospice Care

CAPITULO ONCE
Cuidado en Casa/Hospicio

The patient who receives care in the home generally has a chronic condition. A number of health care providers may provide services to the patient the same day.

El paciente que recive cuidado en casa generalmente tiene una condición crónica. Un número de provedores de salud le puede prestar servicios al paciente el mismo día.

Mr. Roche is 88 years old and has chronic obstructive pulmonary disease. He suffered an embolism 8 days ago. He is being cared for by the home health nurse, the health aide, a physical therapist, and a respiratory therapist.

El Señor Roche tiene ochenta y ocho años y tiene obstrucción pulmonar crónica. Sufrió una embolia hace ocho dias. Lo cuida la enfermera de cuidados en casa, la ayudante, un fisioterapeuta, y un terapeuta de vias respiratorias.

Good morning, Mr. Roche.	Buenos días, Señor Roche.
	(Boo-eh-nohs dee-ahs, Seh-nyohr Roh-cheh)
How are you, today?	¿Cómo está hoy?
	(Koh-moh ehs-tah oh-ee?
I am not well.	No estoy bien.
	(Noh ehs-toh-ee bee-ehn)
What is going on?	¿Qué le pasa?
	(Keh leh pah-sah)
I don't know.	No sé.
	(Noh seh)

Well, let me see.	Bueno, déjeme ver. *(Boo-eh-noh, deh-heh-meh behr)*
I am going to take your blood pressure and the pulse.	Voy a tomar la presión y el pulso. *(Boh-ee ah toh-mahr lah preh-see-ohn ee ehl pool-soh)*
Did you sleep well?	¿Durmió bien? *(Door-mee-oh bee-ehn)*
Did you take your medicines this morning?	¿Tomó las medicinas esta mañana? *(Toh-moh lahs meh-dee-see-nahs ehs-tah mah-nyah-nah)*
Mr. Roche, you are not answering my questions.	Señor Roche, no me contesta las preguntas. *(Seh-nyohr Roh-cheh, noh meh kohn-tehs-tah lahs preh-goon-tahs)*
Blink if you understand me.	Parpadee si me entiende. *(Pahr-pah-dee-eh see meh ehn-tee-ehn-deh)*
I am going to examine you.	Voy a examinarlo. *(Boh-ee ah ehx-ah-mee-nahr-loh)*
I want to hear your heart.	Quiero escuchar el corazón. *(Kee-eh-roh ehs-koo-chahr ehl koh-rah-sohn)*
I want to hear your lungs.	Quiero escuchar los pulmones. *(Kee-eh-roh ehs-koo-chahr lohs pool-moh-nehs)*
I want to hear the abdomen.	Quiero escuchar el abdomen. *(Kee-eh-roh ehs-koo-chahr ehl ahb-doh-mehn)*
Everything sounds good.	Todo se oye bien. *(Toh-doh seh oh-yeh bee-ehn)*

The nurse completes the home health agency's nursing notes. See Figure 11-1 for assessment notes.

La enfermera completa las notas de enfermería de la agencia de cuidados en casa. Vea la Figura 11-1 para la asesoría.

The home health aide arrives to give Mr. Roche a bath and to assist him with breakfast.

La asistente de cuidados en casa llega para bañar al Señor Roche y para asistirlo con el desayuno.

Good morning, Mr. Roche.	Buenos días, Señor Roche. *(Boo-eh-nohs dee-ahs, Seh-nyohr Roh-cheh)*

NURSING NOTES

NOTAS DE ENFERMERIA

PATIENT: _____   DATE: _____
PACIENTE: _____   **FECHA:** _____

VITAL SIGNS	TEMP	AP/R	RESP	BP	
				RA	LA

SIGNOS VITALES	TEMPERATURA	PULSO APICAL	RESPIRACIÓN	PRESIÓN ARTERIAL	
				BRAZO DERECHO	BRAZO IZQUIERDO

HOME BOUND STATUS
☐ Bedbound
☐ O₂ Dependent
☐ IV Therapy
☐ Impaired Vision
☐ Contractures
☐ Other
☐ Medically Contra-Indicated

EN CASA
☐ En Casa
☐ Con Oxígeno
☐ Terapia Intravenosa
☐ Visión Mala
☐ Encogimiento
☐ Otro
☐ Contra Indicado

NEURO
☐ Alert	☐ Syncope	☐ Dysphagia
☐ Oriented	☐ HOH	☐ Blindness
☐ Disoriented	☐ Facial Weakness	☐ Blurred Vision
☐ Numbness	☐ Paralysis	☐ Hallucination
☐ Headache	☐ Dysphasia	☐ Slurred Speech

COMMENTS _____

NEURO
☐ Alerto	☐ Síncope	☐ Disfagia
☐ Orientado	☐ Sordo	☐ Ceguera
☐ Desorientado	☐ Debilidad Facial	☐ Visión Borrosa
☐ Adormecido	☐ Parálysis	☐ Alucinación
☐ Dolor de Cabeza	☐ Disfasia	☐ Lenguaje lento

COMENTARIOS _____

CARDIOVASCULAR
☐ Angina	☐ HTN	☐ Cap. refill good / poor
☐ Tachycardia	☐ Calf Pain	☐ Pulse Bounding /
☐ Bradycardia	☐ Vertigo	weak / strong / reg / irreg
☐ Edema	☐ Hypotension	

Site _____   Size _____   Type _____

COMMENTS _____

CARDIOVASCULAR
☐ Angina	☐ Hypertensión	☐ Relleno capilar bueno / malo
☐ Taquicardia	☐ Dolor del Chamorro	☐ Pulso Débil / fuerte / regular /
☐ Bradicardia	☐ Vértigo	irregular
☐ Edema	☐ Hipotensión	

Area _____   Tamaño _____   Tipo _____

COMENTARIOS _____

Figure 11-1   Nursing notes.
Notas de enfermeria.

Home Health/Hospice Care

RESPIRATORY
- ☐ Breath sounds clear
- ☐ Crackles
- ☐ Rhonchi
- ☐ Wheeze
- ☐ Suctioning
- ☐ SOB rest / amb
- ☐ O₂ _____ L/pm
- ☐ Productive cough
- ☐ Non-productive cough
- ☐ Sputum C / G / Y
- ☐ Trach: Type _____

COMMENTS _____

RESPIRATORIO
- ☐ Sonidos Respiratorios Claros
- ☐ Crujidos
- ☐ Ronquido
- ☐ Resuello sibilante
- ☐ Succión
- ☐ Falta de respiración al descansar/caminar
- ☐ Oxígeno _____ L/pm
- ☐ TOS Productiva
- ☐ TOS No-Productiva
- ☐ Moco claro/verde / amarillo
- ☐ Traqueotomía: Tipo _____

COMENTARIOS _____

MUSCULOSKELETAL
- ☐ Stiffness
- ☐ Muscle Spasms
- ☐ Pain
- ☐ Flaccid
- ☐ Limited ROM UE / LE
- ☐ Spastic
- ☐ Tremors
- ☐ Ataxic gait
- ☐ Shuffling
- ☐ Unsteady
- ☐ Poor Balance
- ☐ Non-ambulatory
- ☐ Walker
- ☐ Cane
- ☐ Crutches
- ☐ Assist (1–2 persons)
- ☐ MAE (moves all extremities)

COMENTS _____

MUSCULOESQUELETAL
- ☐ Duro
- ☐ Espasmos
- ☐ Dolor
- ☐ Flacidés
- ☐ Movimiento Limitado extremidad / brazos/piernas
- ☐ Espástico
- ☐ Temblores
- ☐ Paso atáxico
- ☐ Arrastra los pies
- ☐ Inestable
- ☐ Mal balanceo
- ☐ No ambulatorio
- ☐ Andador
- ☐ Bastón
- ☐ Muletas
- ☐ Asistir (1–2 personas)
- ☐ MTE (mueve todas las extremidades)

COMENTARIOS _____

SKIN
- ☐ Warm
- ☐ Cool
- ☐ Dry
- ☐ Moist
- ☐ Diaphoretic
- ☐ Intact
- ☐ Pale
- ☐ WNL
- ☐ Jaundice
- ☐ Blisters
- ☐ Abrasions
- ☐ Rash
- ☐ Irritation
- ☐ Decubitus
- ☐ Drainage
- ☐ Open wound
- ☐ Circulation Good – Poor
- ☐ Turgor Good – Poor

PIEL
- ☐ Caliente
- ☐ Fría
- ☐ Seca
- ☐ Húmeda
- ☐ Diaforética
- ☐ Intacta
- ☐ Pálida
- ☐ Normal
- ☐ Amarilla
- ☐ Ampollas
- ☐ Abrasiones
- ☐ Erupción
- ☐ Irritación
- ☐ Decúbito
- ☐ Desague
- ☐ Herida abierta
- ☐ Circulación Buena – Mala
- ☐ Turgor Bueno – Malo

Figure 11-1, cont'd.

I am Maria. I will give you a bath.

Yo soy Maria. Voy a bañarlo.
(Yoh soh-ee Mah-ree-ah. Boh-ee ah bah-nyahr-loh)

First, I want to brush your teeth.

Primero, quiero limpiarle los dientes.
(Pree-meh-roh kee-eh-roh leem-pee-ahr-leh lohs dee-ehn-tehs)

You have false teeth.

Tiene dentaduras postizas.
(Tee-eh-neh dehn-tah-doo-rahs pohs-tee-sahs)

The patient responds by blinking or shaking his head.
El paciente responde parpadeando o moviendo la cabeza.

I can help you to sit down.

Le puedo ayudar a sentarse.
(Leh poo-eh-doh ah-yoo-dahr ah sehn-tahr-seh)

Place your arm around my waist.

Ponga su brazo alrededor de mi cintura.
(Pohn-gah soo brah-soh ahl-reh-deh-dohr deh mee seen-too-rah)

The water is warm. Can you feel?

El agua está tibia. ¿Puede sentir?
(Ehl ah-goo-ah ehs-tah tee-bee-ah. Poo-eh-deh sehn-teer)

Lift your right arm.

Levante el brazo derecho.
(Leh-bahn-teh ehl brah-soh deh-reh-choh)

I will lift your left arm.

Le levanto el brazo derecho.
(Leh leh-bahn-toh ehl brah-soh deh-reh-choh)

The aide cooks breakfast. She feeds the patient eggs, ham, toast and coffee.
La ayudante cocina el desayuno. Le da de comer huevos, jamón, pan tostado y café.

Mr. Roche, please open your mouth.

Señor Roche, por favor abra la boca.
(Seh-nyohr Roh-cheh, pohr fah-bohr ah-brah lah boh-kah)

I am going to insert your dentures.

Voy a ponerle la dentadura.
(Boh-ee ah poh-nehr-leh lah dehn-tah-doo-rah)

What would you like to eat first?	¿Qué quiere comer primero? *(Keh kee-eh-reh koh-mehr pree-meh-roh)*
Egg?	Huevo? *(Oo-eh-boh)*
Do you use sugar in the coffee?	¿Usa azúcar en el café? *(Oo-sah ah-soo-kahr ehn ehl kah-feh)*
A teaspoon?	¿Una cucharadita? *(Oo-nah koo-chah-rah-dee-tah)*
Milk?	¿Leche? *(leh-cheh)*
Do you want the toast with butter?	¿Quiere el pan tostado con mantequilla? *(Kee-eh-reh ehl pahn tohs-tah-doh kohn mahn-teh-kee-yah)*
You ate well.	Comió bien. *(Koh-mee-oh bee-ehn)*
I will return tomorrow.	Regreso mañana. *(Reh-greh-soh mah-nyah-nah)*

At 10:30 AM the physical therapist arrives.
A las diez treinta el fisioterapeuta llega.

Good morning, Mr. Roche.	Buenos días, Señor Roche. *(Boo-eh-nohs dee-ahs, Seh-nyohr Roh-cheh)*
I am here to help you with exercises.	Estoy aquí para ayudarlo con ejercicios. *(Ehs-toh-ee ah-kee pah-rah ah-yoo-dahr-loh kohn eh-hehr-see-see-ohs)*
The nurse said that you can't speak very well.	La enfermera dice que no puede hablar bien. *(Lah ehn-fehr-meh-rah dee-seh keh noh poo-eh-deh ah-blahr bee-ehn)*
Move your head to say yes or no.	Mueva la cabeza para decir sí o no. *(Moo-eh-bah lah kah-beh-sah pah-rah deh-seer see oh noh)*
Can you sit up?	¿Puede sentarse? *(Poo-eh-deh sehn-tahr-seh)*
Can you feed yourself?	¿Puede alimentarse? *(Poo-eh-deh ah-lee-mehn-tahr-seh)*
Grab the spoon.	Coja la cuchara. *(Koh-hah lah koo-chah-rah)*

PHYSICAL & OCCUPATIONAL THERAPY REFERRAL FORM
FORMA DE REMISION DE TERAPIA FISICA Y OCUPACIONAL

Agency: _____
Agencia: _____

Referred by: _____
Remitido por: _____

☐ New Patient   ☐ Previous Patient   ☐ Other _____
☐ **Paciente Nuevo**   ☐ **Paciente Previo**   ☐ **Otro** _____

Service Requested   ☐ Physical Therapy   ☐ Occupational Therapy
Servicio Requerido   ☐ **Terapia Física**   ☐ **Terapia Ocupacional**

Ref. Date _____ Record Number: _____ Medicare Number: _____
Fecha de Remisión _____ **Número de Archivo** _____ **Número de Medicare** _____

Last Name: _____ First Name: _____ Phone: _____
Apellido: _____ **Nombre:** _____ **Teléfono:** _____

Address: _____ City: _____ State/Zip: _____
Dirección: _____ **Ciudad:** _____ **Estado/Código Postal** _____

Date of Birth: _____   ☐ Male   ☐ Female   Marital Status: _____
Fecha de Nacimiento: _____   ☐ **Hombre** ☐ **Mujer**   **Estado Civil:** _____

Referring Physician: _____   Phone: _____
Médico Que Remite: _____   **Teléfono:** _____

Address: _____
Dirección: _____

Diagnosis: _____
Diagnóstico: _____

Reason for Referral: _____
Razón de Remisión: _____

Directions to home: _____
Direcciones para llegar a la casa: _____

Name of person receiving referral: _____
Nombre de la persona que remitió: _____

Figure 11-2 Physical and occupational therapy referral form.
Forma de remisión de terapia física y ocupacional.

Put the spoon in your mouth.	Ponga la cuchara en la boca. *(Pohn-gah lah koo-chah-rah ehn lah boh-kah)*
Can you move in bed?	¿Puede moverse en la cama? *(Poo-eh-deh moh-behr-seh ehn lah kah-mah)*
I'm going to test your muscle strength.	Voy a medir la fuerza del músculo. *(Boh-ee ah meh-deer lah foo-ehr sah dehl moos-koo-loh)*
I want to help you stand up.	Quiero ayudarlo a sentarse. *(Kee-eh-roh ah-yoo-dahr-loh ah sehn-tahr-seh)*
Do you have pain?	¿Tiene dolor? *(Tee-eh-neh doh-lohr?*
Let's walk.	Vamos a caminar. *(Bah-mohs ah kah-mee-nahr)*
Let's see how far you can walk.	Vamos a ver que tan lejos puede caminar. *(Bah-mohs a behr keh tahn leh-hos poo-eh-deh kah-mee-nahr)*
I will help you sit in the chair.	Le ayudaré a sentarse en la silla. *(Leh ah-yoo-dah-reh ah sehn-tahr-seh ehn lah see-yah)*
Now, follow my commands.	Ahora, siga mis órdenes. *(Ah-oh-rah see-gah mees ohr-deh-nehs)*
Reach out with your arm.	Alarge el brazo. *(Ah-lahr-geh ehl brah-soh)*
Touch your face with your hand.	Toque la cara con la mano. *(Toh-keh lah kah-rah kohn lah mah-noh)*
Point to your nose.	Apunte a la nariz. *(Ah-poon-teh ah lah nah-rees)*
Make a fist.	Haga un puño. *(Ah-gah oon poo-nyoh)*
I want you to use a cane.	Quiero que use un bastón. *(Kee-eh-roh keh oo-seh oon bahs-tohn)*

The physical therapist talks to Mrs. Roche regarding safety precautions at home.

El físio terapeuta habla con la Señora Roche sobre precauciones en la casa.

There are a few things that you have to keep in mind.	Hay varias cosas que debe recordar. *(Ah-ee bah-ree-ahs koh-sahs keh deh-beh reh-kohr-dahr)*
Remove all throw rugs in the hallway.	Quite todos los tapetes del pasillo. *(Kee-teh toh-dohs lohs tah-peh-tehs dehl pah-see-yoh)*
Place a light in the hallway.	Ponga una luz en el pasillo. *(Pohn-gah oo-nah loos ehn ehl pah-see-yoh)*
Before he sits up in bed, lower the bed.	Antes de que se levante, baje la cama. *(Ahn-tehs deh keh seh leh-bahn-teh, bah-heh lah kah-mah)*
Have someone help your husband to stand up.	Asegure que alguien le ayude a su esposo a levantarse. *(Ah-seh-goo-reh keh ahl-gee-ehn leh ah-yoo-deh ah soo ehs-poh-soh ah leh-bahn-tahr-seh)*
Place the sling on his right arm.	Póngale el cabestrillo en el brazo derecho. *(Pohn-gah-leh ehl kah-behs-tree-yoh ehn ehl brah-soh deh-reh-choh)*
I want him to do each exercise three times a day. Each movement 10 times.	Quiero que haga cada ejercicio tres veces al día. Cada movimiento diez veces. *(Kee-eh-roh keh ah-gah kah-dah eh-hehr-see-see-oh trehs beh-sehs ahl dee-ah. Kah-dah moh-bee-mee-ehn-toh dee-ehs beh-sehs)*
I will return in two days.	Regresaré en dos días. *(Reh-greh-sah-reh ehn dohs dee-ahs)*

The respiratory therapist arrives at 3 PM to check on Mr. Roche's oxygen needs.

El terapeuta de vías respiratorias llega a las tres de la tarde para checar las necesidades de oxígeno del Señor Roche.

Good afternoon, Mr. Roche.	Buenas tardes, Señor Roche. *(Boo-eh-nahs tahr-dehs Señor Roche)*
I am going to check the oxygen tank.	Voy a checar el tanque de oxígeno. *(Boh-ee ah cheh-kahr ehl tahn-keh deh ohx-ee-heh-noh)*

Remember the following precautions:	Recuerde las siguientes precauciones: *(Reh-koo-ehr-deh lahs see-gee-ehn-tehs preh-kah-oo-see-oh-nehs)*
The flow rate should be at $\frac{1}{2}$ liter.	El flujo debe de ser de medio litro. *(Ehl floo-hoh deh-beh sehr deh meh-dee-oh lee-troh)*
Do not smoke in the room when the oxygen is being used.	No fume en el cuarto donde se usa el oxígeno. *(Noh foo-meh ehn ehl koo-ahr-toh dohn-deh seh oo-sah ehl ohx-ee-heh-noh)*
Keep the oxygen equipment at least 10 feet away from stoves, furnaces, and water heaters.	Guarde el equipo de oxígeno retirado al menos diez pies de estufas, calentadores, o calentador de agua. *(Goo-ahr-deh ehl eh-kee-poh deh ohx-ee-heh-noh reh-tee-rah-doh ahl meh-nohs dee-ehs pee-ehs deh ehs-too-fahs, kah-lehn-tah-doh-rehs, o kah-lehn-tah-dohr deh ah-goo-ah)*
Do not use flammable substances.	No use substancias flamables. *(Noh oo-seh soobs-tahn-see-ahs flah-mah-blehs)*
Lotions	Lociones *(Loh-see-oh-nehs)*
Grease	Grasa *(Grah-sah)*
Vaseline	Vaselina *(Bah-seh-lee-nah)*
And others	Y otras *(Ee oh-trahs)*

HOSPICE CARE

CUIDADO HOSPICIO

Many families prefer to keep the terminally ill relative at home. When the care in the hospital is no longer possible, the patient must be monitored at home. Hospice nurses take care of the patient during his terminal illness.

Muchas familias prefieren que el pariente con enfermedad terminal se quede en casa. Cuando el cuidado hospitalario no es posible, el paciente se debe mantener en casa. Las enfermeras del hospicio cuidan al paciente durante su enfermedad terminal.

Good evening, Mrs. Roche.

Buenas noches, Señora Roche.
(Boo-eh-nahs noh-chehs, Seh-nyoh-rah Roh-cheh)

My agency asked me to visit you.

Mi agencia me pidió que la visitara.
(Mee ah-hehn-see-ah meh pee-dee-oh keh lah bee-see-tah-rah)

I am here to care for your husband.

Estoy aquí para cuidar a su esposo.
(Ehs-toh-ee ah-kee pah-rah koo-ee-dahr ah soo ehs-poh-soh)

I want to review our services.

Quiero repasar nuestros servicios.
(Kee-eh-roh reh-pah-sahr noo-ehs-trohs sehr-bee-see-ohs.

We can control the patient's pain and keep him comfortable.

Podemos controlar el dolor del paciente y mantenerlo cómodo.
(Poh-deh-mohs kohn-troh-lahr ehl doh-lohr dehl pah-see-ehn-teh ee mahn-teh-nehr-loh koh-moh-doh)

We can teach you about:

Le podemos dar instrucciones sobre:
(Leh poh-deh-mohs dahr eens-trook-see-ohn-ehs soh-breh:)

Care techniques

Técnicas del cuidado
(Tehk-nee-kahs dehl koo-ee-dah-doh)

Feeding approaches

Métodos de alimentación
(Meh-toh-dohs deh ah-lee-mehn-tah-see-ohn)

Medication management

Régimen de medicamentos
(Reh-hee-mehn deh meh-dee-kah-mehn-tohs)

We are available 24 hours per day.

Damos servicio veinticuatro horas por día.
(Dah-mohs sehr-bee-see-oh beh-een-tee-koo-ah-troh oh-rahs pohr dee-ah)

Your husband will be cared for by the doctor, nurse, social worker, and the priest.

Cuidará a su esposo el doctor, la enfermera, la trabajadora social y el sacerdote.
(Koo-ee-dah-rah ah soo ehs-poh-soh ehl dohk-tohr, lah trah-bah-hah-doh-rah soh-see-ahl, ee ehl sah-sehr-doh-teh)

You must tell us your needs.

Debe decirnos que necesita.
(Deh-beh deh-seer-nohs keh neh-seh-see-tah)

Hospice offers care from admission through death.

El cuidado del hospicio se da desde el ingreso hasta la muerte.
(Ehl koo-ee-dah-doh dehl ohs-pee-see-oh seh dah dehs-deh ehl een-greh-soh ahs-tah lah moo-ehr-teh)

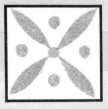

CHAPTER TWELVE
Useful Vocabulary for Home

CAPITULO DOCE
Vocabulario Útil
Sobre la Vivienda

Vocabulary is a group of words from a language. Here we will use the most common or useful words used during an interview or conversation with a patient. This will give us an idea how the patient lives at home or what is available to him.

El vocabulario es un conjunto de palabras de un idioma. En esta ocasión presentaremos las palabras más usuales o útiles en una entrevista o una conversación con el paciente. Esto nos indicará la forma de vivir del paciente.

BATHROOM	**BAÑO**	*(BAH-NYOH)*
basin	lavabo	*(lah-bah-boh)*
hair brush	cepillo de pelo	*(seh-pee-yoh deh peh-loh)*
comb	peine	*(peh-ee-neh)*
cosmetics	cosméticos	*(kohs-meh-tee-kohs)*
deodorant	desodorante	*(deh-soh-doh-rahn-teh)*
razor	navaja de afeitar	*(nah-bah-hah deh ah-feh-ee-tahr)*
shower	regadera/ducha	*(reh-gah-deh-rah/doo-chah)*
soap	jabón	*(hah-bohn)*
toilet	excusado/inodoro	*(ex-koo-sah-doh/ee-noh-doh-roh)*
toothbrush	cepillo de dientes	*(seh-pee-yoh deh dee-ehn-tehs)*
toothpaste	pasta de dientes	*(pahs-tah deh dee-ehn-tehs)*
towel	toalla	*(too-ah-yah)*
BEDROOM	**RECAMARA**	*(REH-KAHM-AH-RAH)*
bed	cama	*(kah-mah)*
bed cover	colcha	*(kohl-chah)*

108

clock	reloj	*(reh-lohj)*
comb	peine	*(peh-ee-neh)*
dresser	aparador	*(ah-pah-rah-dohr)*
hairbrush	cepillo de pelo	*(seh-pee-yoh deh peh-loh)*
mattress	colchón	*(kohl-chohn)*
phone	teléfono	*(teh-leh-foh-noh)*
pillow	almohada	*(ahl-moh-ah-dah)*
radio	radio	*(rah-dee-oh)*
sheets	sábanas	*(sah-bah-nahs)*

DINING ROOM	**COMEDOR**	***(KOH-MEH-DOHR)***
cabinet	gabinete	*(gah-bee-neh-teh)*
chairs	sillas	*(see-yahs)*
drapes	cortinas	*(kohr-tee-nahs)*
table	mesa	*(meh-sah)*

INSIDE HOME	**DENTRO DE LA CASA**	***(DEHN-TROH DEH LAH KAH-SAH)***
air conditioning	aire acondicionado	*(ah-ee-reh ah-kohn-dee-see-oh-nah-doh)*
carpet	alfombra	*(ahl-fohm-brah)*
throw rug	carpeta	*(kahr-peh-tah)*
picture	retrato	*(reh-trah-toh)*
mirror	espejo	*(ehs-peh-hoh)*
room	cuarto	*(koo-ahr-toh)*
heater	calentador	*(kah-lehn-tah-dohr)*
water heater	calentador de agua	*(kah-lehn-tah-dohr deh ah-goo-ah)*

KITCHEN	**COCINA**	***(KOH-SEE-NAH)***
can opener	abrelatas	*(ah-breh-lah-tahs)*
coffee pot	cafetera	*(kah-feh-teh-rah)*
cup	tasa	*(tah-sah)*
dish	plato	*(plah-toh)*
dishwasher	lavaplatos	*(lah-bah-plah-tohs)*
glass	vaso	*(bah-soh)*
hot water	agua caliente	*(ah-goo-ah kah-lee-ehn-teh)*
cold water	agua fría	*(ah-goo-ah free-ah)*
microwave	microondas	*(mee-kroh-ohn-dahs)*
plate	platón	*(plah-tohn)*
pots/pans	trastes/vasijas	*(trahs-tehs/bah-see-hahs)*
refrigerator	refrigerador	*(reh-free-heh-rah-dohr)*
stove	estufa	*(ehs-too-fah)*
table	mesa	*(meh-sah)*

LIVING ROOM	SALA/ESTANCIA	*(SAH-LAH/EHS-TAHN-SEE-AH)*
lamp	lámpara	*(lahm-pah-rah)*
sofa	sofá	*(soh-fah)*

OUTSIDE HOME	EXTERIOR DE CASA	*(EHX-TEH-REE-OHR DEH KAH-SAH)*
address	dirección	*(dee-rehk-see-ohn)*
door	puerta	*(poo-ehr-tah)*
driveway (garage)	entrada para garaje	*(ehn-trah-dah pah-rah gah-rah-heh)*
home	hogar	*(oh-gahr)*
house	casa	*(kah-sah)*
porch/patio	pórtico/patio	*(pohr-tee-koh/pah-tee-oh)*
street/avenue	calle/avenida	*(kah-yeh/ah-beh-nee-dah)*
window	ventana	*(behn-tah-nah)*

OFFICE	OFICINA	*(OH-FEE-SEE-NAH)*
books	libros	*(lee-brohs)*
bookcase	armario/estante	*(ahr-mah-ree-oh/ehs-tahn-teh)*
certificates	certificados	*(sehr-tee-fee-kah-dohs)*
chair	silla	*(see-yah)*
clock	reloj	*(reh-loh)*
computer	computadora	*(kohm-poo-tah-doh-rah)*
copier	fotocopiadora	*(foh-toh-koh-pee-ah-doh-rah)*
desk	escritorio	*(ehs-kree-toh-ree-oh)*
disk	disco	*(dees-koh)*
eraser	borrador	*(boh-rah-dohr)*
fax	fax	*(fahx)*
ink	tinta	*(teen-tah)*
magazine	revista	*(reh-bees-tah)*
monitor	monitor	*(moh-nee-tohr)*
paper	papel	*(pah-pehl)*
pencils	lápices	*(lah-pee-sehs)*
pens	plumas	*(ploo-mahs)*
cartridge	cartucho	*(kahr-too-choh)*
screen	pantalla	*(pahn-tah-yah)*
sharpener	sacapuntas	*(sah-kah-poon-tahs)*
table	mesa	*(meh-sah)*
typewriter	máquina de escribir	*(mah-kee-nah deh ehs-kree-beer)*

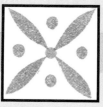

CHAPTER THIRTEEN
The Members of the Family

CAPITULO TRECE
Los Miembros de la Familia

In the past, it was difficult to mention or count all the members of a family. This happened because they were numerous and they lived a long time. One could easily confuse the relationships between members. Today, because families are smaller, one knows who makes up the nuclear family and where we find the best relationships.

En épocas pasadas era tan difícil enumerar o contar a todos los miembros que integraban una familia. Esto sucedía por lo numeroso y por los muchos años que vivían. Fácilmente se podía confundir el parentesco. Ahora, gracias a que las familias son más pequeñas, se pueden conocer mejor los integrantes del núcleo familiar y en dónde encontramos las mejores convivencias.

THE FAMILY	LA FAMILIA	*(LAH FAH-MEE-LEE-AH)*
father	padre	*(pah-dreh)*
dad	papá	*(pah-pah)*
mother	madre	*(mah-dreh)*
mom	mamá	*(mah-mah)*
husband	esposo	*(ehs-poh-soh)*
wife	esposa	*(ehs-poh-sah)*
sister	hermana	*(ehr-mah-nah)*
brother	hermano	*(ehr-mah-noh)*
son	hijo	*(ee-hoh)*
daughter	hija	*(ee-hah)*
niece	sobrina	*(soh-bree-nah)*
nephew	sobrino	*(soh-bree-noh)*
grandmother	abuela	*(ah-boo-eh-lah)*

grandfather	abuelo	*(ah-boo-eh-loh)*
grandparents	abuelos	*(ah-boo-eh-lohs)*
aunt	tía	*(tee-ah)*
uncle	tío	*(tee-oh)*
stepfather	padrastro	*(pah-drahs-troh)*
stepmother	madrastra	*(mah-drahs-trah)*
stepson	hijastro	*(ee-hahs-troh)*
stepdaughter	hijastra	*(ee-hahs-trah)*
children	hijos	*(eeh-hohs)*
great-grandparents	bisabuelos	*(bee-sah-boo-eh-lohs)*
mother-in-law	suegra	*(soo-eh-grah)*
father-in-law	suegro	*(soo-eh-groh)*
sister-in-law	cuñada	*(koo-nyah-dah)*
brother-in-law	cuñado	*(koo-nyah-doh)*
concubine/common law	concubina	*(kohn-koo-bee-nah)*
cousins	primos	*(pree-mohs)*
cousin (female)	prima	*(pree-mah)*
cousin (male)	primo	*(pree-moh)*
grandchildren	nietos	*(nee-eh-tohs)*
godparents	padrinos	*(pah-dree-nohs)*
godfather	padrino	*(pah-dree-noh)*
godmother	madrina	*(mah-dree-nah)*

It is important to determine the family composition soon after you interview the patient. This will give you an idea of the family support for the patient. It may also show potential familial problems. Many problems may be prevented if we know which members of the family have chronic illnesses. See Table 13-1 for common chronic illnesses.

Es muy importante determinar la composición de la familia inmediatamente después de la entrevista. Esto le dará una idea del

TABLE 13-1   Common Chronic Illnesses
TABLA 13-1   Enfermedades Cronicas Comúnes

English	Spanish	Pronunciation
asthma	asma	*ahs-mah*
arthritis	artritis	*ahr-tree-tees*
diabetes	diabetes	*dee-ah-beh-tees*
epilepsy	epilepsia	*eh-pee-lehp-see-ah*
gout	gota	*goh-tah*
hypertension	hipertensión	*ee-pehr-tehn-see-ohn*
obesity	obesidad	*oh-beh-see-dahd*
mental retardation	retraso mental	*reh-trah-soh mehn-tahl*

apoyo de la familia para el paciente. También puede demostrar posibles problemas hereditarios. Muchos problemas se pueden prevenir si sabemos cuáles de los miembros de la familia tienen enfermedades crónico-degenerativas. Vea la tabla 13-1 de enfermedades comúnes.

We must keep in mind that the family composition is changing. A parent may be missing due to death, divorce or abandonment. This means that we must be alert to potential problems, especially when the family has few economic resources, is educationally deprived, or is new to your area.

Debemos considerar que la composición de la familia está evolucionando. El padre o la madre pueden faltar en la familia debido a muerte, divorcio o abandono. Esto nos debe alertar a posibles problemas, especialmente cuando la familia posee escasos recursos económicos, está privada educacionalmente o acaba de integrarse en la comunidad.

Unit 3

Interacting with Health Care Providers

UNIDAD 3

Comunicándose con Proveedores de la Salud

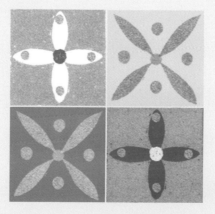

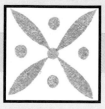

CHAPTER FOURTEEN
A Visit to the Pediatrician

CAPITULO CATORCE
Una Visita al Pediatra

It is important that children visit the pediatrician from infancy in order to evaluate their growth and development and to administer the prescribed immunizations. Mrs. Mora decides to take her two children to the pediatrician. The infant is one month old and the other child is 6 years old.

Es importante que desde los primeros meses de vida, los niños visiten a la pediatra para valorar su desarrollo, crecimiento y vacunación. La señora Mora decide llevar a sus hijos a la consulta: un niño de un mes y el otro de seis años.

Hello, Mrs. Mora.	**Hola, señora Mora.**
	(Oh-lah, seh-nyoh-rah Moh-rah)
How are you?	**¿Cómo está?**
	(Koh-moh ehs-tah)
I am the doctor.	**Yo soy la doctora.**
	(Yoh soh-eeh lah dohk-toh-rah)

A variety of greetings and common expressions will help you to get acquainted with the patients (Table 14-1).

Una variedad de saludos y expresiones comunes le ayudarán a darse a conocer con los pacientes (Tabla 14-1).

I am here to examine the baby.	**Estoy aquí para examinar al bebé.**
	(Ehs-toh-ee ah-kee pah-rah ehx-ah-mee-nahr ahl beh-beh)

TABLE 14-1	Greetings and Common Expressions
TABLA 14-1	Saludos y Expresiones Comúnes

English	Spanish	Pronunciation
Good morning!	¡Buenos días!	*Boo-eh-nohs dee-ahs*
Good evening! Good night!	¡Buenas noches!	*Boo-eh-nahs noh-chehs*
Pardon me!	¡Perdóneme!	*Pehr-doh-neh-meh*
Excuse me!	¡Excúseme!	*Ehx-koo-seh-meh*
Good afternoon!	¡Buenas tardes!	*Boo-eh-nahs tahr-dehs*
Thank you!	¡Gracias!	*Grah-see-ahs*
Please!	¡Por favor!	*Pohr fah-bohr*
Good!	¡Bueno!	*Boo-eh-noh*
Go on!	¡Síga!	*See-gah*

I will start by taking vital signs.	Voy a empezar por tomar los signos vitales. *(Boh-ee ah ehm-peh-sahr pohr toh-mahr lohs seeg-nohs bee-tah-lehs)*
When was he/she born?	¿Cuándo nació? *(Koo-ahn-doh nah-see-oh)*
Where?	¿Dónde? *(Dohn-deh)*
Was the delivery normal?	¿Fué normal el parto? *(Foo-eh nohr-mahl ehl pahr-toh)*

Note that questions in Spanish use the interrogation symbol at the beginning and at the end of the question. It is helpful to memorize some common pronouns used in questions (Table 14-2).

Note que las preguntas en español usan el símbolo interrogativo al principio y al final de la pregunta. Es conveniente memorizar algunos pronombres comúnes que se usan en las preguntas (Tabla 14-2).

Was he premature?	¿Fué prematuro? *(Foo-eh preh-mah-too-roh)*
Has the child been ill?	¿Ha estado enfermo el niño? *(Ah ehs-tah-doh ehn-fehr-moh ehl nee-nyoh)*
Is he/she eating well?	¿Está comiendo bien? *(Ehs-tah koh-mee-ehn-doh bee-ehn)*

TABLE 14-2	Common Interrogative Expressions	
TABLA 14-2	Expresiones Interrogativas Comúnes	

English	Spanish	Pronunciation
Who?	¿Quién?	*Kee-ehn*
Who? (all)	¿Quiénes?	*Kee-ehn-ehs*
What?	¿Qué?	*Keh*
Which?	¿Cuál?	*Koo-ahl*
Which? (ones)	¿Cuáles?	*Koo-ah-lehs*
How many? (m)	¿Cuántos?	*Koo-ahn-tohs*
How many? (f)	¿Cuántas?	*Koo-ahn-tahs*
How much? (m)	¿Cuánto?	*Koo-ahn-toh*
How much? (f)	¿Cuánta?	*Koo-ahn-tah*
How?	¿Cómo?	*Koh-moh*
When?	¿Cuándo?	*Koo-ahn-doh*
Where?	¿Dónde?	*Dohn-deh*
Why?	¿Por qué?	*Pohr keh*
For what?	¿Para qué?	*Pah-rah keh*

Sleeping well?	**¿Durmiendo bien?**	
	(Door-mee-ehn-doh bee-ehn)	
Breast-feeding?	**¿Tomando pecho?**	
	(Toh-mahn-doh peh-choh)	
Taking formula?	**¿Tomando fórmula?**	
	(Toh-mahn-doh fohr-moo-lah)	
What formula does he take?	**¿Qué fórmula toma?**	
	(Keh fohr-moo-lah toh-mah)	
How many ounces does he take?	**¿Cuántas onzas toma?**	
	(Koo-ahn-tahs ohn-sahs toh-mah)	
How often do you feed the baby?	**¿Qué tan a menudo alimenta al bebé?**	
	(Keh tahn ah meh-noo-doh ah-lee-mehn-tah ahl beh-beh)	
Do you feed every three hours?	**¿Le da de comer cada tres horas?**	
	(Leh dah deh koh-mehr kah-dah trehs oh-rahs)	
This is a new formula.	**Esta es una fórmula nueva.**	
	(Ehs-tah ehs oo-nah fohr-moo-lah noo-eh-bah)	

Table 14-3 helps you with the pronunciation of selected words.
La Tabla 14-3 le asiste con la pronunciación de palabras selectas.

| TABLE 14-3 | Pronunciation of Selected Words |
| TABLA 14-3 | Pronunciacion de Palabras Selectas |

English	Spanish	Pronunciation
family	familia	*fah-mee-lee-ah*
nurse	enfermera	*ehn-fehr-meh-rah*
I am	yo soy	*yoh soh-ee*
diaper	pañal	*pah-nyahl*
formula	fórmula	*fohr-moo-lah*
fever	fiebre	*fee-eh-breh*
diarrhea	diarrea	*dee-ah-reh-ah*
sleep	sueño	*soo-eh-nyoh*
colic	cólico	*koh-lee-koh*
cough	tos	*tohs*
medicine	medicina	*meh-dee-see-nah*

Does he/she have fever/diarrhea/colic?
¿Tiene fiebre/diarrea/cólico?
(Tee-eh-neh fee-eh-breh/dee-ah-reh-ah/koh-lee-koh)

Does the baby sleep all night?
¿Duerme el bebé toda la noche?
(Doo-ehr-meh ehl beh-beh toh-dah lah noh-cheh)

How many times does he wake up?
¿Cuántas veces se despierta?
(Koo-ahn-tahs beh-sehs seh dehs-pee-ehr-tah)

Does he cry a lot?
¿Llora mucho?
(Yoh-rah moo-choh)

When was the last time he had a bowel movement?
¿Cuándo fué la última vez que evacuó/hizo del baño?
(Koo-ahn-doh foo-eh lah ool-tee-mah behs keh eh-bah-koo-oh/ee-soh dehl bah-nyoh)

Is he urinating well?
¿Orina bien?
(Oh-ree-nah bee-ehn)

Have you seen blood in the urine?
¿Ha visto sangre en la orina?
(Ah bees-toh sahn-greh ehn lah oh-ree-nah)

How many diapers have you changed since yesterday?
¿Cuántos pañales le ha cambiado desde ayer?
(Koo-ahn-tohs pah-nyah-lehs leh ah kahm-bee-ah-doh dehs-deh ah-yehr)

When did you notice the skin rash?	¿Cuándo se dió cuenta de la piel rosada?
	(Koo-ahn-doh seh dee-oh koo-ehn-tah deh lah pee-ehl roh-sah-dah)
How many times has he vomited?	¿Cuántas veces ha vomitado?
	(Koo-ahn-tahs beh-sehs ah boh-mee-tah-doh)
Is it a lot?	¿Es mucho?
	(Ehs moo-choh)
Does the vomit have blood?	¿Tiene sangre el vómito?
	(Tee-eh-neh sahn-greh ehl boh-mee-toh)
What color?	¿De qué color?
	(Deh keh koh-lohr)
Does it have undigested food?	¿Tiene restos de comida?
	(Tee-eh-neh rehs-tohs deh koh-mee-dah)
Does it smell bad?	¿Huele mal?
	(Oo-eh-leh mahl)
Is he coughing?	¿Está tosiendo?
	(Ehs-tah toh-see-ehn-doh)

Write on an index card some of the common verbs from Table 14-4. They will come in handy in the clinical setting.

TABLE 14-4   Useful Verbs
TABLA 14-4   Verbos Útiles

English	Spanish	Pronunciation
boil	hervir	*ehr-beer*
change	cambiar	*kahm-bee-ahr*
cough	toser	*toh-sehr*
cry	llorar	*yoh-rahr*
dress	vestír	*behs-teer*
drink	beber/tomar	*beh-behr/toh-mahr*
eat	comer	*koh-mehr*
feel	sentír	*sehn-teer*
give	dar	*dahr*
leave	dejar	*deh-hahr*
make	hacer	*ah-sehr*
play	jugar	*hoo-gahr*
see	ver	*behr*
take	tomar/llevar	*toh-mahr/yeh-bahr*

Escriba en una tarjeta algunos verbos comúnes de la Tabla 14-4.
Serán convenientes en el área clínica.

Does he cough only at night?	¿Tose sólo de noche?
	(Toh-seh soh-loh deh noh-cheh)
Is it a dry cough?	¿Es tos seca?
	(Ehs tohs seh-kah)
Moist cough?	¿Tos húmeda?
	(Tohs oo-meh-dah)
Does the cough produce vomit?	¿La tos le produce vómito?
	(Lah tohs leh proh-doo-seh boh-mee-toh)
Dress the baby with few clothes.	Vista al bebé con poca ropa.
	(Bees-tah ahl beh-beh kohn poh-kah roh-pah)
Leave the area uncovered.	Deje el área descubierta.
	(Deh-heh ehl ah-reh-ah dehs-koo-bee-ehr-tah)
Do not put on plastic panties.	No le ponga calzones de plástico.
	(Noh leh pohn-gah kahl-sohn-ehs deh plahs-tee-koh)
Take the temperature rectally.	Tome la temperatura por el recto.
	(Toh-meh lah tehm-peh-rah-too-rah pohr ehl rehk-toh)
Normal rectal temperature should be 100.4 degrees Fahrenheit.	La temperatura normal en el recto es de cien punto cuatro grados Fahrenheit.
	(Lah tehm-peh-rah-too-rah nohr-mahl ehn ehl rehk-toh ehs deh see-ehn poon-toh koo-ah-troh grah-dohs Fah-rehn-heh-eet)
Give him/her the medicine every four hours.	Déle la medicina cada cuatro horas.
	(Deh-leh lah meh-dee-see-nah kah-dah koo-ah-troh oh-rahs)
Boil the water he drinks.	Hierva el agua que toma.
	(Ee-ehr-bah ehl ah-goo-ah keh toh-mah)
Sterilize the bottles.	Esterilice las botellas/los biberones
	(Ehs-teh-ree-lee-seh lahs boh-teh-yahs/lohs bee-beh-roh-nehs)
You can feed him/her solid foods.	Puede darle alimentos sólidos.
	(Poo-eh-deh dahr-leh ah-lee-mehn-tohs soh-lee-dohs)

Wash well all fruits and vegetables.	Lave bien frutas y verduras. *(Lah-beh bee-ehn froo-tahs ee behr-doo-rahs)*
Wash hands before eating.	Lave las manos antes de comer. *(Lah-beh lahs mah-nohs ahn-tehs deh koh-mehr)*
Don't let him put dirt in his mouth.	No deje que se meta tierra en la boca. *(Noh deh-heh keh seh meh-tah tee-eh-rah ehn lah boh-kah)*
Make the baby burp.	Haga que el bebé eructe/repita. *(Ah-gah keh ehl beh-beh eh-rook-teh/reh-pee-tah)*
Keep the baby awake.	Mantenga al bebé despierto. *(Mahn-tehn-gah ahl beh-beh dehs-pee-ehr-toh)*
Don't let the baby sleep more than three hours during the day.	No deje que el bebé duerma más de tres horas durante el día. *(Noh deh-heh keh ehl beh-beh doo-ehr-mah mahs deh trehs oh-rahs doo-rahn-teh ehl dee-ah)*
Watch if he sleeps quietly.	Vigile si su sueño es tranquilo. *(Bee-hee-leh see soo soo-eh-nyoh ehs trahn-kee-loh)*
Watch if he has abnormal movements.	Vigile si presenta movimientos anormales. *(Bee-hee-leh see preh-sehn-tah moh-bee-mee-ehn-tohs ah-nohr-mah-lehs)*
Give the medicine with a dropper.	Dé la medicina con gotero. *(Deh lah meh-dee-see-nah kohn goh-teh-roh)*

It is a good idea to talk to the parents when you examine the baby or older children. Ask direct questions of older children and call them by their names. Also, observe if the parents and the child get along. Table 14-5 has common questions.

Es buena idea hablar con los padres cuando examine al bebé o a niños mayores. Hágales preguntas directamente a los niños mayores y llámeles por su nombre. También observe si los padres y el niño se llevan bien. La Tabla 14-5 tiene preguntas comúnes.

I want to examine the older child.	Quiero examinar al niño mayor. *(Kee-eh-roh ehx-ah-mee-nahr ahl nee-nyoh mah-yohr)*

TABLE 14-5 Simple Questions		
TABLA 14-5 Preguntas Sencillas		
English	**Spanish**	**Pronunciation**
Do you understand?	¿Entiende?	*Ehn-tee-ehn-deh*
What is this?	¿Qué es esto?	*Keh ehs ehs-toh*
Why not?	¿Por qué no?	*Pohr keh noh*
What's going on?	¿Qué pasa?	*Keh pah-sah*
Since when?	¿Desde cuándo?	*Dehs-deh koo-ahn-doh*
For what?	¿Para qué?	*Pah-rah keh*
Never?	¿Nunca?	*Noon-kah*
Are you hungry?	¿Tiene hambre?	*Tee-eh-neh ahm-breh*
Are you thirsty?	¿Tiene sed?	*Tee-eh-neh sehd*
Is that enough?	¿Es suficiente?	*Ehs soo-fee-see-ehn-teh*
Is that too much?	¿Es mucho?	*Ehs moo-choh*
Can you feel this?	¿Siente esto?	*See-ehn-teh ehs-toh*

The one who is 6 years old. — El que tiene seis años.
(Ehl keh tee-eh-neh she-ees ah-nyohs)

Does he go to school? — ¿Va a la escuela?
(Bah ah lah ehs-koo-eh-lah)

Does he sleep well? — ¿Duerme bien?
(Doo-ehr-meh bee-ehn)

Does he wet the bed? — ¿Moja la cama?
(Moh-hah lah kah-mah)

Does he play outdoors? — ¿Juega afuera de la casa?
(Joo-eh-gah ah-foo-eh-rah deh lah kah-sah)

Does he have any friends? — ¿Tiene amigos?
(Tee-eh-neh ah-mee-gohs)

Do any of your children have asthma? — ¿Algunos de sus niños tienen asma?
(Ahl-goo-nohs deh soos nee-nyohs tee-eh-nehn ahs-mah)

Cold/flu? — ¿Resfriado/gripa?
(Rehs-free-ah-doh/gree-pah)

Chickenpox? — ¿Varicela?
(Bah-ree-seh-lah)

Diphtheria? — ¿Difteria?
(Deef-teh-ree-ah)

Measles? — ¿Sarampión?
(Sah-rahm-pee-ohn)

Mumps?	¿Paperas?
	(Pah-peh-rahs)
Pneumonia?	¿Pulmonía?
	(Pool-moh-nee-ah)
Convulsions?	¿Convulsiones?
	(Kohn-bool-see-ohn-ehs)
Nausea and vomiting?	¿Náusea y vómitos?
	(Nah-oo-seh-ah ee boh-mee-tohs)
Hearing defects?	¿Defectos del oído?
	(Deh-fehk-tohs dehl oh-ee-doh)
Delayed speech?	¿Tardío del lenguaje?
	(Tahr-dee-oh dehl lehn-goo-ah-heh)
Visual defects?	¿Defectos de la vista?
	(Deh-fehk-tohs deh lah bees-tah)
Bad coordination?	¿Mala coordinación?
	(Mah-lah kohr-dee-nah-see-ohn)
Is he hyperactive?	¿Es inquieto/latoso?
	(Ehs een-kee-eh-toh/lah-toh-soh)
Does the school have complaints about him?	¿Tiene quejas de la escuela?
	(Tee-eh-neh keh-hahs deh lah ehs-koo-eh-lah)

In general, when speaking to a child, the familiar *you* (tú) is used.

Generalmente se usa la forma familiar de *usted* cuando habla con un niño.

What is your name?	¿Cómo te llamas?
	(Koh-moh teh yah-mahs)
My name is. . .	Mi nombre es. . ./Me llamo. . .
	(Mee nohm-breh ehs/Mee yah-moh)
I would like to talk to you!	¡Me gustaría hablar contigo!
	(Meh goos-tah-ree-ah ah-blahr kohn-tee-goh)
Do you have time?	¿Tienes tiempo?
	(Tee-eh-nehs tee-ehm-poh)
Are you in a hurry?	¿Estás de prisa?
	(Ehs-tahs deh pree-sah)
Do you like going to school?	¿Te gusta ir a la escuela?
	(Teh goos-tah eer ah lah ehs-koo-eh-lah)
What grade are you in?	¿En qué año estás?
	(Ehn keh ah-nyoh ehs-tahs)
What subject do you like best?	¿Qué materia te gusta más?
	(Keh mah-teh-ree-ah teh goos-tah mahs)

What kind of grades do you make?	¿Qué calificaciones sacas? *(Keh kah-lee-fee-kah-see-ohn-ehs sah-kahs)*
Do you play sports?	¿Juegas deportes? *(Joo-eh-gahs deh-pohr-tehs)*
Which kind?	¿Qué clase? *(Keh klah-seh)*
How many friends do you have?	¿Cuántos amigos tienes? *(Koo-ahn-tohs ah-mee-gohs tee-eh-nehs)*
Do you need help with school work?	¿Necesitas ayuda con la tarea? *(Neh-seh-see-tahs ah-yoo-dah kohn lah tah-reh-ah)*
Who helps you?	¿Quién te ayuda? *(Kee-ehn teh ah-yoo-dah)*
Do you have vision problems?	¿Tienes problemas con la visión? *(Tee-eh-nehs proh-bleh-mahs kohn lah bee-see-ohn)*
Do you wear glasses?	¿Usas anteojos/lentes? *(Oo-sahs ahn-teh-oh-hohs/lehn-tehs)*
Can you see the blackboard well?	¿Puedes ver bien el pizarrón? *(Poo-eh-dehs behr bee-ehn ehl pee-sah-rohn)*
Do you miss school a lot?	¿Faltas mucho a la escuela? *(Fahl-tahs moo-choh ah lah ehs-koo-eh-lah)*
Do you get distracted easily?	¿Te distraes fácilmente? *(Teh dees-trah-ehs fah-seel-mehn-teh)*
Who takes you to school?	¿Quién te lleva a la escuela? *(Kee-ehn teh yeh-bah ah lah ehs-koo-eh-lah)*
Do you walk to school?	¿Caminas a la escuela? *(Kah-mee-nahs ah lah ehs-koo-eh-lah)*
Do you eat breakfast/lunch?	¿Tomas desayuno/almuerzo? *(Toh-mahs deh-sah-yoo-noh/ahl-moo-ehr-soh)*
Do you have problems with your teeth?	¿Tienes problemas con los dientes? *(Tee-eh-nehs proh-bleh-mahs kohn lohs dee-ehn-tehs)*
At what time do you go to sleep?	¿A qué hora te acuestas a dormir? *(Ah keh oh-rah teh ah-koo-ehs-tahs ah dohr-meer)*

How many hours do you sleep?	**¿Cuántas horas duermes?** *(Koo-ahn-tahs oh-rahs doo-ehr-mehs)*
Do you wake up at night?	**¿Te despiertas en la noche?** *(Teh dehs-pee-ehr-tahs ehn lah noh-cheh)*
What house chores do you do?	**¿Qué quehaceres haces?** *(Keh keh-ah-seh-rehs ah-sehs)*
How do you feel?	**¿Cómo te sientes?** *(Koh-moh teh see-ehn-tehs)*
Have you been sick?	**¿Has estado enfermo(a)?** *(Ahs ehs-tah-doh ehn-fehr-moh[mah])*
Is there any thing that worries you?	**¿Hay algo que te preocupa?** *(Ah-ee ahl-goh keh teh preh-oh-koo-pah)*
Who do you talk to?	**¿Con quién hablas?** *(Kohn kee-ehn ah-blahs)*
Do you have questions?	**¿Tienes preguntas?** *(Tee-eh-nehs preh-goon-tahs)*
Thank you for talking to me!	**¡Gracias por hablar conmigo!** *(Grah-see-ahs pohr ah-blahr kohn-mee-goh)*
I will talk to your mother again.	**Hablaré con tu mamá otra vez.** *(Ah-blah-reh kohn too mah-mah oh-trah behs)*
Good-bye!	**¡Hasta luego!** *(Ahs-tah loo-eh-goh)*

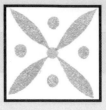

CHAPTER FIFTEEN
A Visit to the Ob-Gyn

CAPITULO QUINCE
Una Visita al Gineco-Obstetra

Mrs. Garcia visits the obstetrician when she finds out that she is pregnant. The doctor orders blood and urine exams to assess the patient's health status. After examining her, he tells her the tentative date of delivery. He also gives her an appointment so she can learn about breast exams.

La señora García visita al gineco-obstetra cuando se entera de que está embarazada. El doctor le ordena los exámenes de sangre y orina para saber el estado de salud de la paciente. Después de examinarla le dice cuál será la fecha del parto. También le da una cita para que acuda a una plática sobre el cáncer.

Mrs. Garcia is a 32-year-old woman who delivered a baby and the doctor is visiting her in her room. He tells her that she will be discharged tomorrow. He also tells her that she must follow directions carefully so that everything turns out all right.

La señora García de 32 años, fué atendida en su parto y el doctor la visita en su cuarto. Le comunica que mañana le dará de alta. También le dice que debe seguir cuidadosamente las recomendaciones que se le den para que todo salga bien.

Mrs. Garcia, tomorrow you will be discharged from the hospital.	Señora García, mañana sale usted del hospital. *(Seh-nyoh-rah Gahr-see-ah, mah-nyah-nah sah-leh oos-tehd dehl ohs-pee-tahl)*

TABLE 15-1	**Discharge Recommendations**	
TABLA 15-1	Recomendaciones al Dar de Alta	

English	Spanish	Pronunciation
recommendations	recomendaciones	*reh-koh-mehn-dah-see-ohn-ehs*
will have	tendrá	*tehn-drah*
keep	guardar	*goo-ahr-dahr*
rest	reposo	*reh-poh-soh*
fats	grasas	*grah-sahs*
hot sauces	picante	*pee-kahn-teh*
wound	herida	*eh-ree-dah*
bleeding	sangrado	*sahn-grah-doh*
go	acuda	*ah-koo-dah*
birth control	control de fertilidad	*kohn-trohl deh fehr-tee-lee-dahd*

I will give you instructions for you and the baby.	Le daré instrucciones para usted y su bebé. *(Leh dah-reh eens-trook-see-ohn-ehs pah-rah oos-tehd ee soo beh-beh)*
You will have to rest at least seven days.	Tendrá que guardar reposo al menos siete días. *(Tehn-drah keh goo-ahr-dahr reh-poh-soh ahl meh-nohs see-eh-teh dee-ahs)*
Your diet should be low in fats and hot sauces.	Su dieta debe ser baja en grasas y picantes. *(Soo dee-eh-tah deh-beh sehr bah-hah ehn grah-sahs ee pee-kahn-tehs)*
Try to have a bowel movement every day.	Procure hacer del baño diariamente. *(Proh-koo-reh ah-sehr dehl bah-nyoh dee-ah-ree-ah-mehn-teh)*
Don't get constipated.	No se deje estreñir. *(Noh seh deh-heh ehs-treh-nyeer)*
Drink a lot of water and juices.	Tome mucha agua y jugos. *(Toh-meh moo-chah ah-goo-ah ee hoo-gohs)*

Watch that your wound doesn't get infected.	Vigile que su herida no se infecte. *(Bee-hee-leh keh soo eh-ree-dah noh seh een-fehk-teh)*
Watch your bleeding.	Vigile su sangrado. *(Bee-hee-leh soo sahn-grah-doh)*
If it is a lot, or there is fever, go to the hospital right away.	Si es abundante, o aparece fiebre, acuda inmediatamente al hospital. *(See ehs ah-boon-dahn-teh, oh ah-pah-reh-seh fee-eh-breh, ah-koo-dah een-meh-dee-ah-tah-mehn-teh ahl ohs-pee-tahl)*
Take a bath every day.	Báñese todos los días. *(Bah-nyeh-seh toh-dohs lohs dee-ahs)*
Clean your breasts thoroughly.	Lave muy bien sus senos/pechos. *(Lah-beh moo-eeh bee-ehn soohs seh-nohs/peh-chohs)*
Sleep at least six hours daily.	Duerma por lo menos seis horas diarias. *(Doo-ehr-mah pohr loh meh-nohs seh-ees oh-rahs dee-ah-ree-ahs)*
As soon as you can, go to your doctor for the birth control plan that you wish to use.	En cuanto pueda, acuda a su doctor para el control de fertilidad que desee. *(Ehn koo-ahn-toh poo-eh-dah, ah-koo-dah ah soo dok-tohr pah-rah ehl kohn-trohl deh fehr-tee-lee-dahd keh deh-seh-eh)*

TABLE 15-2   Useful Words
TABLA 15-2   Palabras Útiles

English	Spanish	Pronunciation
navel	ombligo	*ohm-blee-goh*
burp	repetir/eructar	*reh-peh-teer/eh-rook-tahr*
placing it	colocándolo	*koh-loh-kahn-doh-loh*
loose clothes	ropa cómoda	*roh-pah koh-moh-dah*
vaccinations	vacunas	*bah-koo-nahs*
growth	crecimiento	*kreh-see-mee-ehn-toh*
development	desarrollo	*deh-sah-roh-yoh*
successful	con éxito	*kohn ehx-ee-toh*
I will see you	la veré	*lah beh-reh*

About the baby:	En cuanto al bebé:
	(Ehn koo-ahn-toh ahl beh-beh)
Bathe him every day.	Báñelo diariamente.
	(Bah-nyeh-loh dee-ah-ree-ah-mehn-teh)
Watch the navel.	Vigile el ombligo.
	(Bee-hee-leh ehl ohm-blee-goh)
Clean your nipples before you breast-feed.	Lave sus pezónes antes de dar pecho.
	(Lah-beh soos peh-soh-nehs ahn-tehs deh dahr peh-choh)
Breast-feed or give a bottle every three hours.	Dé pecho o biberón cada tres horas.
	(Deh peh-choh oh bee-beh-rohn kah-dah trehs oh-rahs)
Help him to burp.	Póngalo a repetir/eructar.
	(Pohn-gah-loh ah reh-peh-teer/eh-rook-tahr)
Pat his back gently.	Dé palmaditas en la espalda.
	(Deh pahl-mah-dee-tahs ehn lah ehs-pahl-dah)
Watch his urine and his bowel movements.	Vigile su orina y sus evacuaciones.
	(Bee-hee-leh soo oh-ree-nah ee soos eh-bah-koo-ah-see-oh-nehs)
Watch that his nose is clear.	Vigile que su nariz esté libre.
	(Bee-hee-leh keh soo nah-rees ehs-teh lee-breh)
Dress him with loose clothes.	Póngale ropa cómoda.
	(Pohn-gah-leh roh-pah koh-moh-dah)
Take him for vaccinations at two months.	Llévelo a vacunar a los dos meses.
	(Yeh-beh-loh ah bah-koo-nahr ah lohs dohs meh-sehs)
Watch his growth and development.	Vigile su crecimiento y desarrollo.
	(Bee-hee-leh soo kreh-see-mee-ehn-toh ee deh-sah-roh-yoh)
If you see anything wrong, take him to the doctor.	Si nota algo malo, llévelo a su doctor.
	(See noh-tah ahl-goh mah-loh, yeh-beh-loh ah soo dohk-tohr)

TABLE 15-3	Selected Words
TABLA 15-3	Palabras Selectas

English	Spanish	Pronunciation
classify	clasifique	*klah-see-fee-keh*
classification	clasificación	*klah-see-fee-kah-see-ohn*
detect	descubra	*dehs-koo-brah*
detection	detección	*deh-tehk-see-ohn*
diagnostic	diagnóstico	*dee-ahg-nohs-tee-koh*
illness	enfermedad	*ehn-fehr-meh-dahd*
terminal	terminal	*tehr-mee-nahl*
identified	identificado	*ee-dehn-tee-fee-kah-doh*
classified	clasificado	*klah-see-fee-kah-doh*
characteristics	características	*kah-rahk-teh-rees-tee-kahs*

If you follow these recommendations, everything will be all right.	Si usted sigue estos consejos, todo saldrá con éxito. *(See oos-tehd see-geh ehs-tohs kohn-seh-hohs, toh-doh sahl-drah kohn ehx-ee-toh)*
I will see you, Mrs. Garcia.	Hasta luego, señora García. *(Ahs-tah loo-eh-goh, seh-nyoh-rah Gahr-see-ah)*
I will see you tomorrow.	La veré mañana. *(Lah beh-reh mah-nyah-nah)*

Mrs. Garcia attends a talk that her doctor recommended. The talk is on the subject of cancer.

La señora García acude a la plática que le recomendó el doctor. La plática es sobre el cáncer.

More than 200 diseases have been identified as cancer. They are classified as such because they share common characteristics, progress in similar manner, and are treated similarly. The American Cancer Society defines cancer as a large group of diseases characterized by uncontrolled growth and spread of abnormal cells.

Más de 200 enfermedades se han identificado como cáncer. Se clasifican según sus características comunes, su progresión de manera semejante y su tratamiento similar. La Sociedad Americana de Cáncer, define al cáncer como un grupo grande de enfermedades caracterizadas por un crecimiento anormal de las células.

TABLE 15-4 Selected Words
TABLA 15-4 Palabras Selectas

English	Spanish	Pronunciation
common	común	*koh-moon*
progression	progresión	*proh-greh-see-ohn*
similar	similar	*see-mee-lahr*
growth	crecimiento	*kreh-see-mee-ehn-toh*
abnormal	anormal	*ah-nohr-mahl*
benign	benigno	*beh-neeg-noh*
cancer	cáncer	*kahn-sehr*
chemotherapy	quimioterapia	*kee-mee-oh-teh-rah-pee-ah*
change	cambio	*kahm-bee-oh*
early	temprano	*tehm-prah-no*

Pay attention to the following signs so you can detect cancer early.

Preste atención a las siguientes señas para que detecte el cáncer oportunamente.
(Prehs-teh ah-tehn-see-ohn ah lahs see-gee-ehn-tehs seh-nyahs pah-rah keh deh-tehk-teh ehl kahn-sehr oh-pohr-too-nah-mehn-teh)

1. Change in bowel or bladder habits.

1. Cambio en el hábito de la orina o el excremento.
(Kahm-bee-oh ehn ehl ah-bee-toh deh lah oh-ree-nah oh ehl ehx-kreh-mehn-toh)

2. A sore that does not heal.

2. Un grano que no se cura.
(Oon grah-noh keh noh seh koo-rah)

3. Unusual bleeding or discharge.

3. Sangrado o flujo profuso.
(Sahn-grah-doh oh floo-hoh proh-foo-soh)

4. Lump in breast or elsewhere.

4. Bolita en el pecho o en otra parte.
(Boh-lee-tah ehn ehl peh-choh oh ehn oh-trah pahr-teh)

5. Indigestion or difficulty swallowing.

5. Indigestión o dificultad al tragar.
(Een-dee-hehs-tee-ohn oh dee-fee-kool-tahd ahl trah-gahr)

TABLE 15-5   Selected Words
TABLA 15-5   Palabras Selectas

English	Spanish	Pronunciation
surgery	cirugía	*see-roo-hee-ah*
terms	términos	*tehr-mee-nohs*
tests	pruebas	*proo-eh-bahs*
tissue	tejido	*teh-hee-doh*
treatment	tratamiento	*trah-tah-mee-ehn-toh*
warning	advertencia	*ahd-behr-tehn-see-ah*
tumor	tumor	*too-mohr*
endoscopy	endoscopía	*ehn-dohs-koh-pee-ah*
surgeon	cirujano	*see-roo-hah-noh*

6. Change in wart or mole.

6. Cambio en lunar o verruga.
(Kahm-bee-oh ehn loo-nahr oh beh-roo-gah)

7. Nagging cough or hoarseness.

7. Tos persistente o afónico.
(Tohs pehr-sees-tehn-teh oh ah-foh-nee-koh)

Other recommendations for Mrs. García include:

Otras recomendaciones para la señora García incluyen:
(Oh-trahs reh-koh-mehn-dah-see-oh-nehs pah-rah lah seh-nyoh-rah Gahr-see-ah een-kloo-yehn)

Perform monthly self breast exam.

Haga un autoexamen del pecho cada mes.
(Ah-gah oon ah-oo-toh-ehx-ah-mehn dehl peh-choh kah-dah mehs)

Have a yearly Pap smear.

Haga una prueba de papanicolau cada año.
(Ah-gah oo-nah proo-eh-bah deh pah-pah-nee-koh-lah-oo kah-dah ah-nyoh)

For men: watch urinary problems, evaluate yearly the size of the prostate.

En hombres: vigile los problemas de la orina, haga el examen de la próstata cada año.
(Ehn ohm-brehs: bee-hee-leh lohs proh-bleh-mahs deh lah oh-ree-nah, ah-gah ehl ehx-ah-mehn deh lah prohs-tah-tah kah-dah ah-nyoh)

Some forms of cancer are curable. Methods employed to detect cancer include physical exams, magnetic resonance imaging (MRI), or blood samples. Once the cancer is detected, the type of treatment such as chemotherapy or radiotherapy is initiated. Many factors influence the recovery period. For some people, rehabilitation is difficult.

Algunas formas de cáncer son curables. Los métodos que se emplean para detectar el cáncer incluyen exámenes físicos, la imagen de resonancia magnética y muestras de sangre. Una vez que se detecta el cancer, el tipo de tratamiento tal como la quimioterapia o radioterapia se inicia. Muchos factores influencian el período de recuperación. Para algunas personas la rehabilitación es difícil.

TABLE 15-6	Selected Words
TABLA 15-6	Palabras Selectas

English	Spanish	Pronunciation
emergencies	emergencias	eh-mehr-hehn-see-ahs
examinations	exámenes	ehx-ah-meh-nehs
factors	factores	fahk-toh-rehs
imaging	imagen	ee-mah-hehn
laboratory	laboratorio	lah-boh-rah-toh-ree-oh
magnetic	magnético	muhg-neh-tee-koh
malignant	maligno	mah-leeg-noh
modifiers	modificadores	moh-dee-fee-kah-doh-rehs
oncologic	oncología	ohn-koh-loh-hee-ah
prevention	prevención	preh-behn-see-ohn
radiologic	radiológico	rah-dee-oh-loh-hee-koh
radiotherapy	radioterapia	rah-dee-oh-teh-rah-pee-ah
recovery	recuperación	reh-koo-peh-rah-see-ohn
rehabilitation	rehabilitación	reh-ah-bee-lee-tah-see-ohn
resonance	resonancia	reh-soh-nahn-see-ah
risk	riesgo	ree-ehs-goh
signs	señales	seh-nyah-lehs
sites	sitios	see-tee-ohs
studies	estudios	ehs-too-dee-ohs

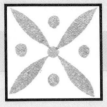

CHAPTER SIXTEEN
A Visit to the Family Medicine Doctor

CAPITULO DIECISEIS
Una Visita al Médico Familiar

Gonzalo Rivera, a 23-year-old male, visits a family doctor for the first time. He is afraid to go into the office. He has questions about his health habits.

Gonzalo Rivera, un hombre de veintitrés años, acude por primera vez al médico familiar. Siente miedo al entrar al consultorio porqué tiene dudas sobre los hábitos de su salud.

Doctor, I think I am infected with AIDS.	Doctor, pienso que estoy infectado de SIDA. *(Dohk-tohr, pee-ehn-so keh ehs-toh-ee een-fek-tah-doh deh see-dah)*

The doctor starts explaining about the disease.

El doctor le da una explicación sobre la enfermedad.

Fear about AIDS comes from ignorance about the true nature of the disease and those who have the virus. The means of transmission are through sexual contact, contact with contaminated blood products and body fluids, or from infected mother to fetus.

El miedo al SIDA proviene de la ignorancia sobre la naturaleza de la enfermedad y los efectos del virus. Los medios de transmisión son: contacto o relaciones sexuales, contacto con productos de la sangre, fluidos del cuerpo contaminados, y madres con la enfermedad que infectan al feto.

The doctor asks the patient:	El doctor le pregunta al paciente: *(Ehl dohk-tohr leh preh-goon-tah ahl pah-see-ehn-teh)*
Have you been exposed to any infectious diseases?	¿Ha estado expuesto a enfermedades infecciosas? *(Ah ehs-tah-doh ehx-poo-ehs-toh ah ehn-fehr-meh-dah-dehs een-fehk-see-oh-sahs)*
Do you have any infectious disease now?	¿Tiene alguna enfermedad infecciosa ahora? *(Tee-eh-neh ahl-goo-nah ehn-fehr-meh-dahd een-fehk-see-oh-sah ah-oh-rah)*
Do you have sexual relations?	¿Tiene relaciones sexuales? *(Tee-eh-neh reh-lah-see-oh-nehs sex-oo-ah-lehs)*
With how many people?	¿Con cuántas personas? *(Kohn koo-ahn-tahs pehr-soh-nahs)*
Do you participate in homosexual relations?	¿Participa en relaciones homosexuales? *(Pahr-tee-see-pah ehn reh-lah-see-ohn-ehs oh-moh-sehx-oo-ah-lehs)*
Do you engage in protective sex?	¿Practica el sexo seguro? *(Prahk-tee-kah ehl sehx-oh seh-goo-roh)*

The doctor explains that AIDS was first reported in 1981. Persons with acquired immune deficiency syndrome develop a defect in their immune system. They are vulnerable to serious infections (referred to as opportunistic infections) that ordinarily pose little threat to an intact immune system. Common problems among AIDS patients are: *Pneumocystis carinii* pneumonia; a type of tumor, Kaposi's sarcoma; problems with the central nervous system that may cause forgetfulness, personality changes, or impaired motor skills. In addition, diarrhea and weight loss are common.

El doctor le explica que el SIDA se reportó por primera vez en 1981. Las personas con este síndrome tienen un defecto en su sistema inmunitario. Ellos son vulnerables a las infecciones serias (llamadas infecciones oportunistas) que amenazan al sistema inmunológico. Los pacientes con SIDA tienen problemas como: neumonía producida por el neumocistis carani; una especie de tumor llamado sarcoma de Kaposi; alteraciones en el sistema nervioso central que pueden causar el olvido de las cosas, cambios en la personalidad, o daños en las habilidades motoras. Adicionalmente, diarreas frecuentes y pérdida de peso son comunes.

TABLE 16-1   Selected Words
TABLA 16-1   Palabras Selectas

English	Spanish	Pronunciation
acquired	adquirida	*ahd-kee-ree-dah*
antibodies	anticuerpos	*ahn-tee-koo-ehr-pohs*
develop	desarrollar	*deh-sah-roh-yahr*
sneeze	estornudo	*ehs-tohr-noo-doh*
ignorance	ignorancia	*eeg-noh-rahn-see-ah*
immunodeficiency	inmunodeficiencia	*een-moo-noh-deh-fee-see-ehn-see-ah*
fear	miedo	*mee-eh-doh*
pneumonia	pulmonía/neumonía	*pool-moh-nee-ah/neh-oo-moh-nee-ah*
nature	naturaleza	*nah-too-rah-leh-sah*
opportunistic	oportunista	*oh-pohr-too-nees-tah*
panic	pánico	*pah-nee-koh*
precaution	precaución	*preh-kah-oo-see-ohn*
preliminary	preliminar	*preh-lee-mee-nahr*
syndrome	síndrome	*seen-droh-meh*
transfusion	transfusión	*trahns-foo-see-ohn*

The patient asks:

What causes AIDS?

A virus known as HIV.

Who is at risk of getting AIDS?

Sexually active homosexual and bisexual males or females.

El paciente pregunta:
(Ehl pah-see-ehn-teh preh-goon-tah)

¿Qué causa el SIDA?
(keh kah-oo-sah ehl see-dah)

El virus causal del SIDA se conoce como VIH.
(Ehl bee-roos kah-oo-sahl dehl see-dah seh koh-noh-seh koh-moh bee-ee-ah-cheh)

¿Quién está en riesgo de contraer el SIDA?
(Kee-ehn ehs-tah ehn ree-ehs-goh deh kohn-trah-ehr ehl see-dah)

Homosexuales activos y hombres o mujeres bisexuales.
(Oh-moh-sehx-oo-ah-lehs ahk-tee-bohs ee ohm-brehs oh moo-heh-rehs bee-sehx-oo-ah-lehs)

Intravenous drug abusers.	Los que abusan de las drogas intravenosas. *(Lohs keh ah-boo-sah deh lahs droh-gahs een-trah-beh-noh-sahs)*
Hemophiliacs and recipients of contaminated blood.	Los hemofílicos y los que reciben transfusión con sangre contaminada. *(Los eh-moh-fee-lee-kohs ee los keh reh-see-behn trahns-foo-see-ohn kohn sahn-greh kohn-tah-mee-nah-dah)*
Fetus of infected mothers.	Fetos de madres contaminadas. *(Feh-tohs deh mah-drehs kohn-tah-mee-nah-dahs)*
If you become infected with HIV, what is the risk of getting AIDS?	Si ha sido infectado con VIH, ¿cuál es el riesgo de contraer el SIDA? *(See ah see-doh een-fehk-tah-doh kohn VIH, koo-ahl ehs ehl ree-ehs-goh deh kohn-trah-ehr ehl see-dah)*
About 31% of infected individuals will develop AIDS within six to seven years.	Cerca del 31 por ciento de individuos infectados desarrollan SIDA dentro de seis a siete años. *(Sehr-kah dehl treh-een-tah ee oon pohr see-ehn-toh deh een-dee-bee-doo-ohs een-fehk-tah-dohs deh-sah-roh-yahn see-dah dehn-troh deh seh-ees ah see-eh-teh ah-nyohs)*
Studies show that many infected persons remain in good health.	Los estudios muestran que muchas personas infectadas quedan con buena salud. *(Lohs ehs-too-dee-ohs moo-ehs-trahn keh moo-chahs pehr-soh-nahs een-fehk-tah-dahs keh-dahn kohn boo-eh-nah sah-lood)*
Infected persons can transmit the virus.	Las personas infectadas pueden transmitir el virus. *(Lahs pehr-soh-nahs een-fehk-tah-dahs poo-eh-dehn trahns-mee-teer ehl bee-roos)*
Can casual contact cause AIDS?	¿Los contactos eventuales pueden causar SIDA? *(Lohs kohn-tahk-tohs eh-behn-too-ah-lehs poo-eh-dehn kah-oo-sahr see-dah)*

HIV is not transmissible by casual contact, nor. . .

El VIH no es transmitido en forma casual, ni por. . .
(Ehl VIH noh ehs trahns-mee-tee-doh ehn fohr-mah kah-soo-ahl, nee pohr:)

Living in same house as infected persons.

Vivir en la misma casa con personas infectadas.
(Bee-beer ehn lah mees-mah kah-sah kohn pehr-soh-nahs een-fehk-tah-dahs)

Eating food handled by persons with AIDS.

Comer comida preparada por personas infectadas con SIDA.
(Koh-mehr koh-mee-dah preh-pah-rah-dah pohr pehr-soh-nahs een-fehk-tah-dahs kohn see-dah)

Coughing, sneezing, kissing, or swimming with infected persons.

Tos, estornudo, besar, o nadar con personas infectadas.
(Tohs, ehs-tohr-noo-doh, beh-sahr, oh nah-dahr kohn pehr-soh-nahs een-fehk-tah-dahs)

Is there a laboratory test for AIDS?

¿Hay pruebas de laboratorio para detectar el SIDA?
(Ah-ee proo-eh-bahs deh lah-boh-rah-toh-ree-oh pah-rah deh-tehk-tahr ehl see-dah)

No, but there is a test for antibodies.

No, pero hay prueba de anticuerpos.
(Noh, peh-roh ah-ee prooh-eh-bah deh ahn-tee-koo-ehr-pohs)

What are the symptoms?

¿Cuáles son los síntomas?
(Koo-ah-lehs sohn lohs seen-toh-mahs)

Most have no symptoms.

La mayoría no tiene síntomas.
(Lah mah-yoh-ree-ah noh tee-eh-neh seen-toh-mahs)

Some develop tiredness, fever, loss of appetite, weight loss, diarrhea, night sweats.

Algunos desarrollan cansansio, fiebre, falta de apetito, pérdida de peso, diarrea, sudor nocturno.
(Ahl-goo-nohs deh-sah-roh-yahn kahn-sahn-see-oh, fee-eh-breh, fahl-tah deh ah-peh-tee-toh, pehr-dee-dah deh peh-soh, dee-ah-reh-ah, soo-dohr nohk-toor-noh)

How is AIDS diagnosed?

¿Cómo se diagnostica el SIDA?
(Koh-moh seh dee-ahg-nohs-tee-kah ehl see-dah)

Diagnosis is based on evaluation of indicators: immune system function and T-cell count, presence of opportunistic diseases, unexplained dementia, and detection of HIV antibodies.

El diagnóstico se basa en la evaluación de indicadores: la función del sistema inmunológico y la cuenta de células T, presencia de enfermedades oportunistas, demencia inexplicada, y el descubrimiento de anticuerpos VIH.

(Ehl dee-ahg-nohs-tee-koh seh bah-sah ehn la eh-bah-loo-ah-see-ohn deh een-dee-kah-doh-rehs: lah foon-see-ohn dehl sees-teh-mah een-moo-noh-loh-hee-koh ee lah koo-ehn-tah deh seh-loo-lahs Teh, preh-sehn-see ah deh ehn-fehr-meh-dah-dehs oh-pohr-too-nees-tahs, deh-mehn-see-ah een-ehx-plee-kah-dah ee ehl dehs-koo-bree-mee-ehn-toh deh ahn-tee-koo-ehr-pohs VIH)

What are some of the diseases affecting persons with AIDS?

¿Cuáles son las enfermedades que aparecen en personas infectadas con SIDA?

(Koo-ah-lehs sohn lahs ehn-fehr-meh-dah-dehs keh ah-pah-reh-sehn ehn pehr-soh-nahs een-fehk-tah-dahs kohn see-dah)

About 85% of AIDS patients have had one or both:

Cerca del 85 por ciento de pacientes con SIDA han tenido una o ambas:

(Sehr-kah dehl oh-chehn-tah ee seen-koh pohr see-ehn-toh deh pah-see-ehn-tehs kohn see-dah ahn teh-nee-doh oo-nah oh ahm-bahs:)

Pneumocystis carinii pneumonia (PCP), and/or Kaposi's sarcoma.

Neumonía por neumocistis carinii (PCP) y/o sarcoma de Kaposi.

(Neh-oo-moh-nee-ah pohr neh-oo-moh-sees-tees kah-ree-nee (PCP) ee/oh sahr-koh-mah deh Kah-poh-sees)

How serious is AIDS?

¿Qué tan serio es el SIDA?

(Keh tahn seh-ree-oh ehs ehl see-dah)

AIDS has a high fatality rate approaching 100%.

El SIDA tiene una tasa cercana al 100 por ciento de mortalidad.
(Ehl see-dah tee-eh-neh oo-nah tah-sah sehr-kah-nah ahl see-ehn pohr see-ehn-toh deh mohr-tah-lee-dahd)

The majority of patients have a life span of about 18–24 months.

La mayoría de los pacientes tienen una sobrevivencia aproximada de dieciocho a veinticuatro meses.
(Lah mah-yoh-ree-ah deh lohs pah-see-ehn-tehs tee-eh-nehn oo-nah soh-breh-bee-behn-see-ah ah-prohx-ee-mah-dah deh dee-eh-see-oh-choh ah veh-een-tee-koo-ah-troh meh-sehs)

Is there a danger from donated blood?

¿Qué peligro hay por sangre donada?
(Keh peh-lee-groh ah-ee pohr sahn-greh doh-nah-dah)

Absolutely not. Blood banks and other centers use sterile equipment and disposable needles.

Absolutamente ningún peligro. Los bancos de sangre y otros centros usan equipos estériles y agujas desechables.
(Ahb-soh-loo-tah-mehn-teh neen-goon peh-lee-groh. Lohs bahn-kohs deh sahn-greh ee oh-trohs sehn-trohs oo-sahn eh-kee-pohs ehs-teh-ree-lehs ee ah-goo-hahs deh-seh-chah-blehs)

What can be done to prevent AIDS?

¿Qué se puede hacer para prevenir el SIDA?
(Keh seh poo-eh-deh ah-sehr pah-rah preh-beh-neer ehl see-dah)

The U.S. Public Health Service recommends:

El Departamento de Salud Pública de los Estados Unidos recomienda:
(Ehl Deh-pahr-tah-mehn-toh deh Sah-lood Poo-blee-kah deh lohs Ehs-tah-dohs Oo-nee-dohs reh-koh-mee-ehn-dah)

1. Know sexual background/ habits of partners.

1. Conozca los hábitos sexuales de su pareja.
(Koh-nohs-kah lohs ah-bee-tohs sehx-oo-ah-lehs deh soo pah-reh-hah)

2. Use contraceptive measures.

3. If your partner is in a high risk group, cease sexual relations.

4. Eliminate multiple sexual partners.

5. Don't use intravenous drugs with contaminated needles; don't share needles or syringes.

2. Use medidas contraceptivas.
(Oo-seh meh-dee-dahs kohn-trah-sehp-tee-bahs)

3. Si su compañera está en el grupo de alto riesgo, suspenda las relaciones sexuales.
(See soo kohm-pah-nyeh-rah ehs-tah ehn ehl groo-poh deh ahl-toh ree-ehs-goh, soos-pehn-dah lahs reh-lah-see-ohn-ehs sehx-oo-ahl-ehs)

4. Elimine múltiples compañeros sexuales.
(Eh-lee-mee-neh mool-tee-plehs kohm-pah-nyeh-rohs sehx-oo-ah-lehs)

5. No use drogas intravenosas con agujas contaminadas; no comparta agujas o jeringas.
(Noh oo-seh droh-gahs een-trah-beh-noh-sahs kohn ah-goo-hahs kohn-tah-mee-nah-dahs; noh kohm-pahr-tah ah-goo-hahs oh heh-reen-gahs)

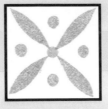

CHAPTER SEVENTEEN
A Visit to the Cardiologist

CAPITULO DIECISIETE
Una Visita al Cardiólogo

Mrs. Ortiz is at the cardiologist's office. She was sent by her family medicine doctor who found heart problems and hypertension.

La Sra. Ortiz está en la oficina del cardiólogo. La envió su médico familiar porqué encontró una alteración en su corazón y en su presión arterial.

Good morning, Mrs. Ortiz!	¡Buenos días, señora Ortiz! *(Boo-eh-nohs dee-ahs seh-nyo-rah ohr-tees)*
Good morning, Doctor.	¡Buenos días, Doctor! *(Boo-eh-nohs dee-ahs Dohk-tohr)*
How old are you?	¿Cuántos años tiene? *(Koo-ahn-tohs ah-nyohs tee-eh-neh)*
Forty-five years old.	Cuarenta y cinco años. *(Koo-ah-rehn-tah ee seen-koh ah-nyohs)*
Do you smoke?	¿Fuma usted? *(Foo-mah oo-stehd)*
Yes.	Sí. *(See)*
How many cigarettes per day?	¿Cuántos cigarrillos al día? *(Koo-ahn-tohs see-gah-ree-yohs ahl dee-ah)*
Fifteen per day.	Quince al día. *(Keen-seh ahl dee-ah)*

Do you have high blood pressure?	¿Tiene la presión alta?
	(Tee-eh-neh lah preh-see-ohn ahl-tah)
Do you have chest pain?	¿Tiene dolor en el pecho?
	(Tee-eh-neh doh-lohr ehn ehl peh-choh)
Occasionally.	Ocasionalmente.
	(Oh-kah-see-ohn-ahl-mehn-teh)
Palpitations?	¿Palpitaciones?
	(Pahl-pee-tah-see-ohn-ehs)
Once in a while.	De vez en cuando.
	(Deh behs ehn koo-ahn-doh)
Have you had pain in the left arm?	¿Ha sentido dolor en el brazo izquierdo?
	(Ah sehn-tee-doh doh-lohr ehn ehl brah-soh ees-kee-ehr-doh)
Yes, last week.	Sí, la semana pasada.
	(See, lah seh-mah-nah pah-sah-dah)
How long did it last?	¿Cuánto duró?
	(Koo-ahn-toh doo-roh)
Only five minutes.	Sólo cinco minutos.
	(Soh-loh seen-koh mee-noo-tohs)
When you have pain, do you get nauseated?	Cuando tiene dolor, ¿le da náuseas?
	(Koo-ahn-doh tee-eh-neh doh-lohr, leh dah nah-oo-seh-ahs)
No/yes.	No/sí.
	(Noh/see)
Do you have relatives with cardiac problems?	¿Tiene familiares con problemas cardíacos?
	(Tee-eh-neh fah-mee-lee-ah-rehs kohn proh-bleh-mahs kahr-dee-ah-kohs)
Yes, my dad.	Sí, mi papá.
	(See, mee pah-pah)
What happened to him?	¿Qué le pasó?
	(Keh leh pah-soh)
He had high cholesterol and he had surgery.	Tenía colesterol alto y le hicieron cirugía.
	(Teh-nee-ah koh-lehs-teh-rohl ahl-toh ee leh ee-see-eh-rohn see-roo-hee-ah)
Have you had rheumatic fever?	¿Ha tenido fiebre reumática?
	(Ah teh-nee-doh fee-eh-breh reh-oo-mah-tee-kah)

No.

No.
(Noh)

Have you had headaches?

¿Ha tenido dolor de cabeza?
(Ah teh-nee-doh doh-lohr deh kah-beh-sah)

Often, two times per week.

Seguido, dos veces por semana.
(Seh-gee-doh, dohs beh-sehs pohr seh-mah-nah)

Have you passed out?

¿Se ha desmayado?
(Seh ah dehs-mah-yah-doh)

No, never.

No, nunca.
(Noh, noon-kah)

Do you have dizzy spells?

¿Tiene mareos?
(Tee-eh-neh mah-reh-ohs)

Swelling of the ankles?

¿Hinchazón en los tobillos?
(Een-chah-sohn ehn lohs toh-bee-yohs)

Yes, in the afternoon.

Sí, por la tarde.
(See, pohr lah tahr-deh)

Are you diabetic?

¿Es diabética?
(Ehs dee-ah-beh-tee-kah)

I am prediabetic. I control it with diet.

Soy prediabética. Me controlo con dieta.
(Soh-ee preh-dee-ah-beh-tee-kah. Meh kohn-troh-loh kohn dee-eh-tah)

Do you drink alcohol?

¿Toma bebidas alcohólicas?
(Toh-mah beh-bee-dahs ahl-koh-lee-kahs)

Only at parties.

Sólo en las fiestas.
(Soh-loh ehn lahs fee-ehs-tahs)

The cardiologist examines Mrs. Ortiz. He finds a blood pressure of 160/100, a splitting of the second heart sound, and jugular pulsation.

El cardiólogo examina a la señora Ortiz. Le encuentra presión de ciento sesenta sobre cien, un desdoblamiento del segundo ruido cardíaco, y leve injurgitación de la yugular.

Mrs. Ortiz, you need to go to the hospital.

Señora Ortiz, necesita ir al hospital.
(Seh-nyoh-rah Ohr-tees, neh-seh-see-tah eer ahl ohs-pee-tahl)

TABLE 17-1 Useful Words
TABLA 17-1 Palabras Utiles

English	Spanish	Pronunciation
palpitations	palpitaciones	*pahl-pee-tah-see-oh-nehs*
rheumatic fever	fiebre reumática	*fee-eh-breh reh-oo-mah-tee-kah*
jugular vein	vena yugular	*beh-nah yoo-goo-lahr*
paralysis	parálisis	*pah-rah-lee-sees*
electrocardiogram	electrocardiograma	*eh-lehk-troh-kahr-dee-oh-grah-mah*
pacemaker	marcapasos	*mahr-kah-pah-sohs*
swollen ankles	tobillos hinchados	*toh-bee-yohs een-chah-dohs*
general chemistry	química general	*kee-mee-kah heh-neh-rahl*
prescription	receta	*reh-seh-tah*
diabetes	diabetes	*dee-ah-beh-tehs*

TABLE 17-2 Useful Words
TABLA 17-2 Palabras Utiles

English	Spanish	Pronunciation
angina	angina	*ahn-hee-nah*
aneurysm	aneurisma	*ah-neh-oo-rees-mah*
arteriosclerosis	arterioesclerosis	*ahr-teh-ree-oh-ehs-kleh-roh-sees*
aorta	aorta	*ah-ohr-tah*
complete blood count	biometría hemática	*bee-oh-meh-tree-ah eh-mah-tee-kah*
thrombus	coágulo	*koh-ah-goo-loh*
dizzy spell	desmayo/mareo	*dehs-mah-yoh/mah-reh-oh*
chest pain	dolor de pecho	*doh-lohr deh peh-choh*
headache	dolor de cabeza	*doh-lohr deh kah-beh-sah*

I am going to order a complete blood count, general chemistry, urine, antistreptolysin, throat culture, electrocardiogram, and chest x-ray.

Voy a ordenar una biometría hemática, química general, orina, antiestreptolicinas, exudado faríngeo, electrocardiograma y radiografía del tórax.
(Boh-ee ah ohr-deh-nahr oo-nah bee-oh-meh-tree-ah eh-mah-tee-kah, kee-mee-kah heh-neh-rahl, oh-ree-nah, ahn-tee-ehs-trehp-toh-lee-see-nahs, ehx-oo-dah-doh fah-reen-heh-oh, eh-lehk-troh-kahr-dee-oh-grah-mah, ee rah-dee-oh-grah-fee-ah dehl toh-rahx)

I will let you know about the exams.

Le avisaré sobre los exámenes.
(Leh ah-bee-sah-reh soh-breh lohs ehx-ah-meh-nehs)

Mrs. Ortiz, take this pill every 8 hours for 10 days.

Señora Ortiz, tome esta pastilla cada ocho horas por diez días.
(Seh-nyoh-rah Ohr-tees, toh-meh ehs-tah pahs-tee-yah kah-dah oh-choh oh-rahs pohr dee-ehs dee-ahs)

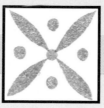

CHAPTER EIGHTEEN
A Visit to the Endocrinologist

CAPITULO DIECIOCHO
Una Visita al Endocrinólogo

The family doctor finds that his patient is a diabetic because of his symptoms and the results of the laboratory exams. He sends him to an endocrinologist who explains the following:

El médico familiar detecta que su paciente es diabético por sus síntomas y los resultados de laboratorio. Lo envía al endocrinólogo quien le explica lo siguiente:

Diabetes mellitus is characterized by the body's inability to utilize glucose.

La diabetes mellitus se caracteriza por la incapacidad del cuerpo para utilizar glucosa.
(Lah dee-ah-beh-tehs meh-lee-toos seh kah-rahk-teh-ree-sah pohr lah een-kah-pah-see-dahd dehl koo-ehr-poh pah-rah oo-tee-lee-sahr gloo-koh-sah)

Diminished amounts of insulin to meet requirements is called non-insulin-dependent DM.

A la disminución de insulina requerida se le llama diabetes no-insulino-dependiente.
(Ah lah dees-mee-noo-see-ohn deh een-soo-lee-nah reh-keh-ree-dah seh leh yah-mah dee-ah-beh-tehs noh-een-soo-lee-noh-deh-pehn-dee-ehn-teh)

It is also an imbalance between the availability and the requirements of insulin.

Es también un desequilibrio entre la disponibilidad y los requerimientos de insulina.
(Ehs tahm-bee-ehn oon deh-seh-kee-lee-bree-oh ehn-treh la dees-poh-nee-bee-lee-dahd ee lohs reh-keh-ree-mee-ehn-tohs deh een-soo-lee-nah)

Absence of insulin in the body is called insulin-dependent DM.

A la ausencia de insulina se le llama diabetes insulino-dependiente.
(Ah lah ah-oo-sehn-see-ah deh een-soo-lee-nah seh leh yah-mah dee-ah-beh-tehs een-soo-lee-noh-deh-pehn-dee-ehn-teh)

The endocrinologist continues to talk to the patient.
El endocrinólogo continúa hablando con el paciente.

I see from your history that weight has always been a problem.

Veo en su historia que su peso siempre ha sido un problema.
(Beh-oh ehn soo ees-toh-ree-ah keh soo peh-soh see-ehm-preh ah see-doh oon proh-bleh-mah)

Is that right?

¿Es cierto?
(Ehs see-ehr-toh)

It has been.

Ha sido.
(Ah see-doh)

I see your sister and grandfather had diabetes.

Veo que su hermana y abuelo tenían diabetes.
(Beh-oh keh soo ehr-mah-nah ee ah-boo-eh-loh teh-nee-ahn dee-ah-beh-tehs)

My grandfather died from complications of an amputation because of DM.

Mi abuelo murió por complicaciones de una amputación debida a DM.
(Mee ah-boo-eh-loh moo-ree-oh pohr kohm-plee-kah-see-oh-nehs deh oo-nah ahm-poo-tah-see-ohn deh-bee-dah ah deh-eh-me)

My sister is now being treated.

Mi hermana está en tratamiento.
(Mee ehr-mah-nah ehs-tah ehn trah-tah-mee-ehn-toh)

How old are you?

¿Cuántos años tiene?
(Koo-ahn-tohs ah-nyohs tee-eh-neh)

I am 44 years old.	Tengo 44 años. *(Tehn-goh koo-ah-rehn-tah ee koo-ah-troh ah-nyohs)*
Are you a smoker?	¿Es fumador? *(Ehs foo-mah-dohr)*
Yes.	Sí. *(See)*
How many packs a day?	¿Cuántas cajetillas al día? *(Koo-ahn-tahs kah-heh-tee-yahs ahl dee-ah)*
One and a half.	Una y media. *(Oo-nah ee meh-dee-ah)*
I want to do some testing.	Quiero hacer una prueba. *(Kee-eh-roh ah-sehr oon-ah proo-eh-bah)*
Have you had a fasting glucose level done?	¿Le han hecho examen de glucosa en ayunas? *(Leh ahn eh-choh ehx-ah-mehn deh gloo-koh-sah ehn ah-yoo-nahs)*
No, I don't think so.	No, no lo creo. *(Noh, noh loh kreh-oh)*
Tomorrow, at 7 AM, go to the lab and have your blood drawn.	Mañana a las siete vaya al laboratorio para tomar una muestra de sangre. *(Mah-nyah-nah ah lahs see-eh- teh bah-yah ahl lah-boh-rah- toh-ree-oh pah-rah toh-mahr oo- nah moo-ehs-trah deh sahn-greh)*

TABLE 18-1   Selected Words
TABLA 18-1   Palabras Selectas

English	Spanish	Pronunciation
dependent	dependiente	*deh-pehn-dee-ehn-teh*
hypoglycemia	hipoglucemia	*ee-poh-gloo-seh-mee-ah*
ketoacidosis	cetoacidosis	*seh-toh-ah-see-doh-sees*
pathophysiology	fisiopatología	*fee-see-oh-pah-toh-loh-gee-ah*
risk	riesgo	*ree-ehs-goh*
disorder	desorden	*deh-sohr-dehn*
utilize	utilizar	*oo-tee-lee-sahr*
absence	ausencia	*ah-oo-sehn-see-ah*
requirements	requerimiento	*reh-keh-ree-mee-ehn-toh*
available	disponible	*dees-poh-nee-bleh*

I can do that.	Puedo hacerlo.
	(Poo-eh-doh ah-sehr-loh)
Be sure not eat or drink anything after 9 PM.	No tome nada después de las nueve de la noche.
	(Noh toh-meh nah-dah dehs-poo-ehs deh lahs noo-eh-beh deh lah noh-cheh)
Sure.	Seguro.
	(Seh-goo-roh)
After the bloodwork, you may have your breakfast.	Después de tomar la muestra, puede desayunar.
	(Dehs-poo-ehs deh toh-mahr lah moo-ehs-trah, poo-eh-deh deh-sah-yoo-nahr)
Great.	Bien.
	(Bee-ehn)
Also, make an appointment for Wednesday.	También, pida cita para el miércoles.
	(Tahm-bee-ehn, pee-dah see-tah pah-rah ehl mee-ehr-koh-lehs)
I will do that.	Lo haré.
	(Loh ah-reh)
Please do the following:	Por favor, haga lo siguiente:
	(Pohr fah-bohr, ah-gah loh see-gee-ehn-teh)
Take the medicines daily.	Tome las medicinas diariamente.
	(Toh-meh lahs meh-dee-see-nahs dee-ah-ree-ah-mehn-teh)

TABLE 18-2   Selected Words
TABLA 18-2   Palabras Selectas

English	Spanish	Pronunciation
nephropathy	nefropatía	*neh-froh-pah-tee-ah*
neuropathy	neuropatía	*neh-oo-roh-pah-tee-ah*
polydipsia	polidipsia	*poh-lee-deep-see-ah*
polyuria	poliuria	*poh-lee-oo-ree-ah*
retinopathy	retinopatía	*reh-tee-noh-pah-tee-ah*
glycosuria	glucosuria	*gloo-koh-soo-ree-ah*
polyphagia	polifagia	*poh-lee-fah-hee-ah*
lipoatrophy	lipotrofia	*lee-poh-troh-fee-ah*

Eat a 1,500 calorie diet.

Lleve la dieta de 1,500 calorías.
*(Yeh-beh lah dee-eh-tah deh
meel-kee-nee-ehn-tahs kah-loh-
ree-ahs)*

Keep a general hygiene:
bath, nail cutting, sleep.

Medidas de higiene general:
baño, recorte de uñas, dormir.
*(Meh-dee-dahs deh ee-hee-eh-
neh heh-neh-rahl: bah-nyoh,
reh-kohr-teh deh oo-nyahs,
dohr-meer)*

Use comfortable clothes and
shoes.

Use ropa y zapatos cómodos.
*(Ooseh roh-pah ee sah-pah-
tohs koh-moh-dohs)*

Avoid scratching or cutting
your skin.

Evite rasguños o heridas en
la piel.
*(Eh-bee-teh rahs-goo-nyohs
oh eh-ree-dahs ehn lah pee-ehl)*

Exercise.

Haga ejercicio.
(Ah-gah eh-hehr-see-see-oh)

Go to the dentist every six
months.

Vaya al dentista cada seis
meses.
*(Bah-yah ahl dehn-tees-tah
kah-dah seh-ees meh-sehs)*

Go to the ophthalmologist
every year.

Vaya al oftalmólogo cada
año.
*(Bah-yah ahl ohf-tahl-moh-
loh-goh kah-dah ah-nyoh)*

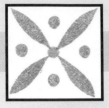

CHAPTER NINETEEN
A Visit to the Surgeon

CAPITULO DIECINUEVE
Una Visita al Cirujano

The surgeon is a doctor that has prepared for many years. He specializes in the treatment of diseases, injuries, and deformities.

El cirujano es un médico que se ha preparado varios años. Se especializa en el tratamiento de enfermedades, lesiones (heridas), y deformidades.

Mr. Garza arrives at doctor Ortega's office.	El señor Garza llega al consultorio del doctor Ortega. *(Ehl seh-nyohr Gahr-sah yeh-gah ahl kohn-sool-toh-ree-oh dehl dohk-tohr Ohr-teh-gah)*
Hello Mr. Garza. What is wrong?	Hola Señor Garza. ¿Qué le pasa. *(Oh-lah seh-nyohr Gahr-sah! Keh leh pah-sah)*
Doctor, I have had pain for the last five hours.	Doctor, desde hace cinco horas tengo dolor. *(Dohk-tohr, dehs-deh ah-seh seen-koh oh-rahs tehn-goh doh-lohr)*
Tell me, where did the pain start?	Dígame, ¿dónde comenzó el dolor? *(Dee-gah-meh, dohn-deh koh-mehn-soh ehl doh-lohr)*

Here, below the sternum.	Aquí, debajo del esternón. *(Ah-kee deh-bah-hoh dehl* *ehs-tehr-nohn)*
Is the pain localized in the same place?	¿El dolor está fijo en el mismo lugar? *(Ehl doh-lohr ehs-tah fee-hoh ehn ehl* *mees-moh loo-gahr)*
No, it moved to the right side.	No, se recorrió al lado derecho. *(Noh, seh reh-koh-ree-oh ahl lah-doh* *deh-reh-choh)*
What other discomfort do you have?	¿Qué otra molestia tiene? *(Keh oh-trah moh-lehs-tee-ah* *tee-eh-neh)*
I have nausea, vomiting, fever, and general malaise.	Tengo náuseas, vómito, fiebre, y malestar general. *(Tehn-goh nah-oo-seh-ahs,* *boh-mee-toh, fee-eh-breh ee* *mahl-ehs-tahr heh-neh-rahl)*
Lay down so I can examine you.	Acuéstese para explorarlo. *(Ah-koo-ehs-teh-seh pah-rah* *ehx-ploh-rahr-loh)*
Tell me if it hurts more when I press or when I let go.	Dígame si le duele más al presionar o al retirar la mano. *(Dee-gah-meh see leh doo-eh-leh* *mahs ahl preh-see-oh-nahr oh ahl* *reh-tee-rahr lah mah-noh)*
When you let go.	Al retirar la mano. *(Ahl reh-tee-rahr lah mah-noh)*
He takes the temperature. It is 100 degrees.	Le toma la temperatura. Es de cien grados. *(Leh toh-mah lah tehm-peh-rah-* *too-rah. Ehs deh see-ehn* *grah-dohs)*
Mr. Garza, you probably have appendicitis.	Señor Garza, probablemente tenga apendicitis. *(Seh-nyohr Gahr-sah, proh-bah-bleh-* *mehn-teh tehn-gah ah-pehn-dee-* *see-tees)*
You must go to the hospital.	Debe ir al hospital. *(Deh-beh eer ahl ohs-pee-tahl)*

At the hospital, Dr. Ortega orders blood and urine samples, and x-rays of the abdomen. The doctor checks the results, finds that the white blood cell (leukocytosis) count is high, and that the x-ray of the abdomen shows blurring of the psoas muscle.

Ya en el hospital el doctor Ortega solicita exámenes de sangre, de orina y radiografías del abdomen. El doctor revisa los resultados de los exámenes y encuentra que en la sangre hay un aumento en los glóbulos blancos (leucocitosis) y la radiografía del abdomen muestra borramiento de los psoas.

Mr. Garza is sent to the anesthesiologist who asks:	El señor Garza es enviado con el anestesiólogo, quien pregunta: *(Ehl seh-nyohr Gahr-sah ehs ehn-bee-ah-doh kohn ehl ah-nehs-teh-see-oh-loh-goh, kee-ehn preh-goon-tah)*
Do you have allergies, asthma, high blood pressure, cardiac problems, diabetes?	¿Tiene alergias, asma, alta presión, problemas cardíacos, diabetes? *(Tee-eh-neh ah-lehr-hee-ahs, ahs-mah, ahl-tah preh-see-ohn, proh-bleh-mahs kahr-dee-ah-kohs, dee-ah-beh-tehs)*
Mr. Garza responds: I am very healthy!	El señor Garza responde: ¡Estoy muy sano! *(Ehl seh-nyohr Gahr-sah rehs-pohn-deh: Ehs-toh-ee moo-ee sah-noh)*

He is sent back to the surgeon who tells him that he must have surgery as soon as possible. He explains to Mr. Garza what the surgery is about.

Se le regresa al cirujano, quien le dice que debe ser operado lo más pronto posible. Le explica en qué consiste la cirugía.

After a few hours, Mr. Garza is taken to his room where he recovers from surgery.

Después de unas horas, el señor Garza es llevado a su cuarto donde se recupera de la cirugía.

How do you feel, Mr. Garza?	¿Cómo se siente, señor Garza? *(Koh-moh seh see-ehn-teh, seh-nyohr Gahr-sah)*
I am fine, Doctor, thank you! I feel like new.	Muy bien, Doctor, gracias. ¡Me siento como nuevo! *(Moo-ee bee-ehn, Dohk-tohr, grah-see-ahs. Meh see-ehn-toh koh-moh noo-eh-boh)*

TABLE 19-1	Useful Words	
TABLA 19-1	Palabras Utiles	
English	**Spanish**	**Pronunciation**
surgeon	cirujano	*see-roo-hah-noh*
problems	problemas	*proh-bleh-mahs*
organs	órganos	*ohr-gah-nohs*
sternum	esternón	*ehs-tehr-nohn*
epigastrium	epigastrio	*eh-pee-gahs-tree-oh*
discomfort	molestia	*moh-lehs-tee-ah*
white cells	glóbulos blancos	*gloh-boo-lohs blahn-kohs*
appendicitis	apendicitis	*ah-pehn-dee-see-tees*
confirm	confirmar	*kohn-feer-mahr*
diagnosis	diagnóstico	*dee-ahg-nohs-tee-koh*
order	solicitar	*sohl-ee-see-tahr*
accept	aceptar	*ah-sehp-tahr*
doctor's office	oficina/consultorio	*oh-fee-see-nah/kohn-sool-toh-ree-oh*
leukocytes	leucocitos	*leh-oo-koh-see-tohs*
sutures	suturas/puntos	*soo-too-rahs/poon-tohs*
infections	infecciones	*een-fehk-see-oh-nehs*
analgesics	analgésicos	*ahn-ahl-heh-see-kohs*
antibiotics	antibióticos	*ahn-tee-bee-oh-tee-kohs*

Well, you are going home tomorrow, but you must return to my office in eight days so I can remove your sutures.

Bueno, mañana se va a su casa, pero debe regresar a mi oficina en ocho días para retirar los puntos de sutura.
(Boo-eh-noh, mah-nyah-nah seh bah ah soo kah-sah, peh-roh deh-beh reh-greh-sahr ah mee oh-fee-see-nah ehn oh-choh dee-ahs pah-rah reh-tee-rahr lohs poon-tohs deh soo-too-rah)

Take this antibiotic to prevent infections and this analgesic for pain.

Tome este antibiótico para evitar infecciones y este analgésico para el dolor.
(Toh-meh ehs-teh ahn-tee-bee-oh-tee-koh pah-rah eh-bee-tahr een-fehk-see-oh-nehs ee ehs-teh ah-nahl-heh-see-koh pah-rah ehl doh-lohr)

Do not lift more than ten pounds of weight.

No levante más de diez libras de peso.
(Noh leh-bahn-teh mahs deh dee-ehs lee-brahs deh peh-soh)

Eat soft foods.

Coma alimentos blandos.
(Koh-mah ah-lee-mehn-tohs blahn-dohs)

If you notice fever or any problems in the incision, go to my office immediately.

Si nota fiebre o problemas en la herida, vaya inmediatamente a mi oficina.
(See noh-tah fee-eh-breh oh proh-bleh-mahs ehn lah eh-ree-dah, bah-yah een-meh-dee-ah-tah-mehn-teh ah mee oh-fee-see-nah)

TABLE 19-2   Useful Phrases
TABLA 19-2   Frases Utiles

English	Spanish	Pronunciation
I have pain.	Tengo dolor.	*Tehn-goh doh-lohr*
The pain is on the side.	El dolor está en el lado/costado.	*Ehl doh-lohr ehs-tah ehn ehl lah-doh/kohs-tah-doh*
The pain is localized, sharp.	El dolor está fijo, agudo.	*Ehl doh-lohr ehs-tah fee-hoh, ah-goo-doh*
The pain is worse.	El dolor es peor.	*Ehl doh-lohr ehs peh-ohr*
I have nausea and fever.	Tengo náusea y fiebre.	*Tehn-goh nah-oo-seh-ah ee fee-eh-breh*
Do you have high blood pressure?	¿Tiene alta presión?	*Tee-eh-neh ahl-tah preh-see-ohn*
Do you have cardiac problems?	¿Tiene problemas cardíacos?	*Tee-eh-neh proh-bleh-mahs kahr-dee-ah-kohs*
Don't lift more than 5 pounds.	No levante más de cinco libras.	*Noh leh-bahn-teh mahs deh seen-koh lee-brahs*
Keep the area clean.	Mantenga el área limpia.	*Mahn-tehn-gah ehl ah-reh-ah leem-pee-ah*
Eat soft foods.	Coma alimentos blandos.	*Koh-mah ah-lee-mehn-tohs blahn-dohs*
You can go back to work in one week.	Puede regresar al trabajo en una semana.	*Poo-eh-deh reh-greh-sahr ahl trah-bah-hoh ehn oo-nah seh-mah-nah*

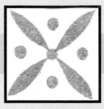

CHAPTER TWENTY
Amputations

CAPITULO VEINTE
Amputaciones

There are approximately 420,000 amputees in the United States, with an annual increase of about 5%. The majority of these amputations are lower extremity amputations. Amputations can be performed through the joint or the bone itself. The term for an amputation through the joint is called *disarticulation*. General sites of the amputation are described by the joint nearest to the location of the amputation (i.e., lower shin or calf amputation is called *below-the-knee amputation*).

Hay aproximadamente 420,000 (cuatrocientos veinte mil) amputados en los Estados Unidos, con un crecimiento anual de aproximadamente cinco por ciento. La mayoría de estas amputaciones son más frecuentes en extremidades inferiores. Se pueden ejecutar amputaciones por las articulaciones o el hueso mismo. El término de una amputación por la articulación se llama *desarticulación*. Los sitios generales de la amputación son descritos por la articulación cercana a la amputación por ejemplo, la operación abajo de la rodilla es llamada *amputación de la pantorrilla*.

Dialogue:	Diálogo:
	(Dee-ah-loh-goh)
Good morning, Doctor!	¡Buenos días, Doctor!
	(Boo-eh-nohs dee-ahs, Dohk-tohr)
I have looked at the information we discussed yesterday.	He revisado la información que discutimos ayer.
	(Heh reh-bee-sah-doh lah een-fohr-mah-see-ohn keh dees-koo-tee-mohs ah-yehr)

Good morning, Ms. Martinez.	Buenos días, Señorita Martínez. *(Boo-eh-nohs dee-ahs, seh-nyoh-ree-tah Mahr-tee-nehs)*
We will start with diagnostic studies to assess how severe your problem might be.	Empezaremos con estudios para evaluar la gravedad de su problema. *(Ehm-peh-sah-reh-mohs kohn ehs-too-dee-ohs pah-rah eh-bah-loo-ahr lah grah-beh-dahd deh soo proh-bleh-mah)*
We will begin with the use of angiography.	Comenzaremos con el estudio de angiografía. *(Koh-mehn-sah-reh-mohs kohn ehl ehs-too-dee-oh deh ahn-hee-oh-grah-fee-ah)*
What is that?	¿Qué es eso? *(Keh ehs eh-soh)*
It is a procedure used to see how open the veins are throughout the leg.	Es un procedimiento para valorar las venas de la pierna. *(Ehs oon proh-seh-dee-mee-ehn-toh pah-rah bah-loh-rahr lahs beh-nahs deh lah pee-ehr-nah)*
How is it done?	¿Cómo se hace? *(Koh-moh seh ah-seh)*
We inject a radioactive dye into the blood vessels and view the flow of blood through the vessels.	Se inyecta un medio de contraste en los vasos sanguíneos y se valora el flujo de la sangre por las venas. *(Seh een-yehk-tah oon meh-dee-oh deh kohn-trahs-teh ehn lohs bah-sohs sahn-ghee-neh-ohs ee seh bah-loh-rah ehl floo-hoh deh lah sahn-greh pohr lahs beh-nahs)*
Can I be poisoned by the radiation?	¿Puedo ser dañada por la radiación? *(Poo-eh-doh sehr dah-nyah-dah pohr lah rah-dee-ah-see-ohn)*
No. We control the amount of radiation you receive. We know which limits to trace throughout your system.	No. Controlamos la cantidad de radiación que recibe. Sabemos qué límites hay que seguir por todo el sistema. *(Noh. Kohn-troh-lah-mohs lah kahn-tee-dahd deh rah-dee-ah-see-ohn keh reh-see-beh. Sah-beh-mohs keh lee-mee-tehs ah-ee keh seh-gheer pohr toh-doh ehl sees-teh-mah)*

TABLE 20-1 Selected Words
TABLA 20-1 Palabras Selectas

English	Spanish	Pronunciation
amputation	amputación	*ahm-poo-tah-see-ohn*
amputee	amputado	*ahm-poo-tah-doh*
care	cuidado	*koo-ee-dah-doh*
clinical	clínico	*klee-nee-koh*
complication	complicación	*kohm-plee-kah-see-ohn*
diagnostic	diagnóstico	*dee-ahg-nohs-tee-koh*
elderly	anciano	*ahn-see-ah-noh*
emergency	emergencia	*eh-mehr-hehn-see-ah*
incidence	incidencia	*een-see-dehn-see-ah*
indications	indicaciones	*een-dee-kah-see-oh-nehs*
interventions	intervenciones	*een-tehr-behn-see-ohn-ehs*
management	manejo	*mah-neh-hoh*
medical	médico	*meh-dee-koh*

I need for you to sign this permission slip so that the procedure might be done.

Necesito que firme usted el permiso, para realizar este estudio.
(Neh-seh-see-toh keh feer-meh oos-tehd ehl pehr-mee-soh, pah-rah reh-ah-lee-sahr ehs-teh ehs-too-dee-oh)

Do you have any further questions?

¿Tiene más preguntas que hacer?
(Tee-eh-neh mahs preh-goon-tahs keh ah-sehr)

Not right now, but I will discuss it with my family.

No por ahora, pero lo discutiré con mi familia.
(Noh pohr ah-oh-rah, peh-roh loh dees-koo-tee-reh kohn mee fah-mee-lee-ah)

If they have further questions, Ms. Brown is your nurse and she will be able to answer them. If you have additional questions, call me and I will return and answer them all.

Si tienen más preguntas que hacer, la señorita Brown es su enfermera y podrá contestarlas. Si tiene preguntas adicionales, llámeme y vendré para contestarlas.

TABLE 20-2	Selected Words	
TABLA 20-2	Palabras Selectas	

English	Spanish	Pronunciation
nurse	enfermera	*ehn-fehr-meh-rah*
patient	paciente	*pah-see-ehn-teh*
phases	fases	*fah-sehs*
postoperative	postoperatorio	*pohst-oh-peh-rah-toh-ree-oh*
preoperative	preoperatorio	*preh-oh-peh-rah-toh-ree-oh*
procedures	procedimientos	*proh-seh-dee-mee-ehn-tohs*
replantation	reimplantación	*reh-eehm-plahn-tah-see-ohn*
surgery	cirugía	*see-roo-hee-ah*
surgical	quirúrgico	*kee-roor-hee-koh*
tests	pruebas	*proo-eh-bahs*
treatment	tratamiento	*trah-tah-mee-ehn-toh*
types	tipos	*tee-pohs*

	(See tee-eh-nehn mahs preh-goon-tahs keh ah-sehr, lah seh-nyoh-ree-tah Brown ehs soo ehn-fehr-meh-rah ee poh-drah kohn-tehs-tahr-lahs. See tee-eh-neh preh-goon-tahs ah-dee-see-oh-nah-lehs, yah-meh-meh ee behn-dreh pah-rah kohn-tehs-tahr-lahs)
Thank you, Doctor.	**Gracias, Doctor.**
	(Grah-see-ahs, Dohk-tohr)
You are welcome.	**De nada.**
	(Deh nah-dah)

Some of the issues that need to be discussed with the patient are listed below.

Algunos de los puntos que se necesitan discutír con el paciente están listados abajo.

Indications and incidence	**Indicaciones e incidencias**
	(Een-dee-kah-see-oh-nehs eh een-see-dehn-see-ahs)

TABLE 20-3	Selected Words	
TABLA 20-3	Palabras Selectas	
English	**Spanish**	**Pronunciation**
anatomic position	posición anatómica	poh-see-see-ohn ah-nah-toh-mee-kah
blood stream	arroyo de la sangre	ah-roh-yoh deh lah sahn-greh
blood flow	circulación sanguínea	seer-koo-lah-see-ohn sahn-gee-neh-ah
broken bone	hueso* roto	oo-eh-soh roh-toh
Colles' fracture	fractura de Colles	frahk-too-rah deh Koh-yehs
comminuted fractures	fracturas conminutas	frahk-too-rahs kohn-mee-noo-tahs
compound fractures	fracturas compuestas	frahk-too-rahs kohm-poo-ehs-tahs
diagnostic tests	pruebas de diagnóstico	proo-eh-bahs deh dee-ahg-nohs-tee-koh
diagnostic procedures	procedimientos de diagnóstico	proh-seh-dee-mee-ehn-tohs deh dee-ahg-nohs-tee-koh
closed reduction	reducción cerrada	reh-dook-see-ohn seh-rah-dah
hip fracture	fractura de cadera	trahk-too-rah deh kah-deh-rah

*Note that the *h* is always silent.

Diagnostic tests and procedures	Pruebas de diagnóstico y procedimientos (Proo-eh-bahs deh dee-ahg-nohs-tee-koh ee proh-seh-dee-mee-ehn-tohs)
Medical and surgical treatment	Tratamiento médico y quirúrgico (Trah-tah-mee-ehn-toh meh-dee-koh ee kee-roor-hee-koh)
Complications	Complicaciones (Kohm-plee-kah-see-oh-nehs)
Nursing care of the patient	Cuidados del paciente (Koo-ee-dah-dohs dehl pah-see-ehn-teh)
Replantation	Reimplantación (Reh-eem-plahn-tah-see-ohn)

Indications

Emergency care

Indicaciones
(Een-dee-kah-see-oh-nehs)
Cuidado de emergencia
*(Koo-ee-dah-doh deh eh-mehr-
hehn-see-ah)*

Nursing care of the patient having replantation surgery is very important to ensure a successful outcome. Listed below are some key goals.

El cuidado de enfermería en el paciente que tiene cirugía de reimplantación es muy importante para asegurar la recuperación. Listadas abajo están algunas metas clave.

TABLE 20-4   Selected Words
TABLA 20-4   Palabras Selectas

English	Spanish	Pronunciation
immature bone	hueso* inmaduro	*oo-eh-soh een-mah-doo-roh*
major complications	complicaciones mayores	*kohm-plee-kah-see-oh-nes mah-yoh-rehs*
mature bone	hueso* maduro	*oo-eh-soh mah-doo-roh*
medical treatment	tratamiento médico	*trah-tah-mee-ehn-toh meh-dee-koh*
open reduction	reducción abierta	*reh-dook-see-ohn ah-bee-ehr-tah*
patient walkers	pacientes con andadera	*pah-see-ehn-tehs kohn ahn-dah-deh-rah*
pelvic fracture	fractura pélvica	*frahk-too-rah pehl-bee-kah*
prolonged stress	tensión prolongada	*tehn-see-ohn proh-lohn-gah-dah*
pulmonary hypertension	hipertensión pulmonar	*ee-pehr-tehn-see-ohn pool-moh-nahr*
therapeutic measures	medidas terapéuticas	*meh-dee-dahs teh-rah-peh-oo-tee-kahs*
tissue damage	daño del tejido	*dah-nyoh dehl teh-hee-doh*
types of fractures	tipos de fracturas	*tee-pohs deh frak-too-rahs*

*Note that the *h* is always silent.

1. Identify clinical indications for amputations.

1. **Identifique las indicaciones clínicas para amputaciones.**
   (Ee-dehn-tee-fee-keh lahs een-dee-kah-see-oh-nehs klee-nee-kahs pah-rah ahm-poo-tah-see-oh-nehs)

2. Describe different types of amputations.

2. **Describa los diferentes tipos de amputaciones.**
   (Dehs-kree-bah lohs dee-feh-rehn-tehs tee-pohs deh ahm-poo-tah-see-oh-nehs)

3. Discuss medical and surgical management of the amputated patient.

3. **Discuta el manejo médico y quirúrgico del paciente amputado.**
   (Dees-koo-tah ehl mah-neh-hoh meh-dee-koh ee kee-roor-hee-koh dehl pah-see-ehn-teh ahm-poo-tah-doh)

4. Identify appropriate nursing interventions during the preoperative and postoperative phases of care.

4. **Identifique las intervenciones y cuidados del paciente en el proceso preoperatorio y postoperatorio.**
   (Ee-dehn-tee-fee-keh lahs een-tehr-behn-see-oh-nehs ee koo-eeh-dah-dohs dehl pah-see-ehn-teh ehn ehl proh-seh-soh preh-oh-peh-rah-toh-ree-oh ee pohst-oh-peh-rah-toh-ree-oh)

5. Use the nursing process to develop a plan of care.

5. **Use el proceso de enfermería para desarrollar un plan de cuidado.**
   (Oo-seh ehl proh-seh-soh deh ehn-fehr-meh-ree-ah pah-rah deh-sah-roh-yahr oon plahn deh koo-ee-dah-doh)

6. Try to ask about the surgery.

6. **Procure pedir informes sobre la cirugía.**
   (Proh-koo-reh peh-deer een-fohr-mehs soh-breh lah see-roo-hee-ah)

7. Ask about rehabilitation.

7. **Pregunte sobre la rehabilitación.**
   (Preh-goon-teh soh-breh lah reh-ah-bee-lee-tah-see-ohn)

8. Ask if you will use devices, prosthesis, or crutches.

8. **Pregunte si va a usar aparatos, prótesis o muletas.**
   (Preh-goon-teh see bah ah oo-sahr ah-pah-rah-tohs, proh-teh-sees, oh moo-leh-tahs)

TABLE 20-5	Selected Words	
TABLA 20-5	Palabras Selectas	

English	Spanish	Pronunciation
alignment	alineación	*ah-lee-neh-ah-see-ohn*
angulation	angulación	*ahn-goo-lah-see-ohn*
assessment	avalúo	*ah-bah-loo-oh*
canes	bastones	*bahs-toh-nehs*
casts	lanzamientos	*lahn-sah-mee-ehn-tohs*
cells	células	*seh-loo-lahs*
complications	complicaciones	*kohm-plee-kah-see-ohn-ehs*
continuity	continuidad	*kohn-tee-noo-ee-dahd*
crutches	muletas	*moo-leh-tahs*
debris	restos	*rehs-tohs*
diagnosis	diagnóstico	*dee-ahg-nohs-tee-koh*
embolism	embolia	*ehm-boh-lee-ah*
etiology	etiología	*eh-tee-oh-loh-hee-ah*
evaluation	evaluación	*eh-bah-loo-ah-see-ohn*
external	externo	*ehx-tehr-noh*
fat	gordura	*gohr-doo-rah*
fixation	fijación	*fee-hah-see-ohn*
fractures	fracturas	*frahk-too-rahs*
fragments	fragmentos	*frahg-mehn-tohs*
goals	metas	*meh-tahs*

9. Assess hemodynamic status.

9. Evalúe el estado hemodinámico.
(*Eh-bah-loo-eh ehl ehs-tah-doh ee-moh-dee-nah-mee-koh*)

10. Administer intravenous fluids and blood.

10. Administre sueros intravenosos y sangre.
(*Ahd-mee-nees-treh soo-eh-rohs een-trah-beh-noh-sohs ee sahn-greh*)

11. Assess circulatory status: color, capillary refill, coolness.

11. Evalúe el estado circulatorio: color, relleno capilar, piel fría.
(*Eh-bah-loo-eh ehl ehs-tah-doh seer-koo-lah-toh-ree-oh: koh-lohr, reh-yeh-noh kah-pee-lahr, pee-ehl free-ah*)

12. Elevate the limb to promote
venous and lymphatic
drainage.

13. Observe blood pressure,
pulse, and the level of
urine.

14. Observe the patient's
mental status.

15. Allow time for ventilation
of feelings.

16. Assure that family is informed
of patient care.

17. Prepare discharge planning.

12. Eleve el miembro para
promover el desagüe venoso y
linfático.
*(Eh-leh-beh ehl mee-ehm-broh
pah-rah proh-moh-behr ehl
deh-sah-goo-eh beh-noh-soh ee
leen-fah-tee-koh)*

13. Observe la presión de la
sangre, el pulso y el nivel de la
orina.
*(Ohb-sehr-beh lah preh-see-ohn deh
lah sahn-greh, ehl pool-soh ee ehl
nee-behl deh lah oh-ree-nah)*

14. Observe el estado mental del
paciente.
*(Ohb-sehr-beh ehl ehs-tah-doh
mehn-tahl dehl pah-see-ehn-teh)*

15. Permita tiempo para ventilar
sentimientos.
*(Pehr-mee-tah tee-ehm-poh pah-rah
behn-tee-lahr sehn-tee-mee-
ehn-tohs)*

16. Asegure que la familia esté
informada sobre el cuidado
del paciente.
*(Ah-seh-goo-reh keh lah fah-mee-
lee-ah ehs-teh een-fohr-mah-dah
soh-breh ehl koo-ee-dah-doh dehl
pah-see-ehn-teh)*

17. Prepare el plan para dar de
alta.
*(Preh-pah-reh ehl plahn pah-rah
dahr deh ahl-tah)*

Below find definitions of procedures that will help you when explaining the surgical interventions or obtaining surgical permits prior to the surgery.

Abajo encuentre definiciones sobre procedimientos que le ayudarán cuando explique las intervenciones quirúrgicas o al obtener permiso para la cirugía.

TABLE 20-6   Selected Words
TABLA 20-6   Palabras Selectas

English	Spanish	Pronunciation
heal	sano	*sah-noh*
healing	curación	*koo-rah-see-ohn*
hip	cadera	*kah-deh-rah*
incision	incisión	*een-see-see-ohn*
infection	infección	*een-fehk-see-ohn*
internal	interior	*een-teh-ree-ohr*
interventions	intervenciones	*een-tehr-behn-see-oh-nehs*
lungs	pulmones	*pool-moh-nehs*
marrow	médula	*meh-doo-lah*
migrate	emigrar	*eh-mee-grahr*

Amputation   Removal of a limb, part of a limb, or an organ; may be done by surgical means or in an accident.
Amputación   Quitar un miembro, parte de un miembro, o un órgano; se puede hacer por medios quirúrgicos o en un accidente.
Amputee   Individual who has undergone an amputation.
Amputado   Individuo que ha sufrido una amputación.
Closed amputation   Amputation in which a limb or part of a limb is removed and surgically closed.
Amputación cerrada   Amputación en la que un miembro o parte de un miembro se quita y se cierra.
Congenital amputation   Deformity or absence of a limb or limbs that occurs during fetal development in the uterus.
Amputación congénita   Deformidad o ausencia de un miembro o miembros que ocurre durante desarrollo fetal en el útero.
Bone remodeling   Process in which immature bone cells are gradually replaced by mature bone cells.
Remodelación del hueso   Proceso en el que se reemplazan gradualmente las células inmaduras del hueso por células maduras.
Closed or simple fracture   Fracture in which the broken bone does not break through the skin.
Fractura simple o cerrada   Es la fractura en la que el hueso no rompe la piel.
Closed reduction or manipulation   Nonsurgical realignment of the bones to their previous anatomic position using traction, angulation, or rotation, or a combination of these.
Manipulación o reducción cerrada   Es la alineación del hueso a su posición anatómica sin cirugía, usando tracción, angulación, o una combinación de éstos.

Compartment syndrome Serious complication of a fracture caused by internal or external pressure to the affected area, resulting in decreased blood flow, pain, and tissue damage.

Síndrome del compartimiento Complicación seria de una fractura causada por una presión interna o externa, que dá como resultado disminución del flujo sanguíneo, dolor, y daño en los tejidos.

Complete fracture Fracture in which the break extends across the entire bone, dividing it into two separate pieces.

Fractura completa Fractura en la que el espacio se extiende por el hueso, dividiéndolo en dos pedazos separados.

Delayed union Fracture healing that does not occur in the normally expected time.

Retardo en la unión La curación de la fractura que no ocurre en el tiempo normalmente esperado.

Fat embolism Condition in which fat globules are released from the marrow of the broken bone into the blood stream, migrate to the lungs, and cause pulmonary hypertension.

Embolia de grasa Condición en la que glóbulos grasosos se desprenden de la médula del hueso roto hacia la corriente sanguínea, emigrando hacia los pulmones, causando hipertensión pulmonar.

Fixation Procedure done during the open reduction surgical procedure to attach the fragments of the broken bone together when reduction alone is not feasible.

Fijación Procedimiento hecho durante la cirugía de reducción abierta para atar juntos los fragmentos del hueso roto cuando sólo la reducción no es factible.

Fracture Break or disruption in the continuity of a bone.

Fractura Descanso o ruptura en la continuidad de un hueso.

Gangrene Necrosis or death of tissue, usually due to a deficient or absent blood supply; may result from inflammatory processes, injury, arteriosclerosis, frostbite, or diabetes mellitus.

Gangrena Necrosis o muerte de tejido, normalmente debido a un suministro deficiente o ausente de sangre; puede resultar de procesos inflamatorios, lesiones, arterioesclerosis, congelamiento o diabetes mellitus.

Guillotine amputation Type of amputation in which a limb or portion of a limb is severed from the body and the wound is left open; a type of open amputation.

Amputación de la guillotina Tipo de amputación en el que un miembro o una porción de un miembro del cuerpo se desarticula y la herida queda abierta; es un tipo de amputación abierta.

Incomplete fracture Fracture in which the bone breaks only partially across, leaving some portion of the bone intact.

Fractura incompleta Fractura en la que el hueso se rompe sólo parcialmente, dejando alguna porción del hueso intacta.

Nonunion   Failure of a fracture to heal.
Sin unión   **Fracaso de una fractura para sanar.**
Open amputation   Amputation that is left open; usually done in cases of infection or necrosis.
Amputación abierta   **Amputación que se queda abierta; normalmente ocurre en casos de infección o necrosis.**
Open or compound fracture   Fracture in which the fragments of the broken bone break through the skin.
Fractura abierta o compuesta   **Fractura en la que los fragmentos del hueso roto salen por la piel.**
Open reduction   Surgical procedure in which an incision is made at the fracture site, usually on patients with open (compound) or comminuted fractures, to cleanse the area of fragments and debris.
Reducción abierta   **Procedimiento quirúrgico en el que se hace una incisión al sitio de la fractura, normalmente en pacientes con fracturas abiertas o conminutas (compuestas), para limpiar el área de fragmentos y restos.**
Phantom limb   Illusion, following an amputation of a limb, that the limb still exists; the sensation that pain exists in removed limb is called *phantom limb pain.*
Miembro fantasma   **Ilusión, el paciente piensa que el miembro todavía existe; la sensación de que duele y existe el miembro amputado se llama *miembro fantasma doloroso.***
Reduction   Process of bringing the ends of the broken bone into proper alignment.
Reducción   **Proceso de traer los extremos del hueso roto en alineación propia.**

TABLE 20-7   Selected Words
TABLA 20-7   Palabras Selectas

English	Spanish	Pronunciation
pain	dolor	*doh-lohr*
pelvis	pelvis	*pehl-bees*
realign	realinear	*reh-ah-lee-nee-ahr*
reduction	reducción	*reh-dook-see-ohn*
rotation	rotación	*roh-tah-see-ohn*
signs	signos/señales	*seeg-nohs/seh-nyah-lehs*
symptoms	síntomas	*seen-toh-mahs*
syndrome	síndrome	*seen-droh-meh*
traction	tracción	*trak-see-ohn*

Replantation   Surgical reattachment of an organ to its original site; reimplantation.

Reimplantación   Reimplante quirúrgico de un órgano a su sitio original.

Staged amputation   Amputation that is done over the course of several surgeries; usually done to control the spread of infection or necrosis.

Amputación progresiva   Amputación que se vuelve hacer en el curso de varias cirugías, normalmente para controlar la propagación de la infección o necrosis.

Stress fracture   Fracture caused by either sudden force or prolonged stress.

Fractura de la tensión   Fractura causada por la fuerza súbita o prolongada.

Stump   The distal portion of an amputated limb.

Muñon   La porción distal donde se amputó el miembro.

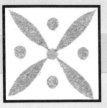

CHAPTER TWENTY-ONE
A Visit to the Psychologist

CAPITULO VEINTIUNO
Una Visita al Psicólogo

ACUTE AND CHRONIC PSYCHOLOGICAL PROBLEMS

PROBLEMAS PSICOLÓGICOS AGUDOS Y CRÓNICOS

In our society, many stressors threaten a person's psychological well-being. Whether at home or at work, as an individual's responsibilities increase, so do his/her stress levels. The many roles that one is called to play on a daily basis provide an open field where stress can flourish.

En nuestra sociedad existen muchos factores estresantes que amenazan el bienestar psicológico de una persona. Ya sea en casa o en el trabajo, el aumento en las responsabilidades de un individuo incrementan el nivel del estrés. La variedad de roles que uno desempeña en la vida diaria proveen un campo libre donde puede florecer el estrés.

| A careful assessment of contributing factors and a thorough psychosocial assessment should assist you in identifying the causes of the imbalance. | Una evaluación cuidadosa de factores y una asesoría psicosocial completa podrá asistirle en la identificación de las causas del problema. |

(Oo-nah eh-bah-loo-ah-see-ohn koo-ee-dah-doh-sah deh fahk-toh-rehs ee oo-nah ah-seh-soh-ree-ah see-koh-soh-see-ahl kohm-pleh-tah poh-drah ahs-ees-teer-leh ehn lah ee-dehn-tee-fee-kah-see-ohn deh lahs kah-oo-sahs dehl proh-bleh-mah)

Very seldom do we visit a psychologist, since this implies that we have to talk about our problems, situations, feelings, and activities. This time, Juan and Roger decide to tell the psychologist about their problems.

Raras veces acudimos a consulta con un psicólogo, ya que implica platicarle nuestros problemas, situaciones, estados de ánimo y actividades. Esta vez Juan y Roger deciden contarle al psicólogo sus problemas.

TABLE 21-1   Selected Words
TABLA 21-1   Palabras Selectas

English	Spanish	Pronunciation
abuse	abuso	*ah-boo-soh*
addictive	adicto	*ah-deek-toh*
analysis	análisis	*ah-nah-lee-sees*
anger	enojo	*eh-noh-hoh*
anxiety	ansiedad	*ahn-see-eh-dahd*
behavior	conducta	*kohn-dook-tah*
bereavement	desamparo	*dehs-ahm-pah-roh*
boredom	fastidio	*fahs-tee-dee-oh*
defense	defensa	*deh-fehn-sah*
dementia	demencia	*deh-mehn-see-ah*
dependence	dependencia	*deh-pehn-dehn-see-ah*
development	desarrollo	*deh-sah-roh-yoh*
diagnosis	diagnóstico	*dee-ahg-nohs-tee-koh*
difficulty	dificultad	*dee-fee-kool-tahd*
disorders	desórdenes	*dehs-ohr-deh-nehs*
evaluation	evaluación	*eh-bah-loo-ah-see-ohn*
findings	hallazgos	*ah-yahs-gohs*

Juan Peña recently changed jobs in order to increase his income. His wife delivered a baby girl one month ago. Two days ago, Juan developed abdominal pains and diarrhea. In addition, he feels short of breath intermittently.

Juan Peña cambió de trabajo recientemente para poder aumentar su salario. Su esposa dió a luz una bebita hace un mes. Hace dos días Juan desarrolló dolores de estómago y diarrea. Además, se siente falto de respiración constantemente.

Tell me, what brought you here?	Dígame ¿qué lo trajo aquí? *(Dee-gah-meh, keh loh trah-hoh ah-kee)*
I feel overwhelmed, anxious.	Me siento abatido, ansioso. *(Meh see-ehn-toh ah-bah-tee-doh, ahn-see-oh-soh)*
What symptoms do you have?	¿Qué síntomas tiene? *(Keh seen-toh-mahs tee-eh-neh)*
I have diarrhea and stomach pains.	Tengo diarrea y dolores de estómago. *(Tehn-goh dee-ah-reh-ah ee doh-loh-rehs deh ehs-toh-mah-goh)*
Has anything changed in your life?	¿Ha cambiado algo en su vida? *(Ah kahm-bee-ah-doh ahl-goh ehn soo bee-dah)*
Well, I just changed jobs.	Bueno, apenas cambié de trabajo. *(Boo-eh-noh, ah-peh-nahs kahm-bee-eh deh trah-bah-hoh)*
Anything else?	¿Alguna otra cosa? *(Ahl-goo-nah oh-trah koh-sah)*
My wife just had a baby.	Mi esposa tuvo un bebé. *(Mee ehs-poh-sah too-boh oon beh-beh)*
Everybody experiences some anxiety.	Todo el mundo pasa por cierta ansiedad. *(Toh-doh ehl moon-doh pah-sah pohr see-ehr-tah ahn-see-eh-dahd)*
Having continuous anxiety may cause serious problems.	El tener ansiedad continua puede llevar a problemas serios. *(Ehl teh-nehr ahn-see-eh-dahd kohn-tee-noo-ah poo-eh-deh yeh-bahr ah proh-bleh-mahs seh-ree-ohs)*
What kinds of problems?	¿Qué clase de problemas? *(Keh klah-seh deh proh-bleh-mahs)*

Problems like ulcers, high blood pressure, and inability to enjoy life and the world.

Problemas como úlceras, alta presión e incapacidad de gozar la vida y el mundo.
(Proh-bleh-mahs koh-moh ool-seh-rahs, ahl-tah preh-see-ohn eh een-kah-pah-see-dahd deh goh-sahr lah bee-dah ee ehl moon-doh)

Do you have trouble making friends at work?

¿En su trabajo tiene dificultad para hacer amistades?
(Ehn soo trah-bah-hoh tee-eh-neh dee-fee-kool-tahd pah-rah ah-sehr ah-mees-tah-dehs)

How do you get along with your peers?

¿Cómo se lleva usted con sus compañeros?
(Koh-moh seh yeh-bah oos-tehd kohn soos kohm-pah-nyeh-rohs)

Do you talk to your wife about your job?

¿Trata de hablar con su esposa acerca de su trabajo?
(Trah-tah deh ah-blahr kohn soo ehs-poh-sah ah-sehr-kah deh soo trah-bah-hoh)

TABLE 21-2 Selected Words
TABLA 21-2 Palabras Selectas

English	Spanish	Pronunciation
hope	esperanza	*ehs-peh-rahn-sah*
hostility	hostilidad	*ohs-tee-lee-dahd*
humanistic	humanístico	*oo-mahn-ees-tee-koh*
implementation	implementación	*eem-pleh-mehn-tah-see-ohn*
implications	implicaciones	*eem-plee-kah-see-oh-nehs*
independence	independencia	*een-deh-pehn-dehn-see-ah*
interaction	interacción	*een-tehr-ahk-see-ohn*
interpersonal	interpersonal	*een-tehr-pehr-soh-nahl*
loneliness	soledad	*soh-leh-dahd*
loss	pérdida	*pehr-dee-dah*
manifestation	manifestación	*mahn-ee-fehs-tah-see-ohn*
manipulation	manipulación	*mahn-ee-poo-lah-see-ohn*
personality	personalidad	*pehr-soh-nah-lee-dahd*
planning	planificación	*plah-nee-fee-kah-see-ohn*
purpose	propósito	*proh-poh-see-toh*
relation	relación	*reh-lah-see-ohn*

Do you have her support in everything?

¿Tiene apoyo de ella en todo?
(Tee-eh-neh ah-poh-yoh deh eh-yah ehn toh-doh)

Do you have insomnia?

¿Tiene insomnio?
(Tee-eh-neh een-sohm-nee-oh)

Do you try to relax to forget your anxiety?

¿Procura distraerse para olvidar su ansiedad?
(Proh-koo-rah dees-trah-ehr-seh pah-rah ohl-bee-dahr soo ahn-see-eh-dahd)

If your behavior changes you must go to a specialist.

Si continúa con cambios en su persona debe acudir con un especialista.
(See kohn-tee-noo-ah kohn kahm-bee-ohs ehn soo pehr-soh-nah deh-beh ah-koo-deer kohn oon ehs-peh-see-ah-lees-tah)

For now, follow these recommendations:

Por ahora, siga estas recomendaciones:
(Pohr ah-oh-rah, see-gah ehs-tahs reh-koh-mehn-dah-see-oh-nehs)

1. Take 30 minutes every day to examine your feelings. Think about what makes you depressed.

1. Tome treinta minutos diariamente para examinar sus sentimientos. Piense qué le causa depresión.
(Toh-meh treh-een-tah mee-noo-tohs dee-ah-ree-ah-mehn-teh pah-rah ehx-ah-mee-nahr soos sehn-tee-mee-ehn-tohs. Pee-ehn-seh keh leh kah-oo-sah deh-preh-see-ohn.

2. Do not deny your feelings.

2. No niege sus sentimientos.
(Noh nee-eh-geh soos sehn-tee-mee-ehn-tohs)

3. If it is something you cannot control, ignore it!

3. Si es algo que no puede controlar, ¡ignórelo!
(See ehs ahl-goh keh noh poo-eh-deh kohn-troh-lahr, eeg-noh-reh-loh)

4. Share your feelings with your wife and one friend.

4. Comparta sus sentimientos con su esposa y un amigo.
(Kohm-pahr-tah soos sehn-tee-mee-ehn-tohs kohn soo ehs-poh-sah ee oon ah-mee-goh)

TABLE 21-3 Selected Words
TABLA 21-3 Palabras Selectas

English	Spanish	Pronunciation
somatization	somatización	*soh-mah-tee-sah-see-ohn*
theories	teorías	*teh-oh-ree-ahs*
trust	confianza	*kohn-fee-ahn-sah*
flexibility	flexibilidad	*flehx-ee-bee-lee-dahd*
grieving	afligir	*ah-flee-heer*
guilt	culpa	*kool-pah*
response	contestación	*kohn-tehs-tah-see-ohn*
rigidity	rigidez	*ree-hee-dehs*
sample	muestra	*moo-ehs-trah*
sociocultural	sociocultural	*soh-see-oh-kool-too-rahl*
cognitive	cognoscitivo	*kohg-noh-see-tee-boh*
concepts	conceptos	*kohn-sehp-tohs*
coping	sobrellevando	*soh-breh-yeh-bahn-doh*
mechanisms	mecanismos	*meh-kah-nees-mohs*
methodology	metodología	*meh-toh-doh-loh-hee-ah*
mistrust	desconfianza	*dehs-kohn-fee-ahn-sah*
victims	víctimas	*beek-tee-mahs*

5. Every day, spend time in exercise or a hobby.

5. Diariamente, tome tiempo para hacer ejercicio o una actividad favorita.
(Dee-ah-ree-ah-mehn-teh, toh-meh tee-ehm-poh pah-rah ah-sehr eh-hehr-see-see-oh oh oo-nah ahk-tee-bee-dahd fah-boh-ree-tah)

6. Make your home pleasant and cheerful.

6. Haga su hogar placentero y alegre.
(Ah-gah soo oh-gahr plah-sehn-teh-roh ee ah-leh-greh)

7. Treat everyone with affection.

7. Trate a todos con afecto.
(Trah-teh ah toh-dohs kohn ah-fehk-toh)

8. Do not isolate yourself.

8. No se aparte.
(Noh seh ah-pahr-teh)

9. When you feel depressed, go for a walk.

9. Cuando se deprima, salga de paseo.
(Koo-ahn-doh seh deh-pree-mah, sahl-gah deh pah-seh-oh)

10. Eat and sleep well.

10. **Aliméntese y duerma bien.**
(Ah-lee-mehn-teh-seh ee doo-ehr-mah bee-ehn)

11. Do not assume others don't understand what you are feeling.

11. **No presuma que otros no entienden lo que está sintiendo.**
(Noh preh-soo-mah keh oh-trohs noh ehn-tee-ehn-dehn loh keh ehs-tah seen-tee-ehn-doh)

Roger is hospitalized in a psychiatric unit. Part of the milieu therapy requires that he participate in activities.

Roger está hospitalizado en una unidad de psiquiatría. Parte del la terapia de medio ambiente requiere que participe en actividades.

TABLE 21-4 Selected Phrases
TABLA 21-4 Frases Selectas

English	Spanish & Pronunciation
our society	**nuestra sociedad** *(noo-ehs-trah soh-see-eh-dahd)*
stressful factors	**factores estresantes** *(fahk-tohr-ehs ehs-treh-sahn-tehs)*
responsibilities and activities	**responsabilidades y actividades** *(rehs-pohn-sah-bee-lee-dah-dehs ee ahk-tee-bee-dah-dehs)*
increase the level	**incrementar el nivel** *(een-kreh-mehn-tahr ehl nee-behl)*
psychosocial evaluation	**asesoría psicosocial** *(ah-seh-soh-ree-ah see-koh-soh-see-ahl)*
identification of the problem	**identificación del problema** *(ee-dehn-tee-fee-kah-see-ohn dehl proh-bleh-mah)*
I feel uneasy constantly	**Me siento abatido constantemente** *(Meh see-ehn-toh ah-bah-tee-doh kohns-tahn-teh-mehn-teh)*
I changed jobs recently	**Cambié de trabajo recientemente** *(Kahm-bee-eh deh trah-bah-hoh reh-see-ehn-teh-mehn-teh)*
certain anxiety	**cierta ansiedad** *(see-ehr-tah ahn-see-eh-dahd)*
incapable of having fun	**incapacidad de gozar** *(een-kah-pah-see-dah deh goh-sahr)*

Roger, it is time to go to
your OT appointment.

Roger, es la hora de ir a su cita
de terapia ocupacional (TO).
*(Roger, ehs lah oh-rah deh eer
ah soo see-tah deh teh-rah-pee-
ah oh-koo-pah-see-oh-nahl [TO])*

I'm not going today.

Hoy no voy a ir.
(Oh-ee noh boh-ee ah eer)

You are not going?

¿Usted no va?
(Oos-tehd noh bah)

No.

No.
(Noh)

You enjoyed working on your
house yesterday.

Disfrutó el trabajar en su casa
ayer.
*(Dees-froo-toh ehl trah-bah-
hahr ehn soo kah-sah ah-yehr)*

No, I did not enjoy working on
my house.

No, no disfruté el trabajar en
mi casa.
*(Noh, noh dees-froo-teh ehl
trah-bah-hahr ehn mee kah-sah)*

It looked as if a professional
had made it.

Parece como si un profesional
lo hubiera hecho.
*(Pah-reh-seh koh-moh see oon
proh-feh-see-oh-nahl loh oo-
bee-eh-rah heh-choh)*

I don't like it.

No me gusta.
(Noh meh goos-tah)

Please keep your appointment.

Por favor, acuda a la cita.
*(Pohr fah-bohr, ah-koo-dah ah
lah see-tah)*

Activities are part of your
treatment plan while you
are here.

Las actividades son parte del
plan de su tratamiento mientras
esté aquí.
*(Lahs ahk-teh-bee-dah-dehs sohn
pahr-teh dehl plahn deh trah-
tah-mee-ehn-toh mee-ehn-trahs
ehs-tee ah-kee)*

I will return in ten minutes, and
we can walk down together.

Volveré en diez minutos, y
podremos caminar juntos.
*(Bohl-beh-reh ehn dee-ehs mee-
noo-tohs ee poh-dreh-mohs kah-
mee-nahr hoon-tohs)*

Ten minutes pass and the nurse returns.
Diez minutos pasaron y la enfermera regresa.

TABLE 21-5	Selected Phrases	
TABLA 21-5	Frases Selectas	

English	Spanish	Pronunciation
try to talk	trate de hablar	*trah-teh deh ah-blahr*
try to have a good time	procure divertirse	*proh-koo-reh dee-behr-teer-seh*
difficulties at work	dificultades en su trabajo	*dee-fee-kool-tah-dehs ehn soo trah-bah-hoh*
therapy for couples	terapia de parejas	*teh-rah-pee-ah deh pah-reh-hahs*
crisis intervention	intervención de la crisis	*een-tehr-behn-see-ohn deh lah kree-sees*
mental patient	enfermo mental	*ehn-fehr-moh mehn-tahl*
nutritional disorders	desórdenes alimenticios	*deh-sohr-deh-nehs ah-lee-mehn-tee-see-ohs*
family therapy	terapia familiar	*teh-rah-pee-ah fah-mee-lee-ahr*
group therapy	terapia de grupo	*teh-rah-pee-ah deh groo-poh*
mental health	salud mental	*sah-lood mehn-tahl*
milieu therapy	terapia de medio ambiente	*teh-rah-pee-ah deh meh-dee-oh ahm-bee-ehn-teh*

It is time to go, Roger.

Es tiempo de ir, Roger.
(Ehs tee-ehm-poh deh eer, Roger)

Roger gets up and moves to the door.

Roger se levanta y va a la puerta.
(Roger seh leh-bahn-tah ee bah ah lah poo-ehr-tah)

Why do you make me do things I don't want to do?

¿Por qué me haces hacer cosas que no quiero?
(Pohr-keh meh ah-sehs ah-sehr koh-sahs keh noh kee-eh-roh?

I wish all of you would leave me alone.

Deseo que todos ustedes me dejen solo.
(Deh-seh-oh keh toh-dohs oos-teh-dehs meh deh-hehn soh-loh)

Are you mad because you are going to OT?

¿Está enojado porque va a TO?
(Ehs-tah eh-noh-hah-doh pohr-keh bah ah TO)

No, I just don't want to go. It's not helping me.

No, sólo que no quiero ir. No me está ayudando.
(Noh, soh-loh keh noh kee-eh-roh eer. Noh meh ehs-tah ah-yoo-dahn-doh)

Roger, age 26, was involved in the preparation for exams when he experienced a profound depression. He tried to commit suicide by slashing his wrists. He was hospitalized for observation.

Roger estaba ocupado preparando para exámenes cuando se deprimió profundamente. Trató de suicidarse cortándose las muñecas. Se le hospitalizó para observarlo.

Roger states: The failure in the exams represents a disappointment for my family.

Roger dice: La falla en los exámenes representa una desilusión para mi familia.
(Roger dee-seh: Lah fah-yah ehn lohs ehx-ah-meh-nehs reh-preh-sehn-tah oo-nah deh-see-loo-see-ohn pah-rah mee fah-mee-lee-ah)

He sees failure as disgrace, an obstacle to future plans, and a blow to his self-esteem.

El ve el fracaso como una desgracia, un obstáculo para sus planes futuros, y un golpe a su autoestima.
(Ehl beh ehl frah-kah-soh koh-moh oo-nah dehs-grah-see-ah, oon obhs-tah-koo-loh pah-rah soos plah-nehs foo-too-rohs ee oon gohl-peh ah soo ah-oo-toh-ehs-tee-mah)

Roger is now undergoing assessment by the psychiatrist, who asks him a number of questions.

Roger se somete a una asesoría por el psiquiatra, quien le hace varias preguntas.

How long have you felt depressed?

¿Desde cuándo se siente deprimido?
(Dehs-deh koo-ahn-doh seh see-ehn-teh deh-pree-mee-doh)

Is this your first suicide attempt?

¿Es éste su primer intento de suicidio?
(Ehs ehs-teh soo pree-mehr een-tehn-toh deh soo-ee-see-dee-oh)

What kind of weapons have you used?

¿Qué clase de armas ha usado?
(Keh klah-seh deh ahr-mahs ah oo-sah-doh)

Did you call anyone?

¿Llamó a alguien?
(Yah-moh ah ahl-ghee-ehn)

What triggered your depression?

¿Qué precipitó su depresión?
(Keh preh-see-pee-toh soo deh-preh-see-ohn)

TABLE 21-6	Selected Phobias
TABLA 21-6	Fobias Selectas

English	Spanish	Pronunciation
acrophobia (height)	acrofobia (altura)	*ah-kroh-foh-bee-ah (ahl-too-rah)*
agoraphobia (open spaces)	agorafobia (espacios abiertos)	*ah-goh-rah-foh-bee-ah (ehs-pah-see-ohs ah-bee-ehr-tohs)*
anthropophobia (people)	antropofobia (personas)	*ahn-troh-poh-foh-bee-ah (pehr-soh-nahs)*
claustrophobia (closed spaces)	claustrofobia (espacios cerrados)	*klah-oos-troh-foh-bee-ah (ehs-pah-see-ohs seh-rah-dohs)*
hydrophobia (water)	hidrofobia (agua)	*ee-droh-foh-bee-ah (ah-goo-ah)*
mikophobia (germs)	micofobia (gérmenes)	*mee-koh-foh-bee-ah (gehr-meh-nehs)*
mysophobia (dirt) (contamination)	misofobia (tierra) (contaminación)	*mee-soh-foh-bee-ah (tee-eh-rah) (kohn-tah-mee-nah-see-ohn)*
nuctophobia (darkness)	nuctofobia (oscuridad)	*nook-toh-foh-bee-ah (ohs-koo-ree-dahd)*
thanatophobia (death)	tanatofobia (muerte)	*tah-nah-toh-foh-bee-ah (moo-ehr-teh)*
zoophobia (animals)	zoofobia (animales)	*soh-oh-foh-bee-ah (ah-nee-mah-lehs)*

Do you take any drugs?	¿Toma drogas? *(Toh-mah droh-gahs)*
What kind?	¿Qué clase? *(Keh klah-seh)*
How do you feel now?	¿Cómo se siente ahora? *(Koh-moh seh see-ehn-teh ah-oh-rah)*
When was the last time you ate?	¿Cuándo fue la última vez que comió? *(Koo-ahn-doh foo-eh lah ool-tee-mah behs keh koh-mee-oh)*
Is your family in the city?	¿Está su familia en la ciudad? *(Ehs-tah soo fah-mee-lee-ah ehn lah see-oo-dahd)*

I will talk to you every day.	**Hablaré con usted todos los días.** *(Ah-blah-reh kohn oos-tehd toh-dohs lohs dee-ahs)*
The nurse will complete the assessment.	**La enfermera completará la evaluación.** *(Lah ehn-fehr-meh-rah kohm-pleh-tah-rah lah eh-bah-loo-ah-see-ohn)*

The nurse initiates the following interventions.
La enfermera inicia las intervenciones siguientes.

Mental status examination.	**Exámen del estado mental.** *(Ehx-ah-mehn dehl ehs-tah-doh mehn-tahl)*
Includes appearance, activity level, mood and affect, speech, thought content, memory and intellectual level.	**Incluye la apariencia, el nivel de actividad, disposición de ánimo y afecto, conversación, contenido de los pensamientos, memoria y nivel intelectual.** *(Een-kloo-yeh lah ah-pah-ree-ehn-see-ah, ehl nee-behl deh ahk-tee-bee-dahd, dees-poh-see-see-ohn deh ah-nee-moh ee ah-fehk-toh, kohn-behr-sah-see-ohn, kohn-teh-nee-doh deh lohs pehn-sah-mee-ehn-tohs, meh-moh-ree-ah ee nee-behl een-teh-lehk-too-ahl)*
Establish a contract so he does not harm himself.	**Establecer un contrato para que no se cause daño.** *(Ehs-tah-bleh-sehr oon kohn-trah-toh pah-rah keh noh seh kah-oo-seh dah-nyoh)*
Help the patient to identify positive aspects.	**Ayudar al paciente a identificar aspectos positivos.** *(Ah-yoo-dahr ahl pah-see-ehn-teh ah ee-dehn-tee-fee-kahr ahs-pehk-tohs poh-see-tee-bohs)*
Plan an adequate diet.	**Planear alimentos adecuados.** *(Plah-neh-ahr ah-lee-mehn-tohs ah-deh-koo-ah-dohs)*
Encourage relaxation exercises.	**Estimular los ejercicios de relajamiento.** *(Ehs-tee-moo-lahr lohs eh-hehr-see-see-ohs deh reh-lah-hah-mee-ehn-toh)*

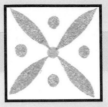

CHAPTER TWENTY-TWO
A Visit to the Dentist

CAPITULO VEINTIDOS
Una Visita al Dentista

Beatriz Madrid Hicks, RDH, MA

Clinical Associate Professor
University of Texas
Health Sciences Center Dental School

Care of the mouth requires frequent visits to the dentist. The condition of the teeth allows for proper chewing and thus assists in digestion of foods. A healthy mouth will always be considered a sign of good health.

El cuidado general de la boca requiere visitas frecuentes al dentista. El buen estado de los dientes permite una buena masticación y por lo tanto la buena digestión de los alimentos. Una boca sana será siempre un signo del buen cuidado personal.

PATIENT MEDICAL HISTORY

Are you under the care of a doctor?

Are you allergic to penicillin or other medications?

LA HISTORIA MÉDICA DEL PACIENTE

¿Está bajo tratamiento con un doctor?
(Ehs-tah bah-hoh trah-tah-mee-ehn-toh kohn oon dohk-tohr)

¿Tiene alergia a la penicilina u otros medicamentos?
(Tee-eh-neh ah-lehr-hee-ah ah lah peh-nee-see-lee-nah oo oh-trohs meh-dee-kah-mehn-tohs)

Have you ever had a heart attack or pains in your heart?	¿Ha tenido ataque al cardiáco o dolor en el pecho?
	(Hah teh-nee-doh ah-tah-keh ahl kahr-dee-ah-koh oh doh-lohr ehn ehl peh-choh)
Rheumatic fever?	¿Fiebre reumática?
	(Fee-eh-breh reh-oo-mah-tee-kah)
Joint replacement?	¿Le han reemplazado alguna articulación?
	(Leh ahn rehm-plah-sah-doh ahl-goo-nah ahr-tee-koo-lah-see-ohn)
Do you have a pacemaker?	¿Tiene marcapaso?
	(Tee-eh-neh mahr-kah-pah-soh)
Have you ever had:	Ha tenido:
	(Ah teh-nee-doh)
Cancer?	¿Cáncer?
	(Kahn-sehr)
Chemotherapy treatment?	¿Tratamiento de quimioterapia?
	(Trah-tah-mee-ehn-toh deh kee-mee-oh-teh-rah-pee-ah)
Allergic reaction to a local anesthetic?	¿Alergia a la anestesia local?
	(Ah-lehr-hee-ah ah lah ah-nehs-teh-see-ah loh-kahl)
Tuberculosis/lung problems?	¿Tuberculosis/problemas con los pulmones?
	(Too-behr-koo-loh-sees/proh-bleh-mahs kohn lohs pool-moh-nehs)
Hepatitis or cirrhosis?	¿Hepatitis o cirrosis?
	(Eh-pah-tee-tees oh see-roh-sees)
A sexually transmitted disease?	¿Enfermedades transmitidas sexualmente?
	(Ehn-fehr-meh-dah-dehs trahns-mee-tee-dahs sehx-oo-ahl-mehn-teh)
Do you have:	Tiene:
	(Tee-eh-neh)
Diabetes?	¿Diabetes?
	(Dee-ah-beh-tehs)
Convulsions?	¿Convulsiones?
	(Kohn-bool-see-oh-nehs)
Any blood disorders such as anemia or leukemia?	¿Problemas de sangre como anemia o leucemia?
	(Proh-bleh-mahs deh sahn-greh koh-moh ah-neh-mee-ah oh loo-seh-mee-ah)

Are you taking:	Está tomando: *(ehs-tah toh-mahn-doh)*
Any medications?	¿Algunas medicinas? *(Ahl-goo-nahs meh-dee-see-nahs)*
Steroids?	¿Esteroides? *(Ehs-teh-roh-ee-dehs)*
Anticoagulants?	¿Anticoagulantes? *(Ahn-tee-koo-ah-goo-lahn-tehs)*
Antidepressants?	¿Antidepresivos? *(Ahn-tee-deh-preh-see-bohs)*
Nitroglycerin?	¿Nitroglicerina? *(Nee-troh-glee-seh-ree-nah)*
Are you pregnant?	¿Está embarazada? *(Ehs-tah ehm-bah-rah-sah-dah)*
(If yes) When is your due date?	Si es así, ¿Cuándo se alivia? *(See ehs ah-see, koo-ahn-doh seh ah-lee-bee-ah)*
Do you smoke or drink alcohol?	¿Fuma o toma alcohol? *(Foo-mah oh toh-mah ahl-kohl)*
Do you have any condition or disease not listed in this questionnaire?	¿Tiene problemas o condiciones de salud que no estén en este cuestionario? *(Tee-eh-neh proh-bleh-mahs oh kohn-dee-see-ohn-ehs deh sah- lood keh noh ehs-tehn ehn ehs- teh koo-ehs-tee-oh-nah-ree-oh)*

It is very important to examine the patient's head and neck before the oral examination.

Es muy importante examinar la cabeza y el cuello del paciente antes de empezar el exámen oral.

ORAL EXAMINATION	**REVISIÓN ORAL** *(Reh-bee-see-ohn oh-rahl)*
Good afternoon, Miss Gonzalez.	Buenas tardes, señorita Gonzalez. *(Boo-eh-nahs tahr-dehs, seh- nyoh-ree-tah Gohn-sah-lehs)*
Come in.	Pase/Entre. *(Pah-seh/Ehn-treh)*
Sit down, please.	Siéntese, por favor. *(See-ehn-teh-seh, pohr fah-bohr)*
What is the matter?	¿Qué le pasa/sucede? *(Keh leh pah-sah/soo-seh-deh)*
When did you see the dentist last?	¿Cuándo vió al dentista la última vez? *(Koo-ahn-doh bee-oh ahl dehn- tees-tah lah ool-tee-mah behs)*

I'm going to check your head, neck, and mouth.

Voy a revisarle su cabeza, cuello, y boca.
(Boh-ee ah reh-bee-sahr-leh soo kah-beh-sah, koo-eh-yoh, ee boh-kah)

I will start the exam by feeling your cheeks.

Voy a empezar por sus mejillas en cada lado.
(Boh-ee ah ehm-peh-sahr pohr soos meh-hee-yahs ehn kah-dah lah-doh)

I will then palpate your jaw. Please open and close your mouth 2 or 3 times.

Voy a palpar su quijada. Por favor abra la boca dos o tres veces.
(Boh-ee ah pahl-pahr soo kee-hah-dah. Pohr fah-bohr ah-brah lah boh-kah dohs oh trehs beh-sehs)

I am going to examine your glands. They are located on your neck and under your chin.

Voy a examinar sus glándulas que están localizadas en su cuello y abajo de su barbilla.
(Boh-ee ah exh-ah-mee-nahr soos glahn-doo-lahs keh ehs-tahn loh-kah-lee-sah-dahs ehn soo koo-eh-yoh ee ah-bah-hoh deh soo bahr-bee-yah)

Now I am going to examine the inside of your mouth.

Ahora voy a examinar adentro de su boca.
(Ah-oh-rah boh-ee ah ehx-ah-mee-nahr ah-dehn-troh deh soo boh-kah)

I am going to feel your lips.

Voy a tocar sus labios.
(Boh-ee ah toh-kahr soos lah-bee-ohs)

I am now going to feel your cheeks and the salivary glands that are on either side.

Voy a tocar cada lado de la mucosa bucal y las glándulas que producen saliva.
(Boh-ee ah toh-kahr kah-dah lah-doh deh lah moo-koh-sah boo-kahl ee lahs glahn-doo-lahs keh proh-doo-sehn sah-lee-bah)

I am now going to examine the floor of your mouth. Please raise your tongue to the roof of your mouth.

Ahora voy a examinar el piso de la boca. Mueva la lengua hacia el paladar.
(Ah-oh-rah boh-ee ah ehx-ah-mee-nahr el pee-soh deh lah boh-kah. Moo-eh-bah la lehn-goo-ah ah-see-ah ehl pah-lah-dahr)

I am now going to examine the tongue. Stick your tongue out so I can examine the sides of the tongue.	**Voy a examinar la lengua. Saque la lengua para examinar los lados.** *(Boh-ee ah ehx-ah-mee-nahr lah lehn-goo-ah. Sah-keh lah lehn-goo-ah parh-rah ehx-ah-mee-nahr lohs lah-dohs.)*
I am now going to examine the roof of your mouth.	**Voy a examinar el paladar.** *(Boh-ee ah ehx-ah-mee-nahr ehl pah-lah-dahr)*
The last thing I will examine is your throat. Open and say, "Ahh."	**La última cosa que voy a examinar es la garganta. Abra la boca y diga "Ahh."** *(Lah ool-tee-mah koh-sah keh boh-ee ah ehx-ah-mee-nahr ehs lah gahr-gahn-tah. Ah-brah lah boh-kah ee dee-gah "ah.")*
Open your mouth, please.	**Abra la boca, por favor.** *(Ah-brah lah boh-kah, pohr fah-bohr)*
I will check your teeth.	**Revisaré sus dientes.** *(Reh-bee-sah-reh soos dee-ehn-tehs)*
I am going to hit gently.	**Voy a darle golpecitos.** *(Boh-ee ah dahr-leh gohl-peh-see-tohs)*
Point when it hurts.	**Señale cuando duela.** *(Seh-nyah-leh koo-ahn-doh doo-eh-lah)*
Bite!	**¡Muerda!** *(Moo-ehr-dah)*
Please open your mouth some more.	**Por favor, abra más la boca.** *(Pohr fah-bohr, ah-brah mahs lah boh-kah)*
I am going to clean your teeth.	**Voy a limpiarle los dientes.** *(Boh-ee ah leem-pee-ahr-leh lohs dee-ehn-tehs)*
Do your gums bleed?	**¿Le sangran las encías?** *(Leh sahn-grahn lahs ehn-see-ahs)*
Are your teeth sensitive to cold?	**¿Tiene sensibilidad al tomar frío?** *(Tee-eh-neh sehn-see-bee-lee-dahd ahl toh-mahr free-oh)*
Shock?	**¿Toques?** *(Toh-kehs)*
Pain?	**¿Dolor?** *¿(Doh-lohr)*

TABLE 22-1   Common Words
TABLA 22-1   Palabras Comúnes

English	Spanish	Pronunciation
air	aire	*ah-ee-reh*
anesthesia	anestesia	*ah-nehs-teh-see-ah*
anticoagulant	anticoagulante	*ahn-tee-koh-ah-goo-lahn-teh*
antibiotic	antibiótico	*ahn-tee-bee-oh-tee-koh*
baby tooth	diente de leche	*dee-ehn-teh deh leh-cheh*
Bite!	¡Muerda!	*Moo-ehr-dah*
chemotherapy	quimioterapia	*kee-mee-oh-teh-rah-pee-ah*
caries	caries	*kah-ree-ehs*
cavity	cavidad	*kah-bee-dahd*
cement	cemento	*seh-mehn-toh*

Do you have bad breath?
¿Tiene mal aliento?
(Tee-eh-neh mahl ah-lee-ehn-toh)

Frequent blisters/ulcerations?
¿Ulceraciones frecuentes?
(Ool-seh-rah-see-oh-nehs freh-koo-ehn-tehs)

Does the wind hurt your teeth?
¿Le molesta el aire?
(Leh moh-lehs-tah ehl ah-ee-reh)

Does it hurt when you chew very hard?
¿Le duele al masticar con fuerza?
(Leh doo-eh-leh ahl mahs-tee-kahr kohn foo-ehr-sah)

Rinse your mouth.
Enjuague su boca.
(Ehn-hoo-ah-geh soo boh-kah)

I am going to take x-rays.
Le tomaré radiografías.
(Leh toh-mah-reh rah-dee-oh-grah-fee-ahs)

I will return shortly.
Regreso en seguida.
(Reh-greh-soh ehn seh-ghee-dah)

I checked your x-rays.
Revisé sus radiografías
(Reh-bee-seh soos rah-dee-oh-grah-fee-ahs)

I have to take out your tooth.
Tengo que extraer/sacar el diente.
(Tehn-goh keh ehx-trah-ehr/sah-kahr ehl dee-ehn-teh)

I am going to use local anesthetic.
Voy a usar anestesia local.
(Boh-ee ah oo-sahr ah-nehs-teh-see-ah loh-kahl)

Tell me when it feels numb.	Avíseme cuando sienta dormido. *(Ah-bee-seh-meh koo-ahn-doh see-ehn-tah dohr-mee-doh)*
Are you OK?	¿Se siente bien? *(Seh see-ehn-teh bee-ehn)*
Does it still hurt?	¿Todavía le duele? *(Toh-dah-bee-ah leh doo-eh-leh)*
I pulled your tooth.	Le saqué el diente. *(Leh sah-keh ehl dee-ehn-teh)*
I am putting in a temporary filling.	Le aplicaré empaste temporal. *(Leh ah-plee-kah-reh ehm-pahs-teh tehm-poh-rahl)*
I will use resins.	Usaré resinas. *(Oo-sah-reh reh-see-nahs)*
I'm going to polish your teeth.	Ahora voy a pulír sus dientes. *(Ah-oh-rah boh-ee a poo-leer soos dee-ehn-tehs)*
You need to brush your teeth better.	Necesita cepillar mejor sus dientes. *(Neh-seh-see-tah seh-pee-yahr meh-hohr soos dee-ehn-tehs)*
Use dental floss.	Use hilo dental. *(Oo-seh ee-loh dehn-tahl)*

TABLE 22-2   Proper Vocabulary
TABLA 22-2   Vocabulario Apropiado

English	Spanish	Pronunciation
dental floss	hilo dental	*ee-loh dehn-tahl*
dental surgeon	cirujano dentista	*see-roo-hah-noh dehn-tees-tah*
dentist	dentista	*dehn-tees-tah*
dentifrice	dentífrico	*dehn-tee-free-koh*
disclosing solution	solución reveladora	*soh-loo-see-ohn reh-beh-lah-doh-rah*
enamel	esmalte	*ehs-mahl-teh*
extract	extraer/sacar	*ehx-trah-ehr/sah-kahr*
eyetooth	diente canino/ colmillo	*dee-ehn-teh kah-nee-noh/ kohl-mee-yoh*
to fill	empastar/rellenar	*ehm-pahs-tahr/reh-yeh-nahr*
fluoride	fluoruro	*floh-roo-roh*

Return in 10 days.	**Regrese en diez días.**
	(Reh-greh-seh ehn dee-ehs dee-ahs)
Please return as needed.	**En caso necesario, puede regresar.**
	(Ehn kah-soh neh-seh-sah-ree-
	oh, poo-eh-deh reh-greh-sahr)
I hope you do well.	**Que siga bien.**
	(Keh see-gah bee-ehn)

It is very important to give oral hygiene instructions to all patients receiving dental care. This prevents future damage and helps preserve the teeth.

Es muy importante dar instrucciones a todos los pacientes que reciben tratamiento dental. Esto evita daños futuros y ayuda a conservar los dientes.

I want to talk about bacterial plaque.	**Quiero platicar acerca de la placa bacteriana.**
	(Kee-eh-roh plah-tee-kahr ah-sehr-kah deh lah plah-kah bahk-teh-ree-ah-nah)
Plaque is a sticky, colorless layer of bacteria.	**La placa es una capa pegajosa sin color y con bacteria.**
	(Lah plah-kah ehs oo-nah kah-pah peh-gah-hoh-sah seen koh-lohr ee kohn bahk-teh-ree-ah)
It causes dental caries.	**Causa caries dental.**
	(Kah-oo-sah kah-ree-ehs dehn-tahl)
It also causes periodontal disease and tooth loss.	**Causa también pérdida de dientes y enfermedad periodontal.**
	(Kah-oo-sah tahm-bee-ehn pehr-dee-dah deh dee-ehn-tehs ee ehn-fehr-meh-dahd peh-ree-oh-dohn-tahl)
Plaque can be prevented by brushing and flossing.	**La placa se evita usando hilo dental y cepillo.**
	(Lah plah-kah seh eh-bee-tah oo-sahn-doh ee-loh dehn-tahl ee seh-pee-yoh)
The only way we can see plaque is by using a solution that stains the teeth.	**La única manera de ver la placa es usar una solución que mancha los dientes.**
	(Lah oo-nee-kah mah-neh-rah deh behr lah plah-kah ehs oo-sahr oo-nah soh-loo-see-ohn keh mahn-chah lohs dee-ehn-tehs)

TABLA 22-3	Common Diseases	
TABLE 22-3	Enfermedades Comúnes	
English	**Spanish**	**Pronunciation**
abscess	absceso	*ahb-seh-soh*
gingivitis	gingivitis	*heen-hee-bee-tees*
dental plaque	placa	*plah-kah*
periodontal	periodontal	*peh-ree-oh-dohn-tahl*
tumor	tumor	*too-mohr*
lesions	lesiones	*leh-see-oh-nehs*
odontalgia/tooth ache	odontalgia/dolor de muela	*oh-dohn-tahl-hee-ah/ doh-lohr deh moo-eh-lah*

English	Spanish
I am going to put some solution around all your teeth.	Voy a poner una solución alrededor de todos sus dientes. *(Boh-ee ah poh-nehr oo-nah soh-loo-see-ohn ahl-reh-deh-dohr deh toh-dohs soos dee-ehn-tehs)*
Here is a glass of water to rinse with.	Aquí está un vaso con agua para que se enjuague. *(Ah-kee ehs-tah oon bah-soh kohn ah-goo-ah pah-rah keh seh ehn-hoo-ah-geh)*
Give the patient a hand mirror and toothbrush.	Déle al paciente un espejo de mano y un cepillo de dientes. *(Deh-leh ahl pah-see-ehn-teh oon ehs-peh-hoh deh mah-noh ee oon seh-pee-yoh deh dee-ehn-tehs)*
If any plaque is present point to the areas saying:	Si hay placa apunte a las áreas y diga: *(See ah-ee plah-kah ah-poon-teh ah lahs ah-reh-ahs ee dee-gah)*
Can you see the places that are stained?	¿Puede ver los lugares que están dañados? *(Poo-eh-deh behr lohs loo-gah-rehs keh ehs-tahn dah-nyah-dohs)*
That is plaque.	Esa es la placa. *(Eh-sah ehs lah plah-kah)*
You will need to brush a little better in these areas.	Necesitará cepillarse mejor en estas áreas. *(Neh-seh-see-tah-rah seh-pee-yahr-seh meh-hohr ehn ehs-tahs ah-reh-ahs)*

Let me show you with your toothbrush a way that will help you remove the plaque.	Déjeme enseñarle con su cepillo una manera que le ayudará a quitar la placa. *(Deh-heh-meh ehn-seh-nyahr-leh kohn soo seh-pee-yoh oo-nah mah-neh-rah keh leh ah-yoo-dah-rah ah kee-tahr lah plah-kah)*

Demonstrate the basic technique first on yourself, making sure the patient can see exactly what you are doing. Next have the patient practice the technique on himself.

Demuestre la técnica básica primero, asegurando que el paciente vea exactamente lo que hace. Luego, haga que el paciente practique la técnica.

Make sure that you point the toothbrush toward the gumline.	Asegure que el cepillo apunte contra la encía. *(Ah-seh-goo-reh keh ehl seh-pee-yoh ah-poon-teh kohn-trah lah ehn-see-ah)*
Using a circular motion, brush one to two teeth at a time.	Usando movimiento circular, cepille uno o dos dientes a la vez. *(Oo-sahn-doh moh-bee-mee-ehn-toh seer-koo-lahr, seh-pee-yeh oo-noh oh dohs dee-ehn-tehs ah lah behs)*
Practice with the brush; make sure you go around all the teeth.	Practique con el cepillo; asegure de cepillar alrededor de todos los dientes. *(Prahk-tee-keh kohn ehl seh-pee-yoh; ah-seh-goo-reh deh seh-pee-yahr ahl-reh-deh-dohr deh toh-dohs lohs dee-ehn-tehs)*
After you finish brushing, we will practice flossing.	Después de terminar de cepillar practicaremos usando el hilo dental. *(Dehs-poo-ehs deh tehr-mee-nahr deh seh-pee-yahr prahk-tee-kah-reh-mohs oo-sahn-doh ehl ee-loh dehn-tahl)*
Plaque gets in between the teeth where the brush cannot reach.	La placa entra en medio de los dientes donde no alcanza el cepillo. *(Lah plah-kah ehn-trah ehn meh-dee-oh deh lohs dee-ehn-tehs dohn-deh noh ahl-kahn-zah ehl seh-pee-yoh)*

TABLE 22-4   Dental Appliances
TABLA 22-4   Aditamentos Dentales

English	Spanish	Pronunciation
complete dentures	dentadura completa	*dehn-tah-doo-rah kohm-pleh-tah*
fixed bridge	puente fijo	*poo-ehn-teh fee-hoh*
movable bridge	puente móvil	*poo-ehn-teh moh-beel*
partial denture	dentadura parcial	*dehn-tah-doo-rah pahr-see-ahl*
gold tooth	diente de oro	*dee-ehn-teh deh oh-roh*
crowns	coronas	*koh-roh-nahs*
braces	abrazaderas	*ah-brah-sah-deh-rahs*
implant	implante	*eem-plahn-teh*
sealant	placa protectora	*plah-kah proh-tehk-toh-rah*

That is why it is important to clean these areas.	Por ello es importante limpiar estas áreas. *(Pohr eh-yoh ehs eem-pohr-tahn-teh leem-pee-ahr ehs-tahs ah-reh-ahs)*
Let me show you the correct way to floss.	Déjeme enseñarle la manera correcta de usar el hilo. *(Deh-heh-meh ehn-seh-nyahr-leh lah mah-neh-rah koh-rehk-tah deh oo-sahr ehl ee-loh)*

Begin demonstration, explaining each step to the patient.
Empieze la demostración, explicando cada paso al paciente.

Wind 18 inches of floss around one middle finger.	Enrede dieciocho pulgadas de hilo alrededor del tercer dedo. *(Ehn-reh-deh dee-eh-see-oh-choh pool-gah-dahs deh ee-loh ahl-reh-deh-dohr dehl tehr-sehr deh-doh)*
Wind the rest around the middle finger of the other hand.	Enrede el resto alrededor del dedo medio de la otra mano. *(Ehn-reh-deh ehl rehs-toh ahl-reh-deh-dohr dehl deh-doh meh-dee-oh deh lah oh-trah mah-noh)*

Use the thumb and forefingers to guide the floss.	Use los dedos gordos y los índices para guiar el hilo. *(Oo-seh lohs deh-dohs gohr-dohs ee lohs een-dee-sehs pah-rah ghee-ahr ehl ee-loh)*
Insert the floss gently between the teeth.	Meta el hilo suavemente en medio de los dientes. *(Meh-tah ehl ee-loh soo-ah-beh-mehn-teh ehn meh-dee-oh deh lohs dee-ehn-tehs)*
Curve the floss into a "C".	Ponga el hilo en forma de "C". *(Pohn-gah ehl ee-loh ehn fohr-mah deh seh)*

Fluoride makes teeth stronger and healthy. It also helps with sensitivity.

El fluoruro ayuda a que los dientes sean fuertes y sanos. También evita la sensibilidad.

Now I am going to give you some fluoride.	Ahora voy a darle fluoruro. *(Ah-oh-rah boh-ee ah dahr-leh floh-roo-roh)*
This is to help your teeth become stronger and if cavities are present it will help slow the process.	Esto ayudará a hacer que los dientes sean más fuertes y si tiene cavidades, ayudará a retardar el proceso. *(Ehs-toh ah-yoo-dah-rah ah ah-sehr keh lohs dee-ehn-tehs seh-ahn mahs foo-ehr-tehs ee see tee-ehn-eh kah-bee-dah-dehs, ah-yoo-dah-rah ah reh-tahr-dahr ehl proh-seh-soh)*
It will also help if you have any teeth that are sensitive.	Ayudará también si los dientes están sensibles. *(Ah-yoo-dah-rah tahm-bee-ehn see lohs dee-ehn-tehs ehs-tahn sehn-see-blehs)*
I will place the trays over the teeth.	Pondré las bandejas sobre los dientes. *(Pohn-dreh lahs bahn-deh-hahs soh-breh lohs dee-ehn-tehs)*
I want you to chew on them for four minutes.	Quiero que las muerda por cuatro minutos. *(Kee-eh-roh keh lahs moo-ehr-dah pohr koo-ah-troh mee-noo-tohs)*

I will place the saliva ejector in between the trays so that you will not swallow any of the fluoride.	**Pondré el extractor de saliva en medio de las bandejas, para que no se trague el fluoruro.** *(Pohn-dreh ehl ehx-trahk-tohr deh sah-lee-bah ehn meh-dee-oh deh lahs bahn-deh-hahs, pah-rah keh noh seh trah-geh ehl floh-roo-roh)*
Do not eat or drink anything for thirty minutes.	**No coma o beba nada por treinta minutos.** *(Noh koh-mah oh beh-bah nah-dah pohr treh-een-tah mee-noo-tohs)*
Please return in six months.	**Por favor regrese en seis meses.** *(Pohr fah-bohr reh-greh-seh ehn seh-ees meh-sehs)*

Unit 4

The Hospital Setting

UNIDAD 4

En el Hospital

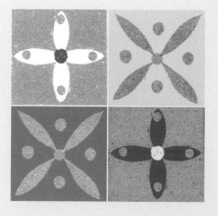

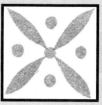

CHAPTER TWENTY-THREE
The Patient's Room

CAPITULO VEINTITRES
El Cuarto del Paciente

Mr. González has been admitted to room 569 (five hundred sixty-nine) of the surgery floor.

Al señor González lo admitieron en el cuarto cinco, seis, nueve (quinientos sesenta y nueve) del piso de cirugía.

Hello Mr. González. I am the nurse in charge.	Hola señor González. Yo soy enfermera encargada. *(Oh-lah seh-nyohr Gohn-sah-lehs. Yoh soh-ee lah ehn-fehr-meh-rah ehn-kahr-gah-dah)*
This is a handout that deals with the hospital's guidelines.	Este es un folleto que trata de las reglas/guías del hospital. *(Ehs-teh ehs oon foh-yeh-toh keh trah-tah deh lahs reh-glahs/gee-ahs dehl ohs-pee-tahl)*
I am going to give you a tour of the floor.	Voy a darle un recorrido por el piso. *(Boh-ee ah dahr-leh oon reh-koh-ree-doh pohr ehl pee-soh)*
This is the lobby.	Esta es la sala de espera. *(Ehs-tah ehs lah sah-lah deh ehs-peh-rah)*
You can bring your family here.	Puede traer a su familia aquí. *(Poo-eh-deh trah-ehr ah soo fah-mee-lee-ah ah-kee)*

This is the service area.	Esta es el área de servicio. *(Ehs-tah ehs ehl ah-reh-ah deh sehr-bee-see-oh)*
You can order coffee here.	Puede ordenar café aquí. *(Poo-eh-deh ohr-deh-nahr kah-feh ah-kee)*
The stairs are at the end of the hallway.	La escalera está al final del pasillo. *(Lah ehs-kah-leh-rah ehs-tah ahl fee-nahl dehl pah-see-yoh)*
The elevators work twenty-four hours.	Los elevadores funcionan las veinticuatro horas. *(Lohs eh-leh-bah-doh-rehs foon-see-oh-nahn lahs beh-een-tee-koo-ah-troh oh-rahs)*
There are bathrooms for guests in the corner.	Hay baños para las vistas en la esquina. *(Hay bah-nyohs pah-rah lahs bee-see-tahs ehn lah ehs-kee-nah)*
In case of fire, take the stairs.	En caso de fuego, use la escalera. *(Ehn kah-soh deh foo-eh-goh, oo-seh lah ehs-kah-leh-rah)*
This is your room.	Este es su cuarto. *(Ehs-teh ehs soo koo-ahr-toh)*

TABLE 23-1   Pronunciation of Selected Words
TABLA 23-1   Pronunciacion de Palabras Selectas

English	Spanish	Pronunciation
bathroom	baño	*bah-nyoh*
corner	esquina	*ehs-kee-nah*
stairs	escalera	*ehs-kah-leh-rah*
room	cuarto	*koo-ahr-toh*
wall	pared	*pah-rehd*
patient	paciente	*pah-see-ehn-teh*
table	mesa	*meh-sah*
bell	campana/timbre	*kahm-pah-nah/teem-breh*
button	botón	*boh-tohn*
window	ventana	*behn-tah-nah*

You cannot hang anything from the ceiling.	No puede colgar nada del techo. *(Noh poo-eh-deh kohl-gahr nah-dah dehl teh-choh)*
You cannot hang anything from the door.	No puede colgar nada en la puerta. *(Noh poo-eh-deh kohl-gahr nah-dah ehn lah poo-ehr-tah)*
You can tape pictures to the wall.	Puede pegar retratos en la pared. *(Poo-eh-deh peh-gahr reh-trah-tohs ehn lah pah-rehd)*
You can put cards on the shelf.	Puede poner tarjetas en el estante. *(Poo-eh-deh poh-nehr tahr-heh-tahs ehn ehl ehs-tahn-teh)*
You can have flowers.	Puede tener flores. *(Poo-eh-deh teh-nehr floh-rehs)*
This chair turns into a bed.	Esta silla se hace cama. *(Ehs-tah see-yah seh ah-seh kah-mah)*
This is the call bell/buzzer.	Esta es la campana/el timbre. *(Ehs-tah ehs lah kahm-pah-nah/ehl teem-breh)*
This button lowers (raises) the headboard.	Este botón baja (sube) la cabecera de la cama. *(Ehs-teh boh-tohn bah-hah [soo-beh] lah kah-beh-seh-rah deh lah kah-mah)*

TABLE 23-2 Useful Verbs
TABLA 23-2 Verbos Útiles

English	Spanish	Pronunciation
can/be/able to	poder	*poh-dehr*
is	es/está	*ehs/ehs-tah*
there is/are	hay	*ah-ee*
to bathe	bañar	*bah-nyahr*
to close	cerrar	*seh-rahr*
to cry	llorar	*yoh-rahr*
to go	ir	*eer*
to hang	colgar	*kohl-gahr*
to have	tener	*teh-nehr*
to speak	hablar	*ah-blahr*

| TABLE 23-3 | Useful Items |
| TABLA 23-3 | Artículos Útiles |

English	Spanish	Pronunciation
cosmetics	cosméticos	*kohs-meh-tee-kohs*
perfume	perfume	*pehr-foo-meh*
toothpaste	pasta de dientes	*pahs-tah deh dee-ehn-tehs*
toothbrush	cepillo de dientes	*seh-pee-yoh deh dee-ehn-tehs*
comb	peine	*peh-ee-neh*
razor	navaja/máquina de afeitar	*nah-bah-hah/mah-kee-nah deh ah-feh-ee-tahr*
drinking glass	vidrio/vaso/	*bee-dree-oh/bah-soh*
nightgown/gown	camisa de dormir/ bata	*kah-mee-sah deh dohr-meer/ bah-tah*
lipstick	lápiz de labios	*lah-pees deh lah-bee-ohs*

Do you need the headboard up?	¿Necesita levantar más la cabecera? *(Neh-seh-see-tah leh-bahn-tahr mahs lah kah-beh-seh-rah)*
The bed has one blanket.	La cama tiene una frazada/colcha. *(Lah kah-mah tee-eh-neh oo-nah frah-sah-dah/kohl-chah)*
If you need more sheets, call the assistant.	Si necesita más sábanas, llame a la/al asistente. *(See neh-seh-see-tah mahs sah-bah-nahs, yah-meh ah lah/ahl ah-sees-tehn-teh)*
Do you need more pillows?	¿Necesita más almohadas? *(Neh-seh-see-tah mahs ahl-moh-ah-dahs)*
You have a private bathroom.	Tiene un baño/inodoro privado. *(Tee-eh-neh oon bah-nyoh/ee-noh-doh-roh pree-bah-doh)*
Keep the siderails up at night.	Mantenga los barandales levantados durante la noche. *(Mahn-tehn-gah lohs bah-rahn-dah-lehs leh-bahn-tah-dohs doo-rahn-teh lah noh-cheh)*
There is a shower.	Hay una ducha/regadera *(Ah-ee oo-nah doo-chah/reh-gah-deh-rah)*

There is also a bathtub/tub.	También hay una bañera/tina. *(Tahm-bee-ehn ah-ee oo-nah bah-nyeh-rah/tee-nah)*
Your clothes go in the closet.	Su ropa va en el closet/ropero. *(Soo roh-pah bah ehn ehl kloh-seht/roh-peh-roh)*
Don't walk barefoot.	No camine descalzo. *(No kah-mee-neh dehs-kahl-soh)*
Use the house shoes; the floor is cold.	Use las pantunflas/chanclas; el piso está frío. *(Oo-seh lahs pahn-toon-flahs/ chahn-klahs; ehl pee-soh ehs-tah free-oh)*
You can make local phone calls.	Puede hacer llamadas locales. *(Poo-eh-deh ah-sehr yah-mah-dahs loh-kah-lehs)*
Dial 9, wait for the tone, then dial the number you want to call.	Marque el nueve, espere el tono, luego marque el número que quiera llamar. *(Mahr-keh ehl noo-eh-beh, ehs-peh-reh ehl toh-noh, loo-eh-goh mahr-keh ehl noo-meh-roh keh kee-eh-rah yah-mahr)*

TABLE 23-4   Clothing Items
TABLA 23-4   Artículos de Vestir

English	Spanish	Pronunciation
skirt	falda	*fahl-dah*
blouse	blusa	*bloo-sah*
suit	traje	*trah-heh*
pants/slacks	pantalones	*pahn-tah-loh-nehs*
dress	vestido	*behs-tee-doh*
coat	abrigo	*ah-bree-goh*
shoes	zapatos	*sah-pah-tohs*
jacket	chaqueta	*chah-keh-tah*
sweater	chamarra/suéter	*chah-mah-rah/soo-eh-tehr*
tie	corbata	*kohr-bah-tah*
underwear	ropa interior	*roh-pah een-teh-ree-ohr*
socks	calcetines/calcetas	*kahl-seh-tee-nehs/kahl-seh-tahs*
hose/stockings	medias	*meh-dee-ahs*

You can call collect.

Puede llamar por cobrar.
(Poo-eh-deh yah-mahr pohr koh-brahr)

If you want to watch TV, you have to pay a fee.

Si quiere ver la televisión, tiene que pagar una cuota.
(See kee-eh-reh behr lah teh-leh-bee-see-ohn, tee-eh-neh keh pah-gahr oo-nah koo-oh-tah)

You cannot smoke in your room.

No puede fumar en el cuarto.
(Noh poo-eh-deh foo-mahr ehn ehl koo-ahr-toh)

You can smoke in the patio.

Puede fumar en el patio.
(Poo-eh-deh foo-mahr ehn ehl pah-tee-oh)

You cannot open the windows.

No puede abrir las ventanas.
(Noh poo-eh-deh ah-breer lahs behn tah-nahs)

Visiting hours are from nine in the morning to nine at night.

Las horas de visita son de las nueve de la mañana a las nueve de la noche.
(Lahs oh-rahs deh bee-see-tah sohn deh lahs noo-eh-beh deh lah mah-nyah-nah ah lahs noo-eh-beh deh lah noh-cheh)

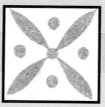

CHAPTER TWENTY-FOUR
The Laboratory

CAPITULO VEINTICUATRO
El Laboratorio

Mrs. Garza is going to have blood drawn in preparation for 24-hour urine collection. The nurse explains the laboratory procedure and the hospital routine.

A la señora Garza le van a tomar muestras de sangre y se prepara para colectar/juntar su orina por veinticuatro horas. La enfermera le explica el procedimiento y la rutina del laboratorio del hospital.

Mrs. Garza, the doctor ordered blood samples.	Señora Garza, el doctor/la doctora ordenó muestras de sangre. *(Seh-nyoh-rah Gahr-sah, ehl dohk-tohr/lah dohk-toh-rah ohr-deh-noh moo-ehs-trahs deh sahn-greh)*
Almost always the technician comes at six in the morning.	Casi siempre el laboratorista viene a las seis de la mañana. *(Kah-see see-ehm-preh ehl lah-boh-rah-toh-rees-tah bee-eh-neh ah lahs seh-ees deh lah mah-nyah-nah)*
Please do not eat after midnight.	Por favor, no coma después de medianoche. *(Pohr fah-bohr, noh koh-mah dehs-poo-ehs deh meh-dee-ah-noh-cheh)*

205

In your case, eat nothing after 8 o'clock.	En su caso, no coma nada después de las ocho de la noche. *(Ehn soo kah-soh, noh koh-mah nah-dah dehs-poo-ehs deh lahs oh-choh deh lah noh-cheh)*
Tomorrow they will give you a special test.	Mañana le harán un examen especial. *(Mah-nyah-nah leh ah-rahn oon ehx-ah-mehn ehs-peh-see-ahl)*
I am going to explain how to collect the urine.	Le voy a explicar cómo juntar la orina. *(Leh boy ah ehx-plee-kahr koh-moh hoon-tahr lah oh-ree-nah)*
I will wake you up in the morning.	La voy a despertar en la mañana. *(Lah boy ah dehs-pehr-tahr ehn lah mah-nyah-nah)*
I will ask you to void.	Le diré que orine. *(Leh dee-reh keh oh-ree-neh)*
Every time you urinate, put it in the container.	Cada vez que orine, póngala en el frasco. *(Kah-dah behs keh oh-ree-neh, pohn-gah-lah ehn ehl frahs-koh)*

TABLE 24-1   Pronunciation of Selected Words
TABLA 24-1   Pronunciacion de Plabras Selectas

English	Spanish	Pronunciation
laboratory	laboratorio	*lah-boh-rah-toh-ree-oh*
technician	técnico	*tehk-nee-koh*
sample	muestra	*moo-ehs-trah*
in the morning	en la mañana	*ehn lah mah-nyah-nah*
tomorrow	mañana	*mah-nyah-nah*
after	después	*dehs-poo-ehs*
explain	explique	*ehx-plee-keh*
every time	cada vez	*kah-dah behs*
bottle	botella	*boh-teh-yah*
remain	quédese	*keh-deh-seh*
next	siguiente	*see-ghee-ehn-teh*
pinprick	picadura	*pee-kah-doo-rah*
tubes	tubos	*too-bohs*
blood	sangre	*sahn-greh*

The container will be kept in a bucket with ice.	El frasco se mantendrá en una tina con hielo. *(Ehl frahs-koh seh mahn-tehn-drah ehn oo-nah tee-nah kohn ee-eh-loh)*
The next day, it will be sent to the laboratory.	Al día siguiente, se mandará al laboratorio. *(Ahl dee-ah see-gee-ehn-teh, seh mahn-dah-rah ahl lah-boh-rah-toh-ree-oh)*
Hello, Mrs. Garza.	Hola, señora Garza. *(Oh-lah, seh-nyoh-rah Gahr-sah)*
Please stay/remain in bed.	Por favor, quédese en la cama. *(Pohr fah-bohr, keh-deh-seh ehn lah kah-mah)*
I am here to draw your blood.	Estoy aquí para tomarle una muestra de sangre. *(Ehs-toh-ee ah-kee pah-rah toh-mahr-leh oo-nah moo-ehs-trah deh sahn-greh)*
I am going to lift your sleeve.	Voy a levantar la manga. *(Boh-ee ah leh-bahn-tahr lah mahn-gah)*
Make a fist.	Cierre la mano. Haga un puño. *(See-eh-reh lah mah-noh/Ah-gah oon poo-nyoh)*
Relax, it will not hurt.	Relájese, no le va a doler. *(Reh-lah-heh-seh, no leh bah ah doh-lehr)*
Open your hand.	Abra la mano. *(Ah-brah lah mah-noh)*
I want to take a sample from your finger.	Quiero tomar una muestra del dedo. *(Kee-eh-roh toh-mahr oo-nah moo-ehs-trah dehl deh-doh)*
I want to see the sugar level.	Quiero ver el nivel de azúcar. *(Kee-eh-roh behr ehl nee-behl deh ah-soo-kahr)*
Do not move.	No se mueva. *(Noh seh moo-eh-bah)*
This is done quickly.	Esto se hace rápido. *(Ehs-toh seh ah-seh rah-pee-doh)*
Have you had blood drawn before?	¿Le han tomado muestras antes? *(Leh ahn toh-mah-doh moo-ehs-trahs ahn-tehs)*

TABLE 24-2	Common Lab Words
TABLA 24-2	Palabras Comúnes en el Laboratorio

English	Spanish	Pronunciation

complete
  blood count
	biometría
	  hemática*
	  completa
		bee-oh-meh-tree-ah
		  heh-mah-tee-kah
		  kohm-pleh-tah

needle	aguja	*ah-goo-hah*
alcohol	alcohol	*ahl-kohl*
syringe	jeringa	*heh-reen-gah*
gloves	guantes	*goo-ahn-tehs*
pathology	patología	*pah-toh-loh-hee-ah*
procedure	procedimiento	*proh-seh-dee-mee-ehn-toh*
STAT/emergency	STAT/emergencia	*ehs-taht/eh-mehr-hehn-see-ah*
reports	reportes	*reh-pohr-tehs*
specimen	muestra	*moo-ehs-trah*
fasting	en ayunas	*ehn ah-yoo-nahs*

*In Spanish, the letter *h* is always silent.

You will feel pain like a pinprick.	Sentirá dolor como una picadura. *(Sehn-tee-rah doh-lohr koh-moh oo-nah pee-kah-doo-rah)*
I need two tubes of blood:	Necesito dos tubos de sangre: *(Neh-seh-see-toh dohs too-bohs deh sahn-greh)*
One tube for a blood count.	Un tubo para una biometría hemática. *(Oon too-boh pah-rah oo-nah bee-oh-meh-tree-ah eh-mah-tee-kah)*
Another for a serology test.	Otro para una prueba serológica. *(Oh-troh pah-rah oo-nah proo-eh-bah seh-roh-loh-hee-kah)*
Take a deep breath.	Respire hondo. *(Rehs-pee-reh ohn-doh)*
Relax, calm down.	Relájese, cálmese. *(Reh-lah-heh-seh, kahl-meh-seh)*
I need to use a tourniquet.	Necesito usar un torniquete. *(Neh-seh-see-toh oo-sahr oon tohr-nee-keh-teh)*

English	Spanish	Pronunciation
	TABLE 24-3 Helpful Verbs	
	TABLA 24-3 Verbos Útiles	
to ask	preguntar	*preh-goon-tahr*
to bend	doblar	*doh-blahr*
to come	venir	*beh-neer*
to go	ir	*eer*
to keep	guardar/mantener	*goo-ahr-dahr/mahn-teh-nehr*
to lift	levantar/elevar	*leh-bahn-tahr/eh-leh-bahr*
to place	poner/colocar	*poh-nehr/koh-loh-kahr*
to wake	despertar	*dehs-pehr-tahr*
to draw	sacar/tirar/dibujar	*sah-kahr/tee-rahr/dee-boo-hahr*
to eat	comer	*koh-mehr*
to drink	beber/tomar	*beh-behr/toh-mahr*

That is all!	¡Es todo!	
	(Ehs toh-doh)	

Please, note that many products' brand names are often not translated, but their pronunciation changes a bit.

Por favor, note que hay muchas marcas de productos que no se traducen, pero la pronunciación cambia un poco.

I am going to put a Band-Aid on you.	Voy a ponerle una cinta adhesiva/un curita/un bandaid. *(Boh-ee ah poh-nehr-leh oo-nah seen-tah ah-deh-see-bah/oo-nah koo-ree-tah/oon bahn-dah-eed).*
Please, bend your arm for about five minutes.	Por favor, doble el brazo por cinco minutos. *(Pohr fah-bohr, doh-bleh ehl brah-soh pohr seen-koh mee-noo-tohs)*
I am through!	¡Ya terminé! *(Yah tehr-mee-neh)*
The nurse wants to talk to you.	La enfermera quiere hablarle. *(Lah ehn-fehr-meh-rah kee-eh-reh ah-blahr-leh)*
Mrs. Garza, I want you to get up and go to urinate.	Señora Garza, quiero que se levante y vaya a orinar. *(Seh-nyoh-rah Gahr-sah, kee-eh-roh keh seh leh-bahn-teh ee bah-yah ah oh-ree-nahr)*

English	Spanish	Pronunciation
TABLE 24-4	Pronunciation of Selected Words	
TABLA 24-4	Pronunciación de Plabras Selectas	

English	Spanish	Pronunciation
additive	aditivo	*ah-dee-tee-boh*
package	paquete	*pah-keh-teh*
limitations	limitaciones	*lee-mee-tah-see-ohn-ehs*
spread	untar/extender	*oohn-tahr/ehx-tehn-dehr*
adhesive	adhesivo	*ah-deh-see-boh*
sterile	estéril	*ehs-teh-reel*
rub	frotar/restregar	*froh-tahr/rehs-treh-gahr*
hematology	hematología*	*eh-mah-toh-loh-hee-ah*
puncture	pinchazo/picadura	*peen-chah-soh/pee-kah-doo-rah*
blood bank	banco de sangre	*bahn-koh deh sahn-greh*
coagulated	coagulado	*koh-ah-goo-lah-doh*

*In Spanish, the letter *h* is always silent.

Void a little, then put urine in this cup.	Orine un poco, luego ponga la orina en esta taza. *(Oh-ree-neh oon poh-koh, loo-eh-goh pohn-gah lah oh-ree-nah ehn ehs-tah tah-sah)*
Remember that you are to urinate and put it in the container.	Recuerde que debe orinar y poner la orina en el frasco. *(Reh-koo-ehr-deh keh deh-beh oh-ree-nahr ee poh-nehr lah oh-ree-nah ehn ehl frahs-koh)*
Remember that you will do this for 24 hours.	Recuerde que hará esto por veinticuatro horas. *(Reh-koo-ehr-deh keh ah-rah ehs-toh pohr beh-een-tee-koo-ah-troh oh-rahs)*
If there is no ice in the bucket, call me.	Si no hay hielo en la tina, llámeme. *(See noh ah-ee ee-eh-loh ehn lah tee-nah, yah-meh-meh)*
I will remind you during the day.	Le recordaré durante el día. *(Leh reh-kohr-dah-reh doo-rahn-teh ehl dee-ah)*
Do you feel all right?	¿Se siente bien? *(Seh see-ehn-teh bee-ehn)*

Are you hungry?	**¿Tiene hambre?**
	(Tee-eh-neh ahm-breh)
Do you want a cup of coffee?	**Quiere una taza de café?**
	(Kee-eh-reh oo-nah tah-sah deh-kah-feh)
Did you understand?	**¿Entendió?**
	(Ehn-tehn-dee-oh)
Tomorrow, bring a specimen of your stool in this container.	**Mañana, traiga una muestra de su excremento en este frasco.**
	(Mah-nyah-nah, trah-ee-gah oo-nah moo-ehs-trah deh soo ehx-kreh-mehn-toh ehn ehs-teh frahs-koh)

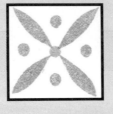

CHAPTER TWENTY-FIVE
The Pharmacy

CAPITULO VEINTICINCO
La Farmacia

The pharmacy provides services as an integral part of total patient care. Drugs are dispensed only upon the order of a physician. The nurse orders the medication from the pharmacy after the doctor has prescribed the treatment for the patient.

La farmacia provee servicios como parte integral del cuidado total del paciente. Los medicamentos son distribuidos solamente por órdenes del doctor. La/el enfermera(o) ordena la medicina a la farmacia después de que el doctor dejó la receta con el tratamiento para el paciente.

The inpatient pharmacy:	La farmacia para pacientes que están internados: *(Lah fahr-mah-see-ah pah-rah pah-see-ehn-tehs keh ehs-tahn een-tehr-nah-dohs)*
It is open from seven AM to one AM.	Está abierta de las siete de la mañana a la una de la mañana. *(Ehs-tah ah-bee-ehr-tah deh lahs see-eh-teh deh lah mah-nyah-nah ah lah oo-nah deh lah mah-nyah-nah)*
The pharmacy is open Monday through Friday.	La farmacia está abierta de lunes a viernes. *(Lah fahr-mah-see-ah ehs-tah ah-bee-ehr-tah deh loo-nehs ah bee-ehr-nehs)*

| TABLE 25-1 | Drug Categories |
| TABLA 25-1 | Categorias de los Medicamentos |

English	Spanish	Pronunciation
analgesic	analgésicos	*ah-nahl-heh-see-kohs*
antacid	antiácidos	*ahn-tee-ah-see-dohs*
antiarrhythmic	antiarritmias	*ahn-tee-ah-reet-mee-ahs*
antianxiety	contra la ansiedad/	*kohn-trah lah ahn-see-eh-dahd/*
	ansiolíticos	*ahn-see-oh-lee-tee-kohs*
antibiotics	antibióticos	*ahn-tee-bee-oh-tee-kohs*
anticonvulsant	anticonvulsivo/	*ahn-tee-kohn-bool-see-boh/*
	antiepiléptico	*ahn-tee-eh-pee-lchp-tee-koh*
antiemetic	antiemético	*ahn-tee-eh-meh-tee-koh*
antiviral	antivirales	*ahn-tee-bee-rah-lehs*
contraceptives	contraceptivos	*kohn-trah-sehp-tee-bohs*
decongestants	descongestionantes	*dehs-kohn-hehs-tee-oh-nahn-tehs*
laxatives	laxantes/purgantes	*lahx-ahn-tehs/poor-gahn-tehs*
narcotics	narcóticos	*nahr-koh-tee-kohs*
sedatives	sedativo/sedantes	*seh-dah-tee-boh/seh-dahn-tehs*

It is open Saturday, Sunday, and holidays.

Está abierta los sábados, domingos, y días festivos.
(Ehs-tah ah-bee-ehr-tah lohs sah-bah-dohs, doh-meen-gohs ee dee-ahs fehs-tee-bohs)

It is open 7:00 AM to 12:00 midnight.

Está abierta de las siete de la mañana a las doce de la noche/a medianoche.
(Ehs-tah ah-bee-ehr-tah deh las see-eh-teh deh lah mah-nyah-nah ah las doh-seh deh lah noh-cheh/ah meh-dee-ah-noh-cheh)

The staff delivers and picks up orders every hour from the floors.

Los empleados recogen y surten órdenes cada hora en los pisos.
(Los ehm-pleh-ah-dohs reh-koh-hehn ee soor-tehn ohr-deh-nehs kah-dah oh-rah ehn lohs pee-sohs)

Nursing staff take STAT orders to the pharmacy.

Las enfermeras llevan órdenes urgentes a la farmacia.
(Lahs ehn-fehr-meh-rahs yeh-bahn ohr-deh-nehs oor-hehn-tehs ah lah fahr-mah-see-ah)

TABLE 25-2   Potential Poisons
TABLA 25-2   Posibilidad de Envenenamiento

English	Spanish	Pronunciation
alcohol	alcohol	*ahl-kohl*
antihistamine	antihistamínico	*ahn-tee-ees-tah-mee-nee-koh*
ammonia	amonia/amoníaco	*ah-moh-nee-ah/ah-moh-nee-ah-koh*
barbiturates	barbitúricos	*bahr-bee-too-ree-kohs*
boric acid	ácido bórico	*ah-see-doh boh-ree-koh*
cocaine	cocaína	*koh-kah-ee-nah*
digitalis	digitálicos	*dee-hee-tah-lee-kohs*
lead	plomo	*ploh-moh*
morphine	morfina	*mohr-fee-nah*
nicotine	nicotina	*nee-koh-tee-nah*
nitroglycerin	nitroglicerina	*nee-troh-glee-seh-ree-nah*
aspirin	aspirina	*ahs-pee-ree-nah*

Nurses control narcotic records
   on the unit.

Las enfermeras controlan
   archivos de narcóticos en el piso.
   (Lahs ehn-fehr-meh-rahs kohn-
      troh-lahn ahr-chee-bohs deh
      nahr-koh-tee-kohs ehn ehl pee-soh)

Expired items on the unit are
   returned to the pharmacy.

Los artículos con fecha vencida
   se devuelven a la farmacia.
   (Lohs ahr-tee-koo-lohs kohn
      feh-chah behn-see-dah seh boo-
      ehl-behn ah lah fahr-mah-see-ah)

Monthly the medication area is
   inspected.

Cada mes se inspecciona el área
   de medicamentos.
   (Kah-dah mehs seh eens-pehk-
      see-ohn-ah ehl ah-reh-ah deh
      meh-dee-kah-mehn-tohs)

Medication carts are checked for quantity, number, and expiration
date on each item.
   Los carros con medicamentos se checan/revisan para anotar la
cantidad, número, y fecha de caducidad en cada artículo.

A standard schedule is used.

Se usa un horario estándar.
   (Seh oo-sah oon oh-rah-ree-oh
      ehs-tahn-dahr)

TABLE 25-3	Apothecary Measures	
TABLA 25-3	Medidas Apotecarias	
English	**Spanish**	**Pronunciation**
ounces	onzas	*ohn-sahs*
grains	granos	*grah-nohs*
pound	libra	*lee-brah*
quart	cuarto	*koo-ahr-toh*
gallon	galón	*gah-lohn*

The pharmacist interprets the physician's order.

El farmacéutico interpreta la orden del doctor.
(Ehl fahr-mah-seh-oo-tee-koh een-tehr-preh-tah lah ohr-dehn dehl dohk-tohr)

Vials, pills, capsules, liquids, and IV fluids are dispensed.

Frascos, pastillas, cápsulas, líquidos, y sueros se surten.
(Frahs-kohs, pahs-tee-yahs, kahp-soo-lahs, lee-kee-dohs, ee soo-eh-rohs seh soor-tehn).

She assigns a dosage schedule in the computer.

Ella asigna el horario de dosis en la computadora.
(Eh-yah ah-seeg-nah ehl oh-rah-ree-oh deh doh-sees ehn lah kohm-poo-tah-doh-rah)

Four times a day.

Cuatro veces al día.
(Koo-ah-troh beh-sehs ahl dee-ah)

TABLE 25-4	Metric Measures	
TABLA 25-4	Medidas Métricas	
English	**Spanish**	**Pronunciation**
grams	gramos	*grah-mohs*
kilogram/kilo	kilogramos/kilo	*kee-loh-grah-mohs/kee-loh*
milliliter	mililitro	*mee-lee-lee-troh*
liter	litro	*lee-troh*
cubic centimeter	centímetro cúbico	*sehn-tee-meh-troh koo-bee-koh*
meter	metro	*meh-troh*
centimeter	centímetro	*sehn-tee-meh-troh*
milligram	miligramo	*mee-lee-grah-moh*

TABLE 25-5　Household Measures
TABLA 25-5　Medidas Caseras

English	Spanish	Pronunciation
drop	gota	*goh-tah*
teaspoon	cucharadita	*koo-chah-rah-dee-tah*
tablespoon	cucharada	*koo-chah-rah-dah*
cup	taza	*tah-sah*
glass	vaso	*bah-soh*

TABLE 25-6　Medication Forms
TABLA 25-6　Formas de los Medicamentos

English	Spanish	Pronunciation
fluid	fluído	*floo-ee-doh*
liquid	líquido	*lee-kee-doh*
gel	gelatina	*heh-lah-tee-nah*
capsule	cápsula	*kahp-soo-lah*
pill	píldora	*peel-doh-rah*
tablet	tableta	*tah-bleh-tah*
solid	sólido	*soh-lee-doh*
inhalant	inhalante	*een-ah-lahn-teh*
solution	solución	*soh-loo-see-ohn*
syrup	jarabe/zumo	*hah-rah-beh/soo-moh*
lotion	loción	*loh-see-ohn*
ointment	ungüento*	*oon-goo-ehn-toh*
topical	tópico	*toh-pee-koh*
rectal suppository	supositorio rectal	*soo-poh-see-toh-ree-oh rehk-tahl*
vaginal suppository	supositorio vaginal	*soo-poh-see-toh-ree-oh bah-hee-nahl*
semi-solid	semisólido	*seh-mee-soh-lee-doh*
diluent	diluyente	*dee-loo-yehn-teh*

*The sign above the *ü* is used to emphasize it.

Three times a day.	Tres veces al día. *(Trehs beh-sehs ahl dee-ah)*
Twice a day.	Dos veces al día. *(Dohs beh-sehs ahl dee-ah)*
Daily.	Diariamente./Una por día./Cada día. *(Dee-ah-ree-ah-mehn-teh/Oo-nah pohr dee-ah/Kah-dah dee-ah)*
Before/after meals.	Antes/después de las comidas. *(Ahn-tehs/dehs-poo-ehs deh lahs koh-mee-dahs)*
At bedtime.	Al acostarse./A la hora de dormir. *(Ahl ah-kohs-tahr-seh/Ah lah oh-rah deh dohr-meer)*
The pharmacist assists with patient education.	El farmacéutico/La farmacéutica asiste con la educación del paciente. *(Ehl fahr-mah-seh-oo-tee-koh/Lah fahr-mah-seh-oo-tee-kah ah-sees-teh kohn lah eh-doo-kah-see-ohn dehl pah-see-ehn-teh)*
In case of a medication error, the doctor is notified.	En caso de error en el medicamento, se notifica al doctor. *(Ehn kah-soh deh eh-rohr ehn ehl meh-dee-kah-mehn-toh, seh noh-tee-fee-kah ahl dohk-tohr)*

TABLE 25-7 Administration Routes
TABLA 25-7 Vías de Administración

English	Spanish	Pronunciation
by mouth	por la boca	*pohr lah boh-kah*
per rectum	por el recto/rectal	*pohr ehl rehk-toh/rehk-tahl*
vaginal	vaginal	*bah-hee-nahl*
intravenous	intravenoso	*een-trah-beh-noh-soh*
intramuscular	intramuscular	*een-trah-moos-koo-lahr*
sublingual	sublingual	*soob-leen-goo-ahl*
patch	parche	*pahr-cheh*
subcutaneous	subcutáneo	*soob-koo-tah-neh-oh*
oral	oral	*oh-rahl*
nasal	nasal	*nah-sahl*
otic	ótico	*oh-tee-koh*
ophthalmic	oftálmico	*ohf-tahl-mee-koh*

TABLE 25-8 Useful Words
TABLA 25-8 Palabras Útiles

English	Spanish	Pronunciation
systemic	sistemático	*sees-teh-mah-tee-koh*
nausea	náusea	*nah-oo-seh-ah*
vomiting	vomitando	*boh-mee-tahn-doh*
lavage	lavabo	*lah-bah-boh*
induce	inducir	*een-doo-seer*
lubricant	lubricante	*loo-bree-kahn-teh*
sterile	estéril	*ehs-teh-reel*

Outpatient prescriptions are also dispensed.

Las recetas para pacientes de consulta externa se surten también.
(Lahs reh-seh-tahs pah-rah pah-see-ehn-tehs deh kohn-sool-tah ehx-tehr-nah seh soor-tehn tahm-bee-ehn)

Include on the label:

Incluya en la etiqueta:
(Een-kloo-yah ehn lah eh-tee-keh-tah)

Name of the patient.

Nombre del paciente.
(Nohm-breh dehl pah-see-ehn-teh)

Date.

Fecha.
(Feh-chah)

Doctor's name.

Nombre del doctor.
(Nohm-breh dehl dohk-tohr)

Name of the drug.

Nombre de la droga/del medicamento.
(Nohm-breh deh lah droh-gah/dehl meh-dee-kah-mehn-toh)

Dosage.

Dosis.
(Doh-sees)

Route.

Vía/ruta.
(Bee-ah/roo-tah)

Volume.

Volumen.
(Boh-loo-mehn)

Total number of pills.

Número total de pastillas.
(Noo-meh-roh toh-tahl deh pahs-tee-yahs)

Lot number.

Número de lote.
(Noo-meh-roh deh loh-teh)

Expiration date.	Caducidad. *(Kah-doo-see-dahd)*
The outpatient pharmacy is open daily from 9 AM to 6 PM.	La farmacia de consulta externa está abierta diariamente de las nueve de la mañana a las seis de la tarde todos los días. *(Lah fahr-mah-see-ah deh kohn-sool-tah ehx-tehr-nah ehs-tah ah-bee-ehr-tah dee-ah-ree-ah-mehn-teh deh las noo-eh-beh deh lah mah-nyah-nah ah las seh-ees deh lah tahr-deh toh-dohs lohs dee-ahs)*
Please, come back in a few minutes.	Por favor, regrese en unos minutos. *(Pohr fah-bohr, reh-greh-seh ehn oon-ohs mee-noo-tohs)*
Wait your turn.	Espere su turno. *(Ehs-peh-reh soo toor-noh)*
You will have to wait.	Tendrá que esperar. *(Tehn-drah keh ehs-peh-rahr)*
Wait several minutes!	¡Espere varios minutos! *(Ehs-peh-reh bah-ree-ohs mee-noo-tohs)*
At least 30 minutes!	¡Al menos treinta minutos! *(Ahl meh-nohs treh-een-tah mee-noo-tohs)*
The prescription will be ready at _____.	La receta estará lista a las _____. *Lah reh-seh-tah ehs-tah-rah lees-tah ah lahs _____)*
Take the medicine with juice.	Tome la medicina con jugo. *(Toh-meh lah meh-dee-see-nah kohn hoo-goh)*
Take it with a full glass of water.	Tómela con un vaso lleno de agua. *(Toh-meh-lah kohn oon bah-soh yeh-noh deh ah-goo-ah)*
Do not drink alcohol with this medicine.	No tome alcohol con esta medicina. *(No toh-meh ahl-kohl kohn ehs-tah meh-dee-see-nah)*
It can cause drowsiness.	Le puede causar sueño. *(Leh poo-eh-deh kah-oo-sahr soo-eh-nyoh)*
Do not drive!	¡No maneje/conduzca! *(Noh mah-neh-heh/kohn-doos-kah)*

Do not operate machinery!	¡No maneje/opere una máquina/una maquinaria! *(Noh mah-neh-heh/oh-peh-reh oo-nah mah-kee-nah/mah-kee-nah-ree-ah)*
This is an antacid.	Este es un antiácido. *(Ehs-teh ehs oon ahn-tee-ah-see-doh)*
This is a sedative.	Este es un sedante. *(Ehs-teh ehs oon seh-dahn-teh)*
This medicine is a pain killer.	Esta medicina quita/alivia el dolor. *(Ehs-tah meh-dee-see-nah kee-tah/ah-lee-bee-ah ehl doh-lohr)*
Take on an empty stomach.	Tómela con el estómago vacío. *(Toh-meh-lah kohn ehl ehs-toh-mah-goh bah-see-oh)*
Take one hour before eating.	Tómela una hora antes de comer. *(Toh-meh-lah oo-nah oh-rah ahn-tehs deh koh-mehr)*

TABLE 25-9   Similar Terms
TABLA 25-9   Términos Similares

English	Spanish	Pronunciation
anemia	anemia	*ah-neh-mee-ah*
angina	angina	*ahn-hee-nah*
cataract	catarata	*kah-tah-rah-tah*
bronchitis	bronquitis	*brohn-kee-tees*
enteritis	enteritis	*ehn-teh-ree-tees*
gangrene	gangrena	*gahn-greh-nah*
hypertension	hipertensión	*ee-pehr-tehn-see-ohn*
laryngitis	laringitis	*lah-reen-hee-tees*
pancreatitis	pancreatitis	*pahn-kreh-ah-tee-tees*
pneumonia	pulmonía/neumonía	*pool-moh-nee-ah/neh-oo-moh-nee-ah*
rubella	rubéola	*roo-beh-oh-lah*
tonsillitis	tonsilitis/amigda litis	*tohn-see-lee-tees/ah-meeg-dah-lee-tees*
vaginitis	vaginitis	*bah-hee-nee-tees*
constipation	constipación/ estreñimiento	*kohns-tee-pah-see-ohn/ehs-treh-nyee-mee-ehn-toh*
cirrhosis	cirrosis	*see-roh-sees*

Take the medicine with food.

Tome la medicina con comida.
(Toh-meh lah meh-dee-see-nah kohn koh-mee-dah)

Avoid sunlight.

Evite asolearse/los rayos del sol.
(Eh-bee-teh ah-soh-leh-ahr-seh/lohs rah-yohs dehl sohl)

Follow the instructions carefully.

Siga las instrucciones con cuidado.
(See-gah lahs eens-trook-see-ohn-ehs kohn koo-ee-dah-doh)

Take two aspirins.

Tome dos aspirinas.
(Toh-meh dohs ahs-pee-ree-nahs)

Sleep at least 8 hours.

Duerma al menos ocho horas.
(Doo-ehr-mah ahl meh-nohs oh-choh oh-rahs)

You can refill _____ times.

Puede surtir _____ veces.
(Poo-eh-deh soor-teer _____ beh-sehs)

Take all the medicine in the prescription.

Tome toda la medicina indicada en la receta.
(Toh-meh toh-dah lah meh-dee-see-nah een-dee-kah-dah ehn lah reh-seh-tah)

This prescription may not be refilled.

Esta receta no se puede surtir de nuevo.
(Ehs-tah reh-seh-tah noh seh poo-eh-deh soor-teer deh noo-eh-boh)

If you react to the medicine call your physician.

Si reacciona mal al medicamento llame a su médico.
(See reh-ahk-see-ohn-ah mahl ahl meh-dee-kah-mehn-toh yah-meh ah soo meh-dee-koh)

Go immediately to the hospital!

¡Vaya inmediatamente/en seguida al hospital!
(Bah-yah een-meh-dee-ah-tah-mehn-teh/ehn seh-ghee-dah ahl ohs-pee-tahl)

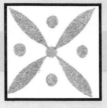

CHAPTER TWENTY-SIX
The X-ray Department

CAPITULO VEINTISEIS
El Departamento de Rayos X

M r. Martinez, a 60-year-old patient, is going to have X-rays. He is scheduled for abdomen and chest X-rays.
Al señor Martínez, paciente de sesenta años, le van a tomar rayos-X. Está en el horario para tomarle rayos X del abdomen y del pecho.

Good morning, Mr. Martínez.	¡Buenos días, señor Martínez! *(Boo-eh-nohs dee-ahs, seh-nyohr Mahr-tee-nehs)*
Transportation is here.	El transporte está aquí. *(Ehl trahns-pohr-teh ehs-tah ah-kee)*
Good morning!	¡Buenos días! *(Boo-eh-nohs dee-ahs)*
Where do I need to go?	¿Adónde tengo que ir? *(Ah-dohn-deh tehn-goh keh eer)*
We are going to x-rays.	Vamos a rayos X. *(Bah-mohs ah rah-yohs eh-kiss)*
I am going to help you lie on the stretcher.	Voy a ayudarlo a acostarse en la camilla. *(Boh-ee ah ah-yoo-dahr-loh ah ah-kohs-tahr-seh ehn lah kah-mee-yah)*
Don't move!	¡No se mueva! *(Noh seh moo-eh-bah)*
We are going to pull the sheet at the count of three.	Vamos a jalar la sábana al contar tres. *(Bah-mohs ah hah-lahr lah sah-bah-nah ahl kohn-tahr trehs)*

One, two, three ...	Uno, dos, tres . . .
	(Oo-noh, dohs, trehs)
Very good!	¡Muy bien!
	(Moo-ee bee-ehn)
Don't hold the rail.	No agarre el barandal.
	(Noh ah-gah-reh ehl bah-rahn-dahl)
I am going to cover you with a sheet.	Voy a cubrirlo con una sábana.
	(Boh-ee ah koo-breer-loh kohn oo-nah sah-bah-nah)
Take your medical file.	Lleve su archivo.
	(Yeh-beh soo ahr-chee-boh)
Take your hospital card.	Lleve su tarjeta del hospital.
	(Yeh-beh soo tahr-heh-tah dehl ohs-pee-tahl)
Remember to bring them back.	Acuérdese de regresarlos.
	(Ah-koo-ehr-deh-seh deh reh-greh-sahr-lohs)
It's not very far.	No está muy lejos.
	(Noh ehs-tah moo-ee leh-hohs)
We are here!	¡Ya llegamos!/¡Estamos Aquí!
	(Yah yeh-gah-mohs/Ehs-tah-mohs ah-kee)
Stay as you are.	Quédese como está.
	(Keh-deh-seh koh-moh ehs-tah)

Mr. Martinez arrives at the department.
El señor Martínez llega al departamento.

Hello, Mr. Martinez.	Hola, señor Martínez.
	(Oh-lah, seh-nyohr Mahr-tee-nehs)
I am the technician.	Yo soy el técnico/la técnica.
	(Yoh soh-ee ehl tehk-nee-koh/lah tehk-nee-kah)
Please, change clothes.	Por favor, cambiese de ropa.
	(Por fah-bohr, kahm-bee-eh-seh deh roh-pah)
I am going to take x-rays of the abdomen first.	Voy a tomar rayos X del abdomen primero.
	(Boh-ee ah toh-mahr rah-yohs eh-kiss dehl ahb-doh-mehn pree-meh-roh)
Lie down.	Acuéstese.
	(Ah-koo-ehs-teh-seh)

I am putting a cassette under your waist.	Estoy poniendo una placa abajo de la cintura. *(Ehs-toh-ee poh-nee-ehn-doh oo-nah plah-kah ah-bah-hoh deh lah seen-too-rah)*
It feels like a board.	Se siente como una tabla. *(Seh see-ehn-teh koh-moh oo-nah tah-blah)*
It has the film inside.	Tiene la película adentro. *(Tee-eh-neh lah peh-lee-koo-lah ah-dehn-troh)*
Don't move!	¡No se mueva! *(Noh seh moo-eh-bah)*
When I tell you, hold your breath.	Cuando le avise, no respire. *(Koo-ahn-doh leh ah-bee-seh, noh rehs-pee-reh)*
Don't breathe!	¡No respire! *(Noh rehs-pee-reh)*
You can breathe now.	Ya puede respirar. *(Yah poo-eh-deh rehs-pee-rahr)*
Breathe out.	Exhale./Respire. *(Ehx-ah-leh/Rehs-pee-reh)*

TABLE 26-1 Common Commands
TABLA 26-1 Ordenes/Mandatos Comúnes

English	Spanish	Pronunciation
Tighten your muscle!	¡Apriete el músculo!	*Ah-pree-eh-teh ehl moos-koo-loh*
Turn on your side!	¡Voltéese de lado!	*Bohl-teh-eh-seh deh lah-doh*
Stand straight!	¡Párese derecho!	*Pah-reh-seh deh-reh-choh*
Keep your feet together!	¡Mantenga los pies juntos!	*Mahn-tehn-gah lohs pee-ehs hoon-tohs*
Turn to the right!	¡Voltee a la derecha!	*Bohl-teh-eh ah lah deh-reh-chah*
Walk straight ahead!	¡Camine derecho!	*Kah-mee-neh deh-reh-choh*
Lift your arms!	¡Levante los brazos!	*Leh-bahn-teh lohs brah-sohs*
Stay as you are!	¡Quédese como está!	*Keh-deh-seh koh-moh ehs-tah*

Turn on your side.	Voltéese de lado.
	(Bohl-teh-eh-seh deh lah-doh)
Turn to the right.	Voltee a la derecha.
	(Bohl-teh-eh ah lah deh-reh-chah)
One more time.	Una vez más.
	(Oo-nah behs mahs)
Hold your breath.	No respire.
	(Noh rehs-pee-reh)
Breathe!	¡Respire!
	(Rehs-pee-reh)
Now I need to x-ray the chest.	Ahora necesito tomar radiografía del pecho.
	(Ah-oh-rah neh-seh-see-toh toh-mahr rah-dee-oh-grah-fee-ah dehl peh-choh)
Stand straight.	Párese derecho.
	(Pah-reh-seh deh-reh-choh)
Keep your feet together.	Ponga los pies juntos.
	(Pohn-gah lohs pee-ehs hoon-tohs)
Lift your arms.	Levante los brazos.
	(Leh-bahn-teh lohs brah-sohs)
Stay like this for a while.	Quédese así por un rato.
	(Keh-deh-seh ah-see pohr oon rah-toh)

TABLE 26-2   Commands
TABLA 26-2   Ordenes/Mandatos

English	Spanish	Pronunciation
Don't hold on!	¡No se agarre!	*Noh seh ah-gahr-reh*
Breathe!	¡Respire!	*Rehs-pee-reh*
Don't breathe!	¡No respire!	*Noh rehs-pee-reh*
Don't move!	¡No se mueva!	*Noh seh moo-eh-bah*
Don't laugh!	¡No se ría!	*Noh seh ree-ah*
Talk!	¡Hable!	*Ah-bleh*
Lie down!	¡Acuéstese!	*Ah-koo-ehs-teh-seh*
Hold your breath!	¡No respire!	*Noh rehs-pee-reh*
Keep quiet!	¡Estése quieto!/	*Ehs-teh-seh kee-eh-toh/*
	¡No se mueva!	*Noh seh moo-eh-bah*
Don't lie down!	¡No se acueste!	*Noh seh ah-koo-ehs-teh*
Press hard!	¡Presione fuerte!	*Preh-see-oh-neh foo-ehr-teh*
Sit down!	¡Siéntese!	*See-ehn-teh-seh*
Stay still!	¡Quédese quieto!	*Keh-deh-seh kee-eh-toh*

Now, turn to the screen.	Ahora, voltee hacia la placa. *(Ah-oh-rah, bohl-teh-eh ah-see-ah lah plah-kah)*
This will feel cold.	Esto se sentirá frío. *(Ehs-toh seh sehn-tee-rah free-oh)*
It will take a minute.	Va a tomar un minuto. *(Bah ah toh-mahr oon mee-noo-toh)*
Are you hurting?	¿Tiene dolor? *(Tee-eh-neh doh-lohr)*
Stop breathing.	No respire. *(Noh rehs-pee-reh)*
You can breathe.	Puede respirar. *(Poo-eh-deh rehs-pee-rahr)*
I am through.	Ya terminé. *(Yah tehr-mee-neh)*
I will return shortly.	Regresaré en seguida. *(Reh-greh-sah-reh ehn seh-gee-dah)*
Please sit down.	Siéntese, por favor. *(See-ehn-teh-seh, pohr fah-bohr)*

TABLE 26-3   Common Questions
TABLA 26-3   Preguntas Comúnes

English	Spanish	Pronunciation
Where do I need to go?	¿Adónde necesito ir?	*Ah dohn-deh neh-seh-see-toh eer*
Do you need help?	¿Necesita ayuda?	*Neh-seh-see-tah ah-yoo-dah*
Have you had x-rays?	¿Le han tomado rayos X?	*Leh ahn toh-mah-doh rah-yohs eh-kiss*
When was the last time?	¿Cuándo fue la última vez?	*Koo-ahn-doh foo-eh lah ool-tee-mah behs*
Do you know why?	¿Sabe por qué?	*Sah-beh pohr keh*
How old are you?	¿Cuántos años tiene?	*Koo-ahn-tohs ah-nyohs tee-eh-neh*
Are you pregnant?	¿Está embarazada?	*Ehs-tah ehm-bah-rah-sah-dah*
Have you had cancer?	¿Ha tenido cáncer?	*Ah teh-nee-doh kahn-sehr*
Family history of cancer?	¿Hay historia de cáncer en la familia?	*Ah-ee ees-toh-ree-ah deh kahn-sehr ehn lah fah-mee-lee-ah*

| English | Spanish | Pronunciation |

Don't change clothes. No se cambie de ropa.
(Noh seh kahm-bee-eh deh roh-pah)

I want to see if the x-rays are good. Quiero ver si las radiografías salieron bien.
(Kee-eh-roh behr see lahs rah-dee-oh-grah-fee-ahs sah-lee-eh-rohn bee-ehn)

I am back. Ya regresé.
(Yah reh-greh-seh)

Now you can change clothes. Ahora se puede cambiar de ropa.
(Ah-oh-rah seh poo-eh-deh kahm-bee-ahr deh roh-pah)

Do you need help? ¿Necesita ayuda?
(Neh-seh-see-tah ah-yoo-dah)

I am going to call the radiologist. Voy a llamar al radiólogo.
(Boh-ee ah yah-mahr ahl rah-dee-oh-loh-goh)

He will talk to you. El hablará con usted.
(Ehl ah-blah-rah kohn oos-tehd)

Dr. Blanco, the radiologist, stands by the door and greets the patient.
El doctor Blanco, radiólogo, se para en la puerta y saluda al paciente.

Good morning! ¡Buenos días!
(Boo-eh-nohs dee-ahs)

TABLE 26-4   Phrases
TABLA 26-4   Frases

English	Spanish	Pronunciation
I am going to help you.	Voy a ayudarlo.	*Boh-ee ah ah-yoo-dahr-loh*
We are going to pull.	Vamos a jalar.	*Bah-mohs ah hah-lahr*
Very good!	¡Muy bien!	*Moo-ee bee-ehn*
Take your medical file.	Lleve su archivo.	*Yeh-beh soo ahr-chee-boh*
Take your hospital card.	Lleve su tarjeta.	*Yeh-beh soo tahr-heh-tah*
It's not very far.	No está muy lejos.	*Noh ehs-tah moo-ee leh-hohs*
We are here.	Estamos aquí.	*Ehs-tah-mohs ah-kee*
Please put this gown on.	Por favor, póngase esta bata.	*Pohr fah-bohr, pohn-gah-seh ehs-tah bah-tah*

I am Dr. Blanco.	Yo soy el doctor Blanco.
	(Yo soh-ee ehl dohk-tohr Blahn-koh)
We need to bring you back.	Necesitamos que regrese.
	(Neh-seh-see-tah-mohs keh reh-greh-seh)
But we will give you something to drink.	Pero le daremos algo que tomar.
	(Peh-roh leh dah-reh-mohs ahl-goh keh toh-mahr)
We will x-ray the abdomen again.	Vamos a tomar otras radiografías del abdomen.
	(Bah-mohs ah toh-mahr oh-trahs rah-dee-oh-grah-fee-ahs dehl ahb-doh-mehn)
Tonight, eat lightly.	Esta noche coma ligero.
	(Ehs-tah noh-cheh koh-mah lee-heh-roh)
Take these pills after your meal.	Tómese estas pastillas después de la cena.
	(Toh-meh-seh ehs-tahs pahs-tee-yahs dehs-poo-ehs deh lah seh-nah)
You can drink water.	Puede tomar agua.
	(Poo-eh-deh toh-mahr ah-goo-ah)
Please, tell the nurse to call me.	Por favor, dígale a la enfermera que me llame.
	(Por fah-bohr, dee-gah-leh ah lah ehn-fehr-meh-rah keh meh yah-meh)

TABLE 26-5   Helpful Phrases
TABLA 26-5   Frases Útiles

English	Spanish	Pronunciation
It feels like a board	Se siente como una tabla	*Seh see-ehn-teh koh-moh oo-nah tah-blah*
One more time	Una vez más	*Oo-nah behs mahs*
It will take a minute	Va a tomar un minuto	*Bah ah toh-mahr oon mee-noo-toh*
I am through	Ya terminé	*Yah tehr-mee-neh*
I will return!	¡Regresaré!	*Reh-greh-sah-reh*
You need to return	Necesita regresar	*Neh-seh-see-tah reh-greh-sahr*
You need to drink water	Necesita tomar agua	*Neh-seh-see-tah toh-mahr ah-goo-ah*
When I tell you	Cuando le diga	*Koo-ahn-doh leh dee-gah*

Do you have any questions?	¿Tiene preguntas? *(Tee-eh-neh preh-goon-tahs)*
I will see you tomorrow at nine.	Lo veré mañana a las nueve. *(Loh beh-reh mah-nyah-nah ah lahs noo-eh-beh)*
Have a good day!	¡Pase un buen día! *(Pah-seh oon boo-ehn dee-ah)*
Transportation will take you back to your room.	Transportación lo regresará a su cuarto. *(Trahns-pohr-tah-see-ohn loh reh-greh-sah-rah ah soo koo-ahr-toh)*

TABLE 26-6   Common Words
TABLA 26-6   Palabras Comúnes

English	Spanish	Pronunciation
division	división	*dee-bee-see-ohn*
nuclear medicine	medicina nuclear	*meh-dee-see-nah noo-kleh-ahr*
ventilation	ventilación	*behn-tee-lah-see-ohn*
thyroid	tiróide/tiroidea	*tee-roh-ee-deh/tee-roh-ee-deh-ah*
irradiate	irradiar	*ee-rah-dee-ahr*
gallbladder	vesícula biliar/hiel	*beh-see-koo-lah bee-lee-ahr/ee-ehl*
liver	hígado	*ee-gah-doh*
contrast	contraste	*kohn-trahs-teh*
laxative	laxante/purgante	*lahx-ahn-teh/poor-gahn-teh*
enema	enema/sonda	*eh-neh-mah/sohn-dah*
ultrasound	ultrasonido	*ool-trah-soh-nee-doh*
bowel	intestino	*een-tehs-tee-noh*
arteriogram	arteriograma	*ahr-teh-ree-oh-grah-mah*

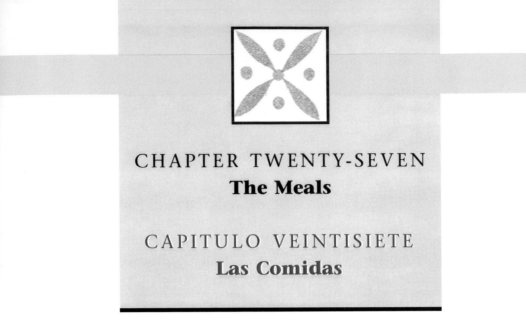

CHAPTER TWENTY-SEVEN
The Meals

CAPITULO VEINTISIETE
Las Comidas

For many patients, meals served in the hospital are not very appetizing. Hispanic patients, in general, prefer foods that are spicy and juicy. They are quite attached to special **"bocadillos,"** *appetizers* that may not be available in the hospital. Please explain to patients what foods they are able to bring from home and assist them with selections that they can make from their menus. Table 27-1 has a list of some diets available in the hospital.

Para muchos pacientes las comidas que se sirven en el hospital no son apetitosas. Los hispanos, en general, prefieren comidas condimentadas y jugosas. Están acostumbrados a comer bocadillos especiales (aperitivos) que a veces no se pueden encontrar en los hospitales. Por favor explíqueles a los pacientes si pueden traer comida de su casa y ayúdeles con las selecciones que pueden hacer en sus menús. La tabla 27-1 tiene una lista de algunas de las dietas que se ofrecen en el hospital.

There are many diets available to patients.	Hay muchas dietas para los pacientes. *(Ah-ee moo-chahs dee-eh-tahs pah-rah lohs pah-see-ehn-tehs)*
The doctor has to prescribe it.	El doctor/La doctora debe de recetarla. *(Ehl dohk-tohr/Lah dohk-tohr(ah) deh-beh deh reh-seh-tahr-lah)*

TABLE 27-1 Types of Diets
TABLA 27-1 Tipos de Dietas

English	Spanish	Pronunciation
regular	regular	*reh-goo-lahr*
diabetic	para diabético	*pah-rah dee-ah-beh-tee-koh*
no salt	sin sal	*seen sahl*
low cholesterol	colesterol bajo	*koh-lehs-teh-rohl bah-hoh*
low fat	poca grasa	*poh-kah grah-sah*
soft	suave	*soo-ah-beh*
liquid	líquida	*lee-kee-dah*

Can you tell me what kind of diet you have?

¿Puede decirme qué dieta tiene?
(Poo-eh-deh deh-seer-meh keh dee-eh-tah tee-eh-neh)

What foods do you like?

¿Qué comidas le gustan?
(Keh koh-mee-dahs leh goos-tahn)

Many patients do not follow a balanced diet because they do not eat a variety of needed foods.

Muchos pacientes no llevan una dieta balanceada porque no comen una variedad de alimentos necesarios.

The following should be included in your diet every day:

Lo siguiente se debe incluir en la dieta todos los días:
(Loh see-gee-ehn-teh seh deh-beh een-kloo-eer ehn soo dee-eh-tah toh-dohs lohs dee-ahs)

2 to 4 servings of milk

Dos a cuatro porciones de leche
(Dohs ah koo-ah-troh pohr-see-ohn-ehs deh leh-cheh)

2 to 3 servings of meat, fish, or poultry

Dos a tres porciones de carne, pescado, o aves de corral
(Dohs ah trehs pohr-see-oh-nehs deh kahr-neh, pehs-kah-doh, oh ah-behs deh ko-rahl)

2 to 4 servings of fruit

dos a cuatro porciones de fruta
(Dohs ah koo-ah-troh pohr-see-ohn-ehs deh froo-tah)

6 to 11 servings of starches	Seis a once porciones de almidones/féculas *(Seh-ees ah ohn-seh pohr-see-oh-nehs deh ahl-mee-doh-nehs/feh-koo-lahs)*
wheat bread and cereals	Pan de trigo y cereales *(Pahn deh tree-goh ee seh-reh-ah-lehs)*
3 to 5 servings of vegetables	Tres a cinco porciones de vegetales *(Trehs ah seen-koh pohr-see-oh-nehs deh beh-heh-tah-lehs)*
I am going to give you a list.	Voy a darle una lista. *(Boh-ee ah dahr-leh oo-nah lees-tah)*
For breakfast:	Para el desayuno: *(Pah-rah ehl deh-sah-yoo-noh)*
eggs	huevos *(oo-eh-bohs)*
toast	pan tostado *(pahn tohs-tah-doh)*
coffee	café *(kah-feh)*
milk	leche *(leh-cheh)*
juice	jugo *(hoo-goh)*
fruit	fruta *(froo-tah)*
How do you like your coffee?	¿Cómo le gusta el café? *(Koh-moh leh goos-tah ehl kah-feh)*
black	negro *(neh-groh)*
with cream	con crema *(kohn kreh-mah)*
with sugar	con azúcar *(kohn ah-soo-kahr)*
What kind of coffee?	¿Qué clase de café? *(Keh klah-seh deh kah-feh)*
regular	regular *(reh-goo-lahr)*
decaffeinated	descafeinado *(dehs-kah-feh-ee-nah-doh)*
instant	instantáneo *(eens-tahn-tah-neh-oh)*
What kind of juices?	¿Qué clase de jugos? *(Keh klah-seh deh joo-gohs)*

orange	naranja *(nah-rahn-hah)*
grape	uva *(oo-bah)*
apple	manzana *(mahn-sah-nah)*
grapefruit	toronja *(toh-rohn-hah)*
prune	ciruela *(see-roo-eh-lah)*
tomato	tomate *(toh-mah-teh)*
How do you like the eggs fixed?	¿Cómo le gustan los huevos? *(Koh-moh leh goos-tahn lohs oo-eh-bohs)*
scrambled	revueltos *(reh-boo-ehl-tohs)*
over easy	volteados *(bohl-teh-ah-dohs)*
fried	fritos *(free-tohs)*
hard-boiled	duros *(doo-rohs)*
with ham	con jamón *(kohn hah-mohn)*
We have cereals.	Tenemos cereales. *(Teh-neh-mohs seh-reh-ah-lehs)*
Do you like them hot/cold?	¿Le gustan calientes/fríos? *(Leh goos-tahn kah-lee-ehn-tehs/free-ohs)*
oatmeal	avena *(ah-beh-nah)*
cream of wheat	crema de trigo *(kreh-mah deh tree-goh)*
corn-flakes	hojitas de maíz/corn-flakes *(oh-hee-tahs deh mah-ees/kohrn fleh-ee-ks)*
We serve lunch at noon.	Servimos la comida al mediodía. *(Sehr-bee-mohs lah koh-mee-dah ahl meh-dee-oh-dee-ah)*
Kitchen personnel bring the food trays.	Los empleados de la cocina traen las bandejas con comida. *(Lohs ehm-pleh-ah-dohs deh lah koh-see-nah trah-ehn lahs bahn-deh-hahs kohn koh-mee-dah)*

| TABLE 27-2 | Common Foods |
| TABLA 27-2 | Comidas Comúnes |

English	Spanish	Pronunciation
desserts	postres	*pohs-trehs*
gelatin	gelatina	*geh-lah-tee-nah*
vinegar	vinagre	*bee-nah-greh*
custard	flan	*flahn*
shrimp	camarones	*kah-mah-roh-nehs*
tuna	atún	*ah-toon*
turkey	pavo/guajolote	*pah-boh/goo-ah-hoh-loh-teh*
lamb	cordero	*kohr-deh-roh*
crab	cangrejos	*kahn-greh-hohs*
tamales	tamales	*tah-mah-lehs*
crackers	galletas saladas	*gah-yeh-tahs sah-lah-dahs*
enchiladas	enchiladas	*ehn-chee-lah-dahs*
cereals	cereales	*seh-reh-ah-lehs*
vegetables	vegetales	*beh-heh-tah-lehs*
coffee	café	*kah-feh*
eggs	huevos	*oo-eh-bohs*

We have meats:	Tenemos carnes:
	(Teh-neh-mohs kahr-nehs)
beef	res
	(rehs)
hamburger	hamburguesa
	(ahm-boor-geh-sah)
steak	bistec
	(bees-tehk)
roast	rostizado
	(rohs-tee-sah-doh)
pork	puerco
	(poo-ehr-koh)
chops	chuletas
	(choo-leh-tahs)
ribs	costillas
	(kohs-tee-yahs)
chicken	pollo
	(poh-yoh)
fried chicken	pollo frito
	(poh-yoh free-toh)
baked chicken	pollo asado
	(poh-yoh ah-sah-doh)

breast	pechuga
	(peh-choo-gah)
leg	pierna
	(pee-ehr-nah)
wings	alas
	(ah-lahs)
fish	pescado
	(pehs-kah-doh)
breaded fish	empanizado
	(ehm-pah-nee-sah-doh)
broiled fish	pescado al horno
	(pehs-kah-doh ahl ohr-noh)
These meats can be substituted.	Estas carnes se pueden substituir.
	(Ehs-tahs kahr-nehs seh poo-eh-dehn soobs-tee-too-eer)
Among the vegetables that we serve are:	Entre los vegetales que servimos hay:
	(Ehn-treh lohs beh-heh-tah-lehs keh sehr-bee-mohs ah-ee)
potatoes	papas
	(pah-pahs)
baked potatoes	papas asadas
	(pah-pahs ah-sah-dahs)
french fries	papas fritas
	(pah-pahs free-tahs)
mashed potatoes	puré de papas
	(poo-reh deh pah-pahs)
green beans	ejotes/habichuelas
	(eh-hoh-tehs/ah-bee-choo-eh-lahs)
peas	chícharos
	(chee-chah-rohs)
corn	maíz/elote
	(mah-ees/eh-loh-teh)
beans	frijoles/habas
	(free-hoh-lehs/ah-bahs)
pinto beans	frijol pinto
	(free-hohl peen-toh)
refried beans	refritos
	(reh-free-tohs)
rice	arroz
	(ah-rohs)
salad	ensalada
	(ehn-sah-lah-dah)
lettuce	lechuga
	(leh-choo-gah)

TABLE 27-3	Pronounciation of Selected Words
TABLA 27-3	Pronunciación de Palabras Selectas

English	Spanish	Pronunciation
alcoholic beverages	alcohólicas/bebidas	*ahl-koh-lee-kahs/ beh-bee-dahs*
minerals	minerales	*mee-neh-rah-lehs*
vitamins	vitaminas	*bee-tah-mee-nahs*
raw	crudo	*kroo-doh*
frozen	helado/congelado	*eh-lah-doh/kohn-heh-lah-doh*
substitutes	substitutos	*soobs-tee-too-tohs*
miscellaneous	miscelánea	*mee-seh-lah-neh-ah*
soups	sopas	*soh-pahs*
cottage cheese	requesón	*reh-keh-sohn*
carbonated drinks	bebidas gaseosas	*beh-bee-dahs gah-seh-oh-sahs*
toothpick	palillo	*pah-lee-yoh*
saccharin	sacarina	*sah-kah-ree-nah*
roast beef	rosbif	*rohs-beef*

We also have desserts.	También tenemos postres. *(Tahm-bee-ehn teh-neh-mohs pohs-trehs)*
ice cream	nieve/helado *(nee-eh-beh/eh-lah-doh)*
vanilla	vainilla *(bah-ee-nee-yah)*
chocolate	chocolate *(choh-koh-lah-teh)*
strawberry	fresa *(freh-sah)*
pies	pasteles *(pahs-teh-lehs)*
pecan	nuez *(noo-ehs)*
apple	manzana *(mahn-sah-nah)*
cookies	galletas *(gah-yeh-tahs)*
candy	dulces *(dool-sehs)*

You can buy canned drinks in the cafeteria.	Puede comprar bebidas envasadas en la cafetería. *(Poo-eh-deh kohm-prahr beh-bee-dahs ehn-bah-sah-dahs ehn lah kah-feh-teh-ree-ah)*
We don't serve drinks like cokes or any canned drinks.	No servimos refrescos como Coca-Cola o bebidas envasadas. *(Noh sehr-bee-mohs reh-frehs-kohs koh-moh Koh-kah Koh-lah oh beh-bee-dahs ehn-bah-sah-dahs)*
You can also ask for snacks:	También puede pedir aperitivos: *(Tahm-bee-ehn poo-eh-deh peh-deer ah-peh-ree-tee-bohs)*
juices	jugos *(joo-gohs)*
fruit	fruta *(froo-tah)*
yogurt	yogurt *(yoh-goor)*
peanut butter sandwich	lonche de crema de cacahuate *(lohn-cheh deh kreh-mah deh kah-kah-oo-ah-teh)*
milk	leche *(leh-cheh)*
breads	panes *(pah-nehs)*
corn bread	maíz/pan de maíz *(mah-ees/pahn deh mah-ees)*
wheat	trigo *(tree-goh)*
white	blanco *(blahn-koh)*
condiments	condimentos *(kohn-dee-mehn-tohs)*
spices	especias *(ehs-peh-see-ahs)*
butter	mantequilla *(mahn-teh-kee-yah)*
mustard	mostaza *(mohs-tah-sah)*
hot sauce	salsa picante *(sahl-sah pee-kahn-teh)*
mayonnaise	mayonesa *(mah-yoh-neh-sah)*

The water is in the glass/pitcher.
El agua está en el vaso/la jarra.
(Ehl ah-goo-ah ehs-tah ehn ehl bah-soh/lah hah-rah)

Do you want water?
¿Quiére agua?
(Kee-eh-reh ah-goo-ah)

Do you need ice?
¿Necesita hielo?
(Neh-seh-see-tah ee-eh-loh)

This is the tray.
Esta es la bandeja.
(Ehs-tah ehs lah bahn-deh-hah)

The fork, spoon, and knife are wrapped in the napkin.
El tenedor, cuchara, y cuchillo están envueltos en la servilleta.
(Ehl teh-neh-dohr, koo-chah-rah ee koo-chee-yoh ehs-tahn ehn-boo-ehl-tohs ehn lah sehr-bee-yeh-tah)

There is a straw.
Hay un popote.
(Ah-ee oon poh-poh-teh)

The salt and pepper are in these packets.
La sal y pimienta están en estos paquetes.
(Lah sahl ee pee-mee-ehn-tah ehs-tahn ehn ehs-tohs pah-keh-tehs)

Sorry, no toothpicks.
Lo siento, no hay palillos.
(Loh see-ehn-toh, noh ah-ee pah-lee-yohs)

The plates are plastic.
Los platos son de plástico.
(Lohs plah-tohs sohn deh plahs-tee-koh)

They can't break.
No se pueden romper.
(Noh seh poo-eh-dehn rohm-pehr)

The cover is hot.
La cubierta está caliente.
(Lah koo-bee-ehr-tah ehs-tah kah-lee-ehn-teh)

It keeps the food warm.
Guarda la comida tibia.
(Goo-ahr-dah lah koh-mee-dah tee-bee-ah)

You can eat in your room or in the visitors' room.
Puede comer en su cuarto o en el cuarto para visitas.
(Poo-eh-deh koh-mehr ehn soo koo-ahr-toh oh ehn ehl koo-ahr-toh pah-rah bee-see-tahs)

Select your foods from the menu after breakfast.
Seleccione las comidas del menú después del desayuno.
(Seh-lehk-see-oh-neh lahs koh-mee-dahs dehl meh-noo dehs-poo-ehs dehl deh-sah-yoo-noh)

You have to choose three meals a day.	Tiene que escoger tres comidas diarias. *(Tee-eh-neh keh ehs-koh-hehr trehs koh-mee-dahs dee-ah-ree-ahs)*
You can order one or two portions.	Puede ordenar una o dos porciones. *(Poo-eh-deh ohr-deh-nahr oo-nah oh dohs pohr-see-oh-nehs)*
We send the menu to the kitchen.	Mandamos el menú a la cocina. *(Mahn-dah-mohs ehl meh-noo ah lah koh-see-nah)*

Some people cannot tolerate gas-producing foods and should avoid eating them.

Algunas personas no toleran comidas que producen gas y deben evitar comerlas.

Gas-producing foods:	Comidas que producen gas: *(Koh-mee-dahs keh proh-doo-sehn gahs)*
onions	cebolla *(seh-boh-yah)*
beans	frijoles *(free-hoh-lehs)*
celery	apio *(ah-pee-oh)*

TABLE 27-4   List of Fruits
TABLA 27-4   Lista de Frutas

English	Spanish	Pronunciation
strawberry	fresa	*freh-sah*
lime	lima	*lee-mah*
cantaloupe	melón	*meh-lohn*
pineapple	piña	*pee-nyah*
cherries	cerezas	*seh-reh-sahs*
watermelon	sandía	*sahn-dee-ah*
plum	ciruelo	*see-roo-eh-loh*
grapefruit	toronja	*toh-rohn-hah*
banana	plátano	*plah-tah-noh*
orange	naranja	*nah-rahn-hah*
pears	peras	*peh-rahs*

carrots	zanahoria *(sah-nah-oh-ree-ah)*
cabbage	col/repollo *(kohl/reh-poh-yoh)*
raisins	pasas *(pah-sahs)*
bananas	plátanos *(plah-tah-nohs)*
prunes	ciruelas *(see-roo-eh-lahs)*

Cholesterol is a type of fat found in the blood. A low cholesterol diet may help to lower your blood cholesterol level if it is too high. Cut down on foods that have high cholesterol content. The following list gives you a general idea of foods you should avoid.

El colesterol es un tipo de grasa en la sangre. Una dieta baja en colesterol le puede ayudar a rebajar el nivel si está muy alto. Reduzca las comidas que tienen contenido muy alto de colesterol. La siguiente lista le da una idea en general de las comidas que debe de evitar.

Foods you may not eat:

Comidas que no debe comer:
(Koh-mee-dahs keh noh deh-beh koh-mehr)

butter	mantequilla *(mahn-teh-kee-yah)*
shortening	manteca *(mahn-teh-kah)*
egg yolks	yema de huevos *(yeh-mah deh oo-eh-bohs)*
biscuits	bisquetes/bizcocho *(bees-keh-tehs/bees-koh-choh)*
pancakes	panqué *(pahn-keh)*
avocados	aguacates *(ah-goo-ah-kah-tehs)*
bacon	tocino *(toh-see-noh)*
sausage	salchicha/chorizo *(sahl-chee-chah/choh-ree-soh)*
hot dog	perro caliente/emparedado de salchicha *(peh-roh kah-lee-ehn-teh/ehm-pah-reh-dah-doh deh sahl-chee-chah)*
whole milk	leche entera *(leh-cheh ehn-teh-rah)*

ice cream	**nieve/helado** *(nee-eh-beh/eh-lah-doh)*
chocolate	**chocolate** *(choh-koh-lah-teh)*
liver	**hígado** *(ee-gah-doh)*
most red meat	**la mayoría de las carnes rojas** *(lah mah-yoh-ree-ah deh lahs kahr-nehs roh-hahs)*
most cookies	**la mayoría de las galletas** *(lah mah-yoh-ree-ah deh lahs gah-yeh-tahs)*

Unit 5

General Vocabulary

UNIDAD 5

Vocabulario General

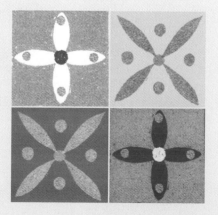

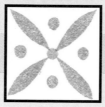

CHAPTER TWENTY-EIGHT
Greetings and Common Expressions

CAPITULO VEINTIOCHO
Saludos y Expresiones Comúnes

Greetings and expressions are used specially to address a person or get someone's attention. Hispanics are generally very friendly and will greet you even when they do not know you. In this chapter we will only provide those greetings that are used most frequently.

Los saludos y expresiones se hacen en forma particular para llamar la atención de la persona. Los hispanos son generalmente muy amigables y saludan aún sin conocer a la persona. En este capítulo sólo hablamos de los saludos que usamos con más frecuencia.

Hi!	¡Hola!
	(Oh-lah)
Good morning.	Buenos días.
	(Boo-eh-nohs dee-ahs)
Good afternoon.	Buenas tardes.
	(Boo-eh-nahs tahr-dehs)
Good evening.	Buenas noches.
	(Boo-eh-nahs noh-chehs)
Good night.	Buenas noches.
	(Boo-eh-nahs noh-chehs)
Do you speak English?	¿Habla inglés?
	(Ah-blah een-glehs)

Yes, I speak English.	Sí, yo hablo inglés.
	(See, yoh ah-bloh een-glehs)
No, I do not speak English.	No, no hablo inglés.
	(Noh, noh ah-bloh een-glehs)
Do you speak Spanish?	¿Habla español?
	(Ah-blah ehs-pah-nyohl)
Yes, I speak Spanish.	Sí, hablo español.
	(See, ah-bloh ehs-pah-nyohl)
No, I do not speak Spanish.	No, no hablo español.
	(Noh, noh ah-bloh ehs-pah-nyohl)
Yes, a little.	Sí, un poco.
	(See, oon poh-koh)
No, I don't understand.	No, no comprendo/no entiendo.
	(Noh, noh kohm-prehn-doh/no ehn-tee-ehn-doh)
Speak slowly, please.	Hable despacio, por favor.
	(Ah-bleh dehs-pah-see-oh, pohr fah-bohr)
Slowly, please.	Despacio, por favor.
	(Dehs-pah-see-oh, pohr fah-bohr)
Thank you!	¡Gracias!
	(Grah-see-ahs)
Thank you very much!	¡Muchas gracias!
	(Moo-chahs grah-see-ahs)
It's nothing/you are welcome.	De nada.
	(Deh nah-dah)
I am. . .	Yo soy. . .
	(Yoh soh-ee)
I am the doctor (male).	Yo soy el doctor.
	(Yoh soh-ee ehl dohk-tohr)
I am the doctor (female).	Yo soy la doctora.
	(Yoh soh-ee lah dohk-tohr-ah)
I am the nurse (female).	Yo soy la enfermera.
	(Yoh soh-ee lah ehn-fehr-meh-rah)
I am the nurse (male).	Yo soy el enfermero.
	(Yoh soh-ee ehl ehn-fehr-meh-roh)
What is your name? (formal)	¿Cómo se llama usted?
	(Koh-moh seh yah-mah oos-tehd)
What is your name? (informal)	¿Cómo te llamas?
	(Koh-moh teh yah-mahs)
My name is. . .	Me llamo. . .
	(Meh yah-moh)
May I join you?	¿Lo/La puedo acompañar?
	(Loh/Lah poo-eh-doh ah-kohm-pah-nyahr)

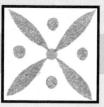

CHAPTER TWENTY-NINE
Commands

CAPITULO VEINTINUEVE
Ordenes o Mandatos

Commands or orders are used in hospitals, private offices, and health care centers. This gives responsibility to patients related to their well-being and state of health. These commands should be given firmly and with confidence. In this manner, the patient is able to understand the outcome of such commands.

Las órdenes o mandatos se usan en los hospitales, las consultas privadas, y los centros de salud. Esto crea en los pacientes una responsabilidad acerca de su bienestar y curación total. Estas órdenes deben darse con mucha firmeza y seguridad. De esta manera el paciente capta en su totalidad la finalidad que se persigue al indicárselas.

Wake up!	¡Despierte!
	(Dehs-pee-ehr-teh)
Get up.	¡Levántese!
	(Leh-bahn-teh-seh)
Do not get up!	¡No se levante!
	(Noh seh leh-bahn-teh)
Sit up!	¡Siéntese!
	(See-ehn-teh-seh)
Walk.	¡Camine!
	(Kah-mee-neh)
Sit on the chair!	Siéntese en la silla.
	(See-ehn-teh-seh ehn lah see-yah)
Stop!	¡Párese!
	(Pah-reh-seh)
Look up/down.	Vea arriba/abajo.
	(Beh-ah ah-ree-bah/ah-bah-hoh)

Move!	¡Muévase! *(Moo-eh-bah-seh)*
Listen!	¡Oiga!/¡Escuche! *(Oh-ee-gah/ehs-koo-cheh)*
Don't talk!	¡No hable! *(Noh ah-bleh)*
Open your mouth.	Abra la boca. *(Ah-brah lah boh-kah)*
Show me your tongue.	Muéstreme la lengua. *(Moo-ehs-treh-meh lah lehn-goo-ah)*
Close your mouth.	Cierre la boca. *(See-eh-reh lah boh-kah)*
Bite!	¡Muerda! *(Moo-ehr-dah)*
Talk.	Hable. *(Ah-bleh)*
Breathe deeply!	¡Respire hondo/profundo! *(Rehs-pee-reh ohn-doh/proh-foon-doh)*
Don't breathe!	¡No respire! *(Noh rehs-pee-reh)*
Turn!	¡Voltee! *(Bohl-teh-eh)*
Take a bath.	Báñese. *(Bah-nyeh-seh)*
Wash your face!	¡Lávese la cara! *(Lah-beh-seh lah kah-rah)*
Brush your teeth!	¡Cepíllese los dientes! *(Seh-pee-yeh-seh lohs dee-ehn-tehs)*
Bend over.	Agáchese. *(Ah-gah-cheh-seh)*
Kneel down.	Póngase de rodillas. *(Pohn-gah-seh deh roh-dee-yahs)*
Open your eyes!	¡Abra los ojos! *(Ah-brah lohs oh-hohs)*
Close your eyes!	¡Cierre los ojos! *(See-eh-reh lohs oh-hohs)*
Lie down!	¡Acuéstese! *(Ah-koo-ehs-teh-seh)*
Eat!	¡Coma! *(Koh-mah)*
Swallow!	¡Trague! *(Trah-gheh)*
Drink.	Beba./Tome. *(Beh-bah/Toh-meh)*

Relax!	¡Relaje!/¡Descanse! *(Reh-lah-heh/Dehs-kahn-seh)*
Run!	¡Corra! *(Koh-rah)*
Wait!	¡Espere! *(Ehs-peh-reh)*
Don't sit.	No se siente. *(Noh seh see-ehn-teh)*
Bend your knee!	¡Doble su rodilla! *(Doh-bleh soo roh-dee-yah)*
Move your eyes.	Mueva sus ojos. *(Moo-eh-bah soos oh-hohs)*
Squeeze my hand.	Apriete mi mano. *(Ah-pree-eh-teh mee mah-noh)*
Cough!	¡Tosa! *(Toh-sah)*
Don't push!	¡No haga esfuerzo! *(Noh ah-gah ehs-foo-ehr-soh)*
Watch your bleeding!	¡Vigile su sangrado! *(Bee-hee-leh soo sahn-grah-doh)*
Take care of yourself!	¡Cuídese mucho! *(Koo-ee-deh-seh moo-choh)*

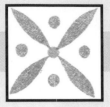

CHAPTER THIRTY
Simple Questions, Interrogatives, Exclamations

CAPITULO TREINTA
Preguntas Sencillas, Interrogativas, Exclamaciones

S imple questions and exclamations are used most frequently. They are used in short form to ask a question or give a command. Note than in the Spanish language the questions must be accompanied by an inverted mark before (¿) and a regular one after it (?). We use questions to let the patient tell us what they know or how they feel. The exclamation points indicate emotion or the mood that the patient is in and are used before and after the statement (¡ !).

Las preguntas sencillas y exclamaciones son las que usamos con mayor frecuencia. Se usan en forma corta ya sea interrogando o exclamando. Note que las preguntas en la lengua española se deben de acompañar por signo de interrogación invertido al inicio (¿) y al final como lo conocemos (?). Las interrogativas son preguntas que se hacen para que nos respondan lo que saben o sienten en ese momento. Las exclamaciones reflejan una emoción o estado de ánimo de la persona y se usan antes y después de la expresión (¡ !).

What?	¿Qué?/¿Qué tal?	*(Keh/keh tahl)*
When?	¿Cuándo?	*(Koo-ahn-doh)*
Where?	¿Dónde?	*(Dohn-deh)*
Why?	¿Por qué?	*(Pohr keh)*
For whom?	¿Para quién?	*(Pah-rah kee-ehn)*
For what?	¿Para qué?	*(Pah-rah keh)*

Which?	¿Cuál?	*(Koo-ahl)*
Who?	¿Quién?	*(Kee-ehn)*
How many?	¿Cuántos?	*(Koo-ahn-tohs)*
How much?	¿Cuánto?	*(Koo-ahn-toh)*
What is it?	¿Qué es?	*(Keh ehs)*
What happens?	¿Qué pasa?	*(Keh pah-sah)*
What's going on?	¿Qué pasa?	*(Keh pah-sah)*
Why not?	¿Por qué no?	*(Pohr keh noh)*
Since when?	¿Desde cuándo?	*(Dehs-deh koo-ahn-doh)*
Do you understand?	¿Comprende? ¿Entiende?	*(Kohm-prehn-deh) (Ehn-tee-ehn-deh)*
Always!	¡Siempre!	*(See-ehm-preh)*
Never!	¡Nunca!	*(Noon-kah)*
None!	¡Ninguno!	*(Neen-goo-noh)*
Do you want the bedpan?	¿Quiere el pato/ el bacín?	*(kee-eh-reh ehl pah-toh/ehl bah-seen)*
Do you wish to pass urine?	¿Quiere orinar?	*(Kee-eh-reh oh-ree-nahr)*
Do you wish to have a bowel movement?	¿Quiere evacuar/hacer del baño?	*(Kee-eh-reh eh-bah-koo-ahr/ah-sehr dehl bah-nyoh)*
Do you want:	¿Quiere:	*(Kee-eh-reh)*
A glass of water?	Un vaso de agua?	*(Oon bah-soh deh ah-goo-ah)*
A glass of juice?	Un vaso de jugo?	*(Oon bah-soh deh hoo-goh)*
Do you want:	¿Quiere:	*(Kee-eh-reh:*
Something to eat?	Algo de comer?	*(Ahl-goh deh koh-mehr)*
Something to drink?	Algo de tomar/beber?	*(Ahl-goh deh toh-mahr/ beh-behr)*
Something to read?	Algo de leer?	*(Ahl-goh deh leh-ehr)*
Are you cold?	¿Tiene frío?	*(Tee-eh-neh free-oh)*
Are you hot?	¿Tiene calor?	*(Tee-eh-neh kah-lohr)*
Are you hungry?	¿Tiene hambre?	*(Tee-eh-neh ahm-breh)*
Are you sleepy?	¿Tiene sueño?	*(Tee-eh-neh soo-eh-nyoh)*
Are you thirsty?	¿Tiene sed?	*(Tee-eh-neh sehd)*
Is that enough?	¿Es suficiente?	*(Ehs soo-fee-see-ehn-teh)*
Is that a lot?	¿Es mucho?	*(Ehs moo-choh)*

Is that too much?	¿Es demasiado?	*(Ehs-deh-mah-see-ah-doh)*
Are you comfortable?	¿Está cómoda?	*(Ehs-tah koh-moh-dah)*
Can you feel this?	¿Siente esto?	*(See-ehn-teh ehs-toh)*
Don't worry!	¡No se preocupe!	*(Noh seh preh-oh-koo-peh)*
Be patient!	¡Tenga paciencia!	*(Tehn-gah pah-see-ehn-see-ah)*

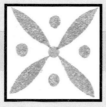

CHAPTER THIRTY-ONE
Phrases

CAPITULO
TREINTA Y UNO
Frases

Phrases consist of a series of words that add "feeling" to a short conversation. They can also mean more than what is expressed. For example, if you ask a person, "How are you?" and he/she replies, "Marvelous," we should understand that this individual feels well and is happy.

Las frases son una serie de palabras que le dan "sentido" a una conversación corta. Significan más de lo que se expresa en ellas. Por ejemplo, al preguntarle a una persona, "¿Cómo se siente?" y nos contesta "Maravilloso(a)" debemos entender que este individuo se siente muy bien y está contento.

to find out. . .   descubrir. . .
(dehs-koo-breehr)

from time to time. . .   de vez en cuando. . .
(deh behs ehn koo-ahn-doh)

for the most part. . .   por la mayor parte. . .
(pohr lah mah-yohr pahr-teh)

deal with. . .   tratar. . .
(trah-tahr)

Don't be afraid!   ¡No tenga miedo!
(Noh tehn-gah mee-eh-doh)

call for. . .   llamar. . .
(yah-mahr)

as a whole. . .   en conjunto. . . /en todo. . .
(ehn kohn-hoon-toh/ehn toh-doh)

according to. . .	de acuerdo con. . . *(deh ah-koo-ehr-doh kohn)*
to go through. . .	atravesar. . . /cruzar. . . *(ah-trah-beh-sahr/kroo-sahr)*
to go by. . .	pasar. . . *(pah-sahr)*
gain by. . .	ganar con. . . *(gah-nahr kohn)*
helpful. . .	útil. . . *(oo-teel)*
in addition. . .	además. . . *(ah-deh-mahs)*
in large part. . .	en gran parte. . . *(ehn grahn pahr-teh)*
in the middle of. . .	a mediados de. . . *(ah meh-dee-ah-dohs deh)*
all of a sudden. . .	de golpe. . . *(deh gohl-peh)*
to keep up. . .	continuar. . . *(kohn-tee-noo-ahr)*
to leave behind. . .	abandonar. . . *(ah-bahn-doh-nahr)*
to meet with. . .	encontrarse con. . . *(ehn-kohn-trahr-seh kohn)*
Never mind.	No importa. *(Noh eem-pohr-tah)*
nonetheless. . .	sin embargo. . . *(seen ehm-bahr-goh)*
not at all. . .	de ningún modo. . . *(deh neen-goon moh-doh)*
Of course.	Desde luego. *(Dehs-deh loo-eh-goh)*
registered/on record. . .	registrado. . . *(reh-hees-trah-doh)*
over a period. . .	durante un período. . . *(doo-rahn-teh oon peh-ree-oh-doh)*
On the one hand. . .	Por un lado. . . *(Pohr oon lah-doh)*
to point out. . .	señalar. . ./apuntar. . . *(seh-nyah-lahr/ah poon-tahr)*
modern/present day. . .	moderno. . . *(moh-dehr-noh)*
each hour. . .	cada hora. . . *(kah-dah oh-rah)*
every 2 hours. . .	cada dos horas. . . *(kah-dah dohs oh-rahs)*

four times. . .	cuatro veces. . . *(koo-ah-troh beh-sehs)*
recall. . .	recordar. . . *(reh-kohr-dahr)*
rather than. . .	más bien que. . . *(mahs bee-ehn keh)*
rely on. . .	confiar. . . *(kohn-fee-ahr)*
Say it again.	Dígalo otra vez./Repita. *(Dee-gah-loh oh-trah behs/ Reh-pee-tah)*
so far/until now. . .	hasta ahora. . . *(ahs-tah ah-oh-rah)*
select. . .	seleccionar. . . *(seh-lehk-see-oh-nahr)*
sort out. . .	escoger. . . *(ehs-koh-hehr)*
such as. . .	tal como. . . *(tahl koh-moh)*
thought to be/considering. . .	considerando. . . *(kohn-see-deh-rahn-doh)*
to some extent. . .	hasta cierto punto. . . *(ahs-tah see-ehr-toh poon-toh)*
Try again!	¡Pruebe otra vez! *(Proo-eh-beh oh-trah behs)*
buzzing in the ears. . .	zumbido en los oídos. . . *(soom-bee-doh ehn lohs oh-ee-dohs)*
sore throat. . .	dolor de garganta. . . *(doh-lohr deh gahr-gahn-tah)*
toothache. . .	dolor de muelas. . . *(doh-lohr deh moo-eh-lahs)*
difficulty in swallowing. . .	dificultad al tragar. . . *(dee-fee-kool-tahd ahl trah-gahr)*
I am continuously. . .	Continuamente estoy. . . *(Kohn-tee-noo-ah-mehn-teh ehs-toh-ee)*
Have you had this happen before?	¿Le ha pasado esto antes? *(Leh ha pah-sah-doh ehs-toh ahn-tehs)*
Don't worry.	No se preocupe. *(Noh seh preh-oh-koo-peh)*
See you later!	¡Hasta luego! *(Ahs-tah loo-eh-goh)*

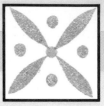

CHAPTER THIRTY-TWO
Numbers

CAPITULO
TREINTA Y DOS
Números

Numbers are as important as nouns and verbs. Everybody needs numbers to buy, sell, mention dates, indicate hours of the day, determine temperature, and state measurements and quantities. Numbers are also needed to make phone calls, to use in all the sciences and thousands of other things. There is a difference between knowing the numbers and how to use them. In medicine, especially, errors can be made if we do not take numbers seriously.

Los números son tan importantes como los nombres y los verbos. Todas las personas necesitamos números para comprar, vender, mencionar fechas, indicar la hora del día, determinar la temperatura y expresar medidas y cantidades. También los números son necesarios para telefonear, para todas las ciencias y para miles de cosas más. Hay diferencia entre saber los números y el saber usarlos. Especialmente en la medicina, se pueden cometer muchos errores si no tomamos en serio a los números.

1	one	uno	(oo-noh)
2	two	dos	(dohs)
3	three	tres	(trehs)
4	four	cuatro	(koo-ah-troh)
5	five	cinco	(seen-koh)
6	six	seis	(seh-ees)
7	seven	siete	(see-eh-teh)
8	eight	ocho	(oh-choh)
9	nine	nueve	(noo-eh-beh)

10	ten	diez	*(dee-ehs)*
11	eleven	once	*(ohn-seh)*
12	twelve	doce	*(doh-seh)*
13	thirteen	trece	*(treh-seh)*
14	fourteen	catorce	*(kah-tohr-seh)*
15	fifteen	quince	*(keen-seh)*
16	sixteen	dieciséis	*(dee-ehs-ee-seh-ees)*
17	seventeen	diecisiete	*(dee-ehs-ee-see-eh-teh)*
18	eighteen	dieciocho	*(dee-ehs-ee-oh-choh)*
19	nineteen	diecinueve	*(dee-ehs-ee-noo-eh-beh)*
20	twenty	veinte	*(beh-een-teh)*

After number 20, use the root of the number (20) and add the first nine numbers in order. See Table 32-1.

Después del número veinte, use la raíz del número (*veinte*) y agregue los primeros nueve números en orden. Vea la Tabla 32-1.

30	thirty	treinta	*(treh-een-tah)*
40	forty	cuarenta	*(koo-ah-rehn-tah)*
50	fifty	cincuenta	*(seen-koo-ehn-tah)*
60	sixty	sesenta	*(seh-sehn-tah)*
70	seventy	setenta	*(seh-tehn-tah)*
80	eighty	ochenta	*(oh-chehn-tah)*
90	ninety	noventa	*(noh-behn-tah)*
100	one hundred	cien	*(see-ehn)*

When forming hundreds, you will use 2, 3, 4, 6, 8 numbers and add the word **cientos**. See Table 32-2.

TABLE 32-1 Add the Roots
TABLA 32-1 Agregue la raíz

English	Spanish	Pronunciation
twenty-one	veintiuno	*beh-een-tee-oo-noh*
twenty-two	veintidós	*beh-een-tee-dohs*
twenty-three	veintitrés	*beh-een-tee-trehs*
twenty-four	veinticuatro	*beh-een-tee-koo-ah-troh*
twenty-five	veinticinco	*beh-een-tee-seen-koh*
twenty-six	veintiséis	*beh-een-tee-seh-ees*
twenty-seven	veintisiete	*beh-een-tee-see-eh-teh*
twenty-eight	veintiocho	*beh-een-tee-oh-choh*
twenty-nine	veintinueve	*beh-een-tee-noo-eh-beh*

TABLE 32-2	In the Hundreds
TABLA 32-2	En los Cientos

English	Spanish	Pronunciation
two hundred	doscientos	*doh-see-ehn-tohs*
three hundred	trescientos	*treh-see-ehn-tohs*
four hundred	cuatrocientos	*koo-ah-troh-see-ehn-tohs*
five hundred	quinientos	*kee-nee-ehn-tohs*
six hundred	seiscientos	*seh-ee-see-ehn-tohs*
seven hundred	setecientos	*seh-teh-see-ehn-tohs*
eight hundred	ochocientos	*oh-choh-see-ehn-tohs*
nine hundred	novecientos	*noh-beh-see-ehn-tohs*

Cuando se forman números en los cientos, usará 2, 3, 4, 6, 8 y agregue la palabra "cientos". Vea la Tabla 32-2.

Larger numbers are easier to deal with. You add the first nine numbers before or after. See below.

Los números mayores ofrecen menos problemas. A la raíz se le agregan los primeros números antes o después. Vea abajo.

1000	one thousand	mil	*(meel)*
1001	one thousand one	mil uno	*(meel oo-noh)*
2000	two thousand	dos mil	*(dohs meel)*
2002	two thousand two	dos mil dos	*(dohs meel dohs)*

In medicine we use fractions. It is necessary to know exact quantities since dosages vary, especially for children. See below.

En medicina usamos números fraccionados. Es necesario saber las cantidades exactas ya que las dosis varían mucho, especialmente para niños. Vea abajo.

$\frac{1}{3}$	one third	un tercio	*(oon tehr-see-oh)*
$\frac{1}{4}$	one fourth	un cuarto	*(oon koo-ahr-toh)*
$\frac{1}{2}$	one half	un medio	*(oon meh-dee-oh)*
$\frac{3}{4}$	three fourths	tres cuartos	*(trehs koo-ahr-tohs)*

When there is a need to emphasize degree or a category of items or persons, you must use ordinal numbers as listed below.

Cuando hay necesidad de enfatizar ciertos grados o categorías se deben usar los números ordinales como se enlistan abajo. ·

1st	first	**primero(a)**	*(pree-meh-roh[rah])*
2nd	second	**segundo(a)**	*(seh-goon-doh[dah])*
3rd	third	**tercero(a)**	*(tehr-seh-roh[rah])*
4th	fourth	**cuarto(a)**	*(koo-ahr-toh[tah])*
5th	fifth	**quinto(a)**	*(keen-toh[tah])*
6th	sixth	**sexto(a)**	*(sehx-toh[tah])*
7th	seventh	**séptimo(a)**	*(sehp-tee-moh[mah])*
8th	eighth	**octavo(a)**	*(ohk-tah-boh[bah])*
9th	ninth	**noveno(a)**	*(noh-beh-noh[nah])*
10th	tenth	**décimo(a)**	*(deh-see-moh[mah])*

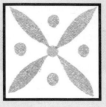

CHAPTER THIRTY-THREE
Time

CAPITULO
TREINTA Y TRES
Tiempo

Time is so important throughout the world that all of us want to know "What time is it?," "At what time do we eat?," "At what time do we go to the movies?" and millions of other questions. Time varies depending on the country where you reside. There are places where time schedules are very different. So, if we wish to travel to far-away places, we must consult our travel agent or a time chart that shows the standard times in various parts of the world with reference to a specified place. In hospitals, time is of the essence, since we can save or lose a life in seconds.

El tiempo es tan importante en el mundo entero que todos queremos saber "¿Qué hora es?," "¿A qué horas comemos?," "¿A qué horas nos vamos al cine?" y un millón de otras preguntas. El tiempo varía de acuerdo al país donde nos encontremos. Hay lugares en los que el horario es muy diferente. Por lo tanto, debemos consultar con nuestro agente de viajes o un esquema que muestre la hora estándar oficial en varias partes del mundo con referencia a un lugar específico. En los hospitales, el tiempo es la esencia, ya que una vida se puede salvar o perder en segundos.

In many hospitals standard time is used. In others, military time is used after noon. See below to compare.

En muchos hospitales se usa la hora estándar. En otros se usa el horario militar después del mediodía. Vea abajo para comparar.

TIME	STANDARD	MILITARY (PM hours)
one o'clock	la una *(lah oo-nah)*	las trece horas *(lahs treh-seh oh-rahs)*
two o'clock	las dos *(lahs dohs)*	las catorce horas *(lahs kah-tohr-seh oh-rahs)*
three o'clock	las tres *(lahs trehs)*	las quince horas *(lahs keen-seh oh-rahs)*
four o'clock	las cuatro *(lahs koo-ah-troh)*	las dieciséis horas *(lahs dee-ehs-ee-seh-ees oh-rahs)*
five o'clock	las cinco *(lahs seen-koh)*	las diecisiete horas *(lahs dee-ehs-ee-see-eh-teh oh-rahs)*
six o'clock	las seis *(lahs seh-ees)*	las dieciocho horas *(lahs dee-ehs-ee-oh-choh oh-rahs)*
seven o'clock	las siete *(lahs see-eh-teh)*	las diecinueve horas *(lahs dee-ehs-ee-noo-eh-beh oh-rahs)*
eight o'clock	las ocho *(lahs oh-choh)*	las veinte horas *(lahs beh-een-teh oh-rahs)*
nine o'clock	las nueve *(lahs noo-eh-beh)*	las veintiuna horas *(lahs beh-een-tee-oo-nah oh-rahs)*
ten o'clock	las diez *(lahs dee-ehs)*	las veintidós horas *(lahs beh-een-tee-dohs oh-rahs)*
eleven o'clock	las once *(lahs ohn-seh)*	las veintitrés horas *(lahs beh-een-tee-trehs oh-rahs)*
noon/midnight	las doce *(lahs doh-seh)*	las cero horas *(lahs seh-roh oh-rahs)*

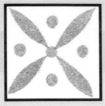

CHAPTER THIRTY-FOUR
The Colors, the Seasons

CAPITULO
TREINTA Y CUATRO
Los Colores,
las Estaciones del Año

COLORS

COLORES

Colors are used frequently in medicine. In daily care, the physician notes the condition of the patient through observation of the color of the skin, hair, eyes, tongue, lips, etc. Colors also assist in making a medical diagnosis. For example, when one notices a reddish tint in the urine, one thinks that it may be caused by kidney problems.

Los colores se utilizan a menudo en el área médica. En el cuidado diario, el médico observa la condición del paciente y vigila el color de la piel, pelo, ojos, lengua, labios, etc. Los colores también apoyan el diagnóstico médico. Por ejemplo, al notar una orina color rojizo, esto indica que hay problemas de riñón.

yellow	amarillo	*(ah-mah-ree-yoh)*
amber	ámbar	*(ahm-bahr)*
clear	claro	*(klah-roh)*
white	blanco	*(blahn-koh)*
albino	albino	*(ahl-bee-noh)*
brown	café	*(kah-feh)*
brown (skin tone)	moreno	*(moh-reh-noh)*

hazel	castaño	*(kahs-tah-nyoh)*
gold	dorado	*(doh-rah-doh)*
emerald	esmeralda	*(ehs-meh-rahl-dah)*
gray	gris	*(grees)*
grayish-white	canoso	*(kah-noh-soh)*
orange	naranja	*(nah-rahn-hah)*
black	negro	*(neh-groh)*
blue	azul	*(ah-sool)*
red	rojo	*(roh-hoh)*
pink	rosa	*(roh-sah)*
blonde	rubio	*(roo-bee-oh)*
green	verde	*(behr-deh)*
violet	violeta	*(bee-oh-leh-tah)*

THE SEASONS

LAS ESTACIONES DEL AÑO

We also use the seasons of the year to guide us during our practice. The human body reacts differently when exposed to temperature variations: cold, warm, hot. These variations cause the skin to be sweaty, dry, or warm. One can detect potential dangers such as dehydration or burns caused by very low temperatures.

También usamos las estaciones del año para guiar nuestra práctica. El cuerpo humano reacciona de manera diferente cuando se expone a variaciones en la temperatura, tales como el frío, a

TABLE 34-1 Descriptive Words
TABLA 34-1 Palabras Descriptivas

English	Spanish	Pronunciation
opaque	opaco	*oh-pah-koh*
transparent	transparente	*trahns-pah-rehn-teh*
grayish	grisáseo	*gree-sah-seh-oh*
icteric	ictérico	*eek-teh-ree-koh*
pinkish	rosado	*roh-sah-doh*
amber	ambarino	*ahm-bah-ree-noh*
orangy	anaranjado	*ah-nah-rahn-hah-doh*
bluish	azuloso	*ah-soo-loh-soh*
cianotic	cianótico/violáceo	*see-ah-noh-tee-koh/bee-oh-lah-se-oh*
pale	pálido	*pah-lee-doh*

humedad o el calor. Estas variaciones causan que la piel se sienta caliente, húmeda, fría, o seca. Uno puede detectar posibles peligros tales como la deshidratación por el calor durante el verano, o las quemaduras causadas por una temperatura muy baja en el invierno.

SEASON	ESTACIÓN	*(EHS-TAH-SEE-OHN)*
spring	primavera	*(pree-mah-beh-rah)*
summer	verano	*(beh-rah-noh)*
fall	otoño	*(oh-toh-nyoh)*
winter	invierno	*(een-bee-ehr-noh)*

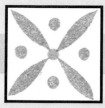

CHAPTER THIRTY-FIVE
The Months, the Days,
the Cardinal Points

CAPITULO
TREINTA Y CINCO
Los Meses, los Días,
Puntos Cardinales

THE MONTHS

LOS MESES

Months become important during a pregnancy, since one can calculate a tentative delivery date. One can program the instruction for the mother and prepare her for the birth date. Also, months help us watch the growth and development of babies since they require scheduled vaccinations at specific times in their lives. In our personal lives, the months indicate all the dates that are important to us when we plan vacations, celebrations, and anniversaries.

Los meses son importantes durante el embarazo, ya que se puede calcular una fecha probable de parto. Se puede entonces programar la educación de la madre y prepararla para el evento del parto. También los meses nos ayudan a vigilar el desarrollo de los bebés ya que ellos requieren de vacunación en cierto tiempo de su vida. Los meses indican, en la vida personal, todas las fechas y eventos que tienen importancia y por los cuales disfrutamos de vacaciones, festejos, y aniversarios.

MONTH	MES	(MEHS)
January	enero*	(eh-neh-roh)
February	febrero	(feh-breh-roh)
March	marzo	(mahr-soh)
April	abril	(ah-breel)
May	mayo	(mah-yoh)
June	junio	(hoo-nee-oh)
July	julio	(hoo-lee-oh)
August	agosto	(ah-gohs-toh)
September	septiembre	(sehp-tee-ehm-breh)
October	octubre	(ohk-too-breh)
November	noviembre	(noh-bee-ehm-breh)
December	diciembre	(dee-see-ehm-breh)

THE DAYS OF THE WEEK

LOS DIAS DE LA SEMANA

The use of days is indispensable in a hospital. We use them in all the medical records, appointments, visits to the laboratory, x-ray department, rehabilitation, or home visits. The days serve as a control. We use the number of hospital days to determine the cost of a hospitalization.

El uso de los días es indispensable en un hospital. Se usan en todas las notas de evolución de los pacientes, citas en el laboratorio, departamento de rayos X, rehabilitación o visitas comunitarias. Los días sirven para controlar la estancia del paciente en el hospital. Se usa el número de días de estancia para determinar el costo de la hospitalización.

DAY	DIA	(DEE-AH)
Monday	lunes*	(loo-nehs)
Tuesday	martes	(mahr-tehs)
Wednesday	miércoles	(mee-ehr-koh-lehs)
Thursday	jueves	(hoo-eh-behs)
Friday	viernes	(bee-ehr-nehs)
Saturday	sábado	(sah-bah-doh)
Sunday	domingo	(doh-meen-goh)

*The names of months and days of the week are not capitalized in Spanish.

CARDINAL POINTS

PUNTOS CARDINALES

Cardinal points serve as orientation, especially when one asks for directions.

Los puntos cardinales sirven de orientación, especialmente cuando uno requiere direcciones.

North	norte	*(nohr-teh)*
South	sur	*(soor)*
East	este	*(ehs-teh)*
West	oeste	*(oh-ehs-teh)*

UNIT 6

Grammar

UNIDAD 6

La Gramática

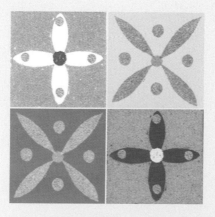

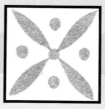

CHAPTER THIRTY-SIX
Alphabet

CAPITULO
TREINTA Y SEIS
Abecedario

The alphabet consists of a series of letters in a language in alphabetical order. It is also used as a manual for deaf and mute persons who use it with finger signals so they can be understood. In 1994 authors at the Royal Spanish Academy omitted the separate use of Ch, Ll, and Rr and incorporated them into the C, L, and R sections in dictionaries. These letters are included here only to facilitate their pronunciation.

El abecedario es una serie de letras de un idioma en orden alfabético. También se usa como un manual en personas sordomudas que lo emplean con signos en los dedos de sus manos para darse a entender con las personas. En 1994 los autores de la Real Academia Española omitieron el uso separado de las letras Ch, L, y Rr y las incorporaron a las secciones C, L, y R en los diccionarios. Estas letras se incluyen aquí sólo para facilitar la pronunciación.

A	**B**	**C**	**Ch**	**D**	**E**
ah	*beh*	*seh*	*Cheh*	*deh*	*eh*
(arm)	(bell)	(casette)	(change)	(day)	(bet)

F	**G**	**H**	**I**	**J**	**K**
eh-feh	*heh*	*ah-cheh*	*ee*	*hoh-tah*	*kah*
(efeminate)	(hen)		(dear)	(holly)	(car)

L	**Ll**	**M**	**N**	**Ñ**	**O**
eh-leh	*eh-yeh*	*eh-meh*	*eh-neh*	*eh-nyeh*	*oh*
(electric)		(emeritus)	(energy)		(opera)

P	Q	R	Rr	S	T
peh	*koo*	*eh-reh*	*doh-bleh*	*eh-seh*	*teh*
(pay)	(cook)	(air)	*eh-reh*	(essence)	(tell)

U	V	W	X	Y	Z
oo	*beh*	*doh-bleh-*	*eh-kees*	*ee gree-eh-gah*	*seh-tah*
(oo)	(verdict)	oo			(gazette)

RULES FOR PRONUNCIATION

REGLAS PARA LA PRONUNCIACIÓN

Spanish is pronounced as it is written. Pay special attention to the five vowel sounds:

El español se escribe como se pronuncia. Ponga atención particularmente a los cinco sonidos de las vocales:

A (ah)	asma *(ahs-mah)*	asthma
E (eh)	vena *(beh-nah)*	vein
I (ee)	herida *(eh-ree-dah)*	wound
O (oh)	obeso *(oh-beh-soh)*	fat
U (oo)	úlcera *(ool-seh-rah)*	ulcer

Now pay attention to the consonants.
Ahora ponga atención a las consonantes.

C	célula *(seh-loo-lah)*	cell
C	ciencia *(see-ehn-see-ah)*	science
C	cama *(kah-mah)*	bed
C	comer *(koh-mehr)*	to eat
C	cuerpo *(koo-ehr-poh)*	body
C	crisis *(kree-sees)*	crisis
CH	chancro *(chahn-kroh)*	chancre
D	dosis *(doh-sees)*	dose
F	fiebre *(fee-eh-breh)*	fever
G	genital *(heh-nee-tahl)*	genital
G	gingivitis *(heen-hee-bee-tees)*	gingivitis
G	gangrena *(gahn-greh-nah)*	gangrene
G	gota *(goh-tah)*	gout
G	gusto *(goos-toh)*	taste
G	glaucoma *(glah-oo-koh-mah)*	glaucoma
H*	hernia *(ehr-nee-ah)*	hernia
J	jeringa *(heh-reen-gah)*	syringe

*Note that the *h* is always silent.

K	**kilogramo** *(kee-loh-grah-moh)*	kilogram
L	**laringitis** *(lah-reen-hee-tees)*	laryngitis
LL	**llorar** *(yoh-rahr)*	to cry
M	**meningitis** *(meh-neen-hee-tees)*	meningitis
N	**náuseas** *(nah-oo-seh-ahs)*	nausea
Ñ	**baño** *(bah-nyoh)*	bath
P	**palpitación** *(pahl-pee-tah-see-ohn)*	palpitation
Q	**quejar** *(keh-hahr)*	to complain
R	**curar** *(koo-rahr)*	to cure
RR	**carro** *(kah-roh)*	car
	hemorragia *(eh-moh-rah-hee-ah)*	hemorrhage
S	**síntomas** *(seen-toh-mahs)*	symptoms
T	**tensión** *(tehn-see-ohn)*	tension
V	**vértigo** *(behr-tee-goh)*	vertigo
W	**watusi** *(oo-ah-too-see)*	watusi
X	**extra** *(ehx-trah)*	extra
Y	**y** *(ee)*	and
Y	**yodo** *(yoh-doh)*	iodine
Z	**zumbido** *(soom-bee-doh)*	buzzing

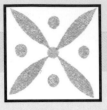

CHAPTER THIRTY-SEVEN
Verbs

CAPITULO
TREINTA Y SIETE
Verbos

Verbs are to a sentence what the spinal cord is to the body. Verbs give structure to a sentence because they tell us what is being done and when it is being done; for example: I *talk* to the nurse (present), I *talked* to the nurse (past), I will *talk* to the nurse (future).

Los verbos son para una oración lo que la espina dorsal es para el cuerpo. Los verbos dan estructura a una oración al indicar qué es lo que se está haciendo y cuándo se está haciendo; por ejemplo: Yo *hablo* con la enfermera (presente), Yo *hablé* con la enfermera ayer (pasado), Yo *hablaré* con la enfermera mañana (futuro).

Regular verbs end in *ar, er,* or *ir* in Spanish. They are easy to conjugate because you usually take the stem of the verb and add the endings *o, as, a, amos, an.* See Table 37-1.

Los verbos regulares tienen la terminación *ar, er, ir* en español. Son fáciles de conjugarse ya que usualmente se toma la raíz del verbo y se le agrega la terminación *o, as, a, amos, an.* Vea la tabla 37-1.

to name	nombrar	*(nohm-brahr)*
to call	llamar	*(yah-mahr)*
to hear/listen	escuchar/oír	*(ehs-koo-chahr/oh-eer)*
to see	ver	*(behr)*
to operate	operar	*(oh-peh-rahr)*
to examine	examinar	*(ehx-ah-mee-nahr)*
to revise	revisar	*(reh-bee-sahr)*
to auscultate	auscultar	*(ah-oos-kool-tahr)*
to palpate	palpar	*(pahl-pahr)*

TABLE 37-1 Regular Verb
TABLA 37-1 Verbo Regular

Verb	Stem	Endings	Persons
	viv-	o	yo vivo *yoh bee-boh*
	viv-	es	tú vives *too bee-behs*
to live			
vivir *(bee-beer)*	viv-	e	el/ella vive *ehl/eh-yah bee-beh*
	viv-	imos	nosotros vivimos *noh-soh-trohs bee-bee-mohs*
	viv-	en	ellos/ellas viven *eh-yohs/eh-yahs bee-behn*

to heal	sanar	*(sah-nahr)*
to get better	mejorar	*(meh-hoh-rahr)*
to become ill	enfermar	*(ehn-fehr-mahr)*
to hurt	doler	*(doh-lehr)*
to vomit	vomitar	*(boh-mee-tahr)*
to die	morir	*(moh-reer)*
to be born	nacer	*(nah-sehr)*
to live	vivir	*(bee-beer)*
to leave (behind)	dejar	*(deh-hahr)*
to eat	comer	*(koh-mehr)*
to bring near	acer car	*(ah-sehr-kahr)*
to remain	quedar	*(keh-dahr)*
to come	venir	*(beh-neer)*
to reach	alcanzar	*(ahl-kahn-sahr)*
to take out	sacar	*(sah-kahr)*
to finish	acabar	*(ah-kah-bahr)*
to walk	caminar	*(kah-mee-nahr)*
to go out	salir	*(sah-leer)*
to let go	soltar	*(sohl-tahr)*
to stop	parar	*(pah-rahr)*
to need	necesitar	*(neh-seh-see-tahr)*
to agree	acordar	*(ah-kohr-dahr)*
to bore	aburrir	*(ah-boo-reer)*
to deserve	merecer	*(meh-reh-sehr)*

| TABLE 37-2 | Present and Past Tense |
| TABLA 37-2 | Tiempo Presente y Pasado |

VERB: to eat   comer *(koh-mehr)*

Present Tense		Tiempo Presente
I eat	yo como	*yoh koh-moh*
you eat	tú comes	*too koh-mehs*
he/she eats	el/ella come	*ehl/eh-yah koh-meh*
we eat	nosotros comemos	*noh-soh-trohs koh-meh-mohs*
they eat	ellos/ellas comen	*eh-yohs/eh-yahs koh-mehn*

Past Tense		Tiempo Pasado
I ate	yo comí	*yoh koh-mee*
you ate	tú comiste	*too koh-mees-teh*
he/she ate	él/ella comió	*ehl/eh-yah koh-mee-oh*
we ate	nosotros comimos	*noh-soh-trohs koh-mee-mohs*
they ate	ellos/ellas comieron	*eh-yohs/eh-yahs koh-mee-eh-rohn*

Personal pronouns designate who is performing the action. Many times it is not necessary to include the personal pronouns when conjugating a verb or using it in a sentence.

Los pronombres personales designan a las personas. Muchas veces no es necesario usar la persona al conjugar verbos o al usarlos en una oración.

PERSONAL PRONOUNS

PRONOMBRES PERSONALES

I	yo	*(yoh)*
you (informal)	tú	*(too)*
he/she/you	él/ella/usted	*(ehl/eh-yah/oos-tehd)*
we	nosotros	*(noh-soh-trohs)*
they/you (plural)	ellos/ellas/ustedes	*(eh-yohs/eh-yahs/ oos-teh-dehs)*

TO FEEL	**SENTIR**	***(SEHN-TEER)***
I feel	siento	*(see-ehn-toh)*
you feel	sientes	*(see-ehn-tehs)*
he/she feels/you feel	siente	*(see-ehn-teh)*
we feel	sentimos	*(sehn-tee-mohs)*
they feel	sienten	*(see-ehn-tehn)*

TO SIT DOWN	**SENTARSE**	**(SEHN-TAHR-SEH)**
I sit	me siento	(meh see-ehn-toh)
you sit	te sientas	(teh see-ehn-tahs)
he/she sits; you sit	se sienta	(seh see-ehn-tah)
we sit	nos sentamos	(nohs sehn-tah-mohs)
they sit	se sientan	(seh see-ehn-tahn)

The reflexive pronouns change the verb's action.
Los pronombres reflexivos cambian la acción del verbo.

Mover (to move)

Action on self	Action on object
yo me muevo	yo muevo
(yoh meh moo-eh-boh)	(yoh moo-eh-boh)
tú te mueves	tú mueves
(too teh moo-eh-behs)	(too moo-eh-behs)
él/ella se mueve	el/ella mueve
(ehl/eh-yah seh moo-eh-beh)	(ehl/eh-yah moo-eh-beh)
nosotros nos movemos	nosotros movemos
(noh-soh-trohs nohs moh-beh-mohs)	(noh-soh-trohs moh-beh-mohs)
ellos/ellas se mueven	ellos/ellas mueven
(eh-yohs/eh-yahs seh moo-eh-behn)	(eh-yohs/eh-yahs moo-eh-behn)

to advise	aconsejar	(ah-kohn-seh-hahr)
to deny	negar	(neh-gahr)
to remember	acordar	(ah-kohr-dahr)
to thank for	agradecer	(ah-grah-deh-sehr)
to loose	perder	(pehr-dehr)
to turn off	apagar	(ah-pah-gahr)
to step	pisar	(pee-sahr)
to drink	beber	(beh-behr)
to take	tomar	(toh-mahr)
to change	cambiar	(kahm-bee-ahr)
to go to bed/to lay down	acostar	(ah-kohs-tahr)
to sleep	dormir	(dohr-meer)
to get up, raise	levantar	(leh-bahn-tahr)
to sit	sentar	(sehn-tahr)
to feel	sentir	(sehn-teer)
to jump	saltar	(sahl-tahr)
to wash	lavar	(lah-bahr)
to clean	limpiar	(leem-pee-ahr)
to bathe	bañar	(bah-nyahr)
to turn	voltear	(bohl-teh-ahr)
to go	ir	(eer)
to do/make	hacer	(ah-sehr)

to promise	prometer	*(proh-meh-tehr)*
to ask	preguntar	*(preh-goon-tahr)*
to communicate	comunicar	*(koh-moo-nee-kahr)*
to respond	responder	*(rehs-pohn-dehr)*
to embrace	abrazar	*(ah-brah-sahr)*
to kiss	besar	*(beh-sahr)*
to believe	creer	*(kreh-ehr)*
to recognize	reconocer	*(reh-koh-noh-sehr)*
to confuse	confundir	*(kohn-foon-deer)*
to remember	recordar	*(reh-kohr-dahr)*
to discover, find	descubrir	*(dehs-koo-breer)*
to joke, kid	bromear	*(broh-meh-ahr)*
to complain	quejar	*(keh-hahr)*
to cry	llorar	*(yoh-rahr)*
to want	querer	*(keh-rehr)*
to wish	desear	*(deh-seh-ahr)*
to give	dar	*(dahr)*
to marry	casar	*(kah-sahr)*
to hunt	cazar	*(kah-sahr)*
to paint	pintar	*(peen-tahr)*
to cook	cocinar	*(koh-see-nahr)*
to build	construir	*(kohns-troo-eer)*
to receive	recibir	*(reh-see-beer)*
to start	comenzar	*(koh-mehn-sahr)*
to conduct	conducir	*(kohn-doo-seer)*
to fix	componer	*(kohm-poh-nehr)*
to destroy	destruir	*(dehs-troo-eer)*
to disappear	desaparecer	*(deh-sah-pah-reh-sehr)*
to find	hallar	*(ah-yahr)*
to break	romper	*(rohm-pehr)*
to cut	cortar	*(kohr-tahr)*
to carry	llevar	*(yeh-bahr)*
to return	regresar	*(reh-greh-sahr)*
to know	conocer	*(koh-noh-sehr)*
to cover	cubrir	*(koo-breer)*
to point	señalar	*(seh-nyah-lahr)*
to serve	servir	*(sehr-beer)*
to eat breakfast	desayunar	*(deh-sah-yoo-nahr)*
to suffer	sufrir	*(soo-freer)*
to shake	temblar	*(tehm-blahr)*
to be afraid	temer	*(teh-mehr)*
to scream	gritar	*(gree-tahr)*
to speak	hablar	*(ah-blahr)*
to employ	emplear	*(ehm-pleh-ahr)*
to take	tomar	*(toh-mahr)*
to work	trabajar	*(trah-bah-hahr)*

TABLE 37-3 Verb Tenses
TABLA 37-3 Tiempo de Los Verbos

Verb	Present Tense	Tiempo Presente
speak	hablar	*ah-blahr*
I speak	yo hablo	*yoh ah-bloh*
you speak	tú hablas	*too ah-blahs*
he/she speaks	el/ella habla	*ehl/eh-yah ah-blah*
we speak	nosotros hablamos	*noh-soh-trohs ah-blah-mohs*
they speak	ellos/ellas hablan	*eh-yohs/eh-yahs ah-blahn*

	Past Tense	Tiempo Pasado
I spoke	yo hablé	*yoh ah-bleh*
you spoke	tú hablaste	*too ah-blahs-teh*
he/she spoke	el/ella habló	*ehl/eh-yah ah-bloh*
we spoke	nosotros hablamos	*noh-soh-trohs ah-blah-mohs*
they spoke	ellos/ellas hablaron	*eh-yohs/eh-yahs ah-blah-rohn*

	Future Tense	Tiempo Futuro
I will speak	yo hablaré	*yoh ah-blah-reh*
you will speak	tú hablarás	*too ah-blah-rahs*
he/she will speak	el/ella hablará	*ehl/eh-yah ah-blah-rah*
we will speak	nosotros hablaremos	*noh-soh-trohs ah-blah-reh-mohs*
they will speak	ellos/ellas hablarán	*eh-yohs/eh-yahs ah-blah-rahn*

to have	haber	*(ah-behr)*
to try	tratar	*(trah-tahr)*
to sell	vender	*(behn-dehr)*
to see	ver	*(behr)*
to boil	hervir	*(ehr-beer)*
to fly	volar	*(boh-lahr)*
to return	volver	*(bohl-behr)*
to fill	llenar	*(yeh-nahr)*
to beat, knock	golpear	*(gohl-peh-ahr)*
to hit	pegar	*(peh-gahr)*
to bleed	sangrar	*(sahn-grahr)*
to activate	activar	*(ahk-tee-bahr)*
to present	presentar	*(preh-sehn-tahr)*
to administer	administrar	*(ahd-mee-nees-trahr)*
to provoke	provocar	*(proh-boh-kahr)*

to authorize	autorizar	*(ah-oo-toh-ree-sahr)*
to reduce	reducir	*(reh-doo-seer)*
to protect	proteger	*(proh-teh-hehr)*
to evaluate	evaluar	*(eh-bah-loo-ahr)*
to accept	aceptar	*(ah-sehp-tahr)*
to write	escribir	*(ehs-kree-beer)*
to interpret	interpretar	*(een-tehr-preh-tahr)*
to control	controlar	*(kohn-troh-lahr)*
to conserve	conservar	*(kohn-sehr-bahr)*
to inform	informar	*(een-fohr-mahr)*
to select	seleccionar	*(seh-lehk-see-oh-nahr)*
to revise	revisar	*(reh-bee-sahr)*
to separate	separar	*(seh-pah-rahr)*
to suspend	suspender	*(soos-pehn-dehr)*

The verbs *ser* and *estar* both translate in English as *to be,* but they are not interchangeable. Both are irregular in the present and the past tense.

Los verbos *ser* y *estar* se traducen al inglés *to be,* pero no se intercambian. Los dos verbos son irregulares en el tiempo presente y en el pasado.

	SER	**ESTAR**
I am	yo soy *(yo soh-ee)*	yo estoy *(yoh ehs-tohy)*
you are	usted es/tú eres *(oos-tehd ehs/too eh-rehs)*	usted está/tú estás *(oos-tehd ehs-tah/ too ehs-tahs)*
he/she/it is	el/ella/eso es *(ehl/eh-yah/eh-soh ehs)*	el/ella/eso está *(ehl/eh-yah/eh-soh ehs-tah)*
we are	nosotros somos *(noh-soh-trohs soh- mohs)*	nosotros estamos *(noh-soh-trohs ehs- tah-mohs)*
they are	ellos/ellas son *(eh-yohs/eh-yahs sohn)*	ellos/ellas están *(eh-yohs/eh-yahs ehs-tahn)*

USES OF *SER*

USOS DE *SER*

Ser expresses a relatively permanent quality.

age:	You are old.	Usted *es* viejo.
characteristic:	The snow is cold.	La nieve *es* fría.

color:	The urine is yellow.	La orina *es* amarilla.
shape:	The glass is round.	El vaso *es* redondo.
size:	You are tall.	Usted *es* alto.
possession:	The pencil is mine.	El lápiz *es* mío.
wealth:	The man is rich.	El hombre *es* rico.

Ser is used with predicate nouns, pronouns, or adjectives.

He is a dentist.	El *es* dentista.
Who am I?	¿Quién *soy* yo?
We are protestant.	Nosotros *somos* protestantes.

Ser indicates material, origin, or ownership.

material:	The needle is metal.	La aguja *es* de metal.
origin:	The doctor is from Texas.	El doctor *es* de Texas.
ownership:	The dentures are mine.	Las dentaduras *son* mías.

Ser tells time.

| It is one o'clock. | *Es* la una. |
| It is 10 o'clock. | *Son* las diez. |

USES OF *ESTAR*

USOS DE *ESTAR*

Estar expresses location (permanent and temporary).

| Dallas is in Texas. | Dallas *está* en Texas. |
| I am in the room. | Yo *estoy* en el cuarto. |

Estar expresses status of health.

How are you?	¿Cómo *está* usted?
I am fine.	*Estoy* bien.
We are sick.	*Estamos* enfermos.

Estar expresses a temporary characteristic or quality.

He is nervous.	El *está* nervioso.
I am ready.	*Estoy* lista.
You are far away.	Usted *está* lejos.

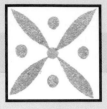

CHAPTER THIRTY-EIGHT
Gender of Nouns

CAPITULO
TREINTA Y OCHO
Género de los
Sustantivos (Nombres)

In Spanish, the gender of a noun corresponds to sex. The name of any male being is masculine, that of a female being is feminine. The grammatical gender of an inanimate object must simply be memorized: *bone* (**el hueso**) is masculine, *head* (**la cabeza**) is feminine, and so on.

En español, el género de los sustantivos (nombres) corresponde al sexo. El nombre de un hombre es masculino, el de una mujer es femenino. El género gramatical de un objeto inanimado se debe memorizar: *hueso* es masculino, *cabeza* es femenina y así sucesivamente.

All Spanish nouns must be masculine or feminine.

En español, todos los sustantivos (nombres) deben ser masculinos o femeninos.

The definite article *the* has the following singular and plural forms in Spanish:

El artículo definitivo *el* tiene las siguientes formas en singular y plural:

el (singular masculine)   la (singular feminine)
los (plural masculine)   las (plural feminine)

The indefinite article *a* or *an* has the following forms in Spanish:

El artículo indefinido *un* tiene las siguientes formas en español:

un (singular masculine)   una (singular feminine)
unos (plural masculine)   unas (plural feminine)

Masculine nouns require a masculine article, feminine nouns require a feminine article.

Los nombres masculinos requieren un artículo masculino, los nombres femeninos requieren un artículo femenino.

the man	el hombre	*(ehl ohm-breh)*
the woman	la mujer	*(lah moo-hehr)*
the boy	el muchacho	*(ehl moo-chah-choh)*
the back	la espalda	*(lah ehs-pahl-dah)*
the friend	el amigo	*(chl ah-mee-goh)*
a rib	una costilla	*(oo-nah kohs-tee-yah)*
the eye	el ojo	*(ehl oh-hoh)*
the bladder	la vejiga	*(lah beh-hee-gah)*
a skeleton	un esqueleto	*(oon ehs-keh-leh-toh)*
the clavicle	la clavícula	*(lah klah-bee-koo-lah)*

An important exception is **la mano**. Note that in spite of the ending *o*, **la mano** is feminine.

Una excepción importante es *la mano*. Note que a pesar de la terminación en *o*, *la mano* es femenina.

Nouns ending in **al, ante, ador**, and **on** are usually masculine.

Los nombres con terminación en *al, ante, ador, y on* son masculinos usualmente.

the hospital	el hospital	*(ehl ohs-pee-tahl)*
the tranquilizer	el tranquilizante	*(ehl trahn-kee-lee-sahn-teh)*
the worker	el trabajador	*(ehl trah-bah-hah-dohr)*
the heart	el corazón	*(ehl koh-rah-sohn)*

The days of the week, months of the year, and the names of languages are masculine.

Los días de la semana, meses del año, y los nombres de los idiomas son masculinos.

Spanish	el español	*(ehl ehs-pah-nyohl)*
Wednesday	el miércoles	*(ehl mee-ehr-koh-lehs)*
the month of April	el mes de abril	*(ehl mehs deh ah-breel)*

Nouns ending in **tad, dad, ción, sión, ez, ie, ud**, and **umbre** are usually feminine.

Los nombres con terminación *tad, dad, ción, sión, ez, ie, ud,* y *umbre* son femeninos usualmente.

the dehydration	la deshidratación	*(lah deh-see-drah-tah-see-ohn)*
the habit	la costumbre	*(lah kohs-toom-breh)*
the age	la edad	*(lah eh-dahd)*
the friendship	la amistad	*(lah ah-mees-tahd)*
the series	la serie	*(lah seh-ree-eh)*
the health	la salud	*(lah sah-lood)*

Nouns ending in *o and a* should be memorized with the definite article.

Los nombres con terminación en *o* y *a* deben memorizarse con el artículo definitivo.

the blood	la sangre	*(lah sahn-greh)*
the penis	el pene	*(ehl peh-neh)*

PLURAL OF NOUNS

EL PLURAL DE LOS SUSTANTIVOS (NOMBRES)

A noun ending in a vowel forms the plural by *s*; those ending in a consonant add *es*.

Para formar el plural de un nombre que termina en una vocal se le agrega una *s*; a los que terminan en una consonante se les agrega *es*.

the physician	el médico	*(ehl meh-dee-koh)*
the physicians	los médicos	*(lohs meh-dee-kohs)*
the doctor	el doctor	*(ehl dohk-tohr)*
the doctors	los doctores	*(lohs dohk-toh-rehs)*

A noun ending in *z* changes to *c* and then adds *es*.

Un nombre que termina en *z* se cambia a una *c* y se le agrega *es*.

the nose	la nariz	*(lah nahr-ees)*
the noses	las narices	*(lahs nahr-ee-sehs)*

Nouns ending in a stressed vowel form the plural by adding *es*.

A los nombres que terminan con énfasis en una vocal se les agrega *es*.

the ruby	el rubí	*(ehl roo-bee)*
the rubies	los rubíes	*(lohs roo-bee-ehs)*

Nouns ending in unstressed *es* or *is* are considered to be both singular and plural. Number is expressed by the article.

Los nombres que terminan sin énfasis en *es* o *is* se consideran singulares y plurales. El número se expresa por el artículo.

Thursday	el jueves	*(ehl hoo-eh-behs)*
Thursdays	los jueves	*(lohs hoo-eh-behs)*

SPECIAL USES OF THE ARTICLES

USOS ESPECIALES DE LOS ARTICULOS

The definite article is used in Spanish, but omitted in English as follows.

El artículo definitivo se usa en español, pero se omite en inglés como sigue:

1. Before the names of languages, except after **hablar, en**, or **de**:
1. Antes de los nombres de idiomas, excepto después de *hablar, en,* o *de*:

Spanish is important.	El español es importante.
	(Ehl ehs-pah-nyohl ehs eem-pohr-tahn-teh)
My friend speaks French.	Mi amigo habla francés.
	(Mee ah-mee-goh ah-blah frahn-sehs)
The whole book is in German.	Todo el libro está en alemán.
	(Toh-doh ehl lee-broh ehs-tah ehn ah-leh-mahn)

2. Before titles, except when addressing the person.
2. Antes de títulos, excepto cuando se dirige a una persona.

Mr. Gomez left yesterday.	El señor Gómez salió ayer.
	(Ehl seh-nyohr Goh-mehs sah-lee-oh ah-yehr)
How are you, Mrs. Garcia?	¿Cómo está, señora García?
	(Koh-moh ehs-tah, seh-nyoh-rah Gahr-see-ah)

The article is omitted before **don, doña, Santo, Santa, San.**

El artículo se omite antes de *don, doña, Santo, Santa, San.*

3. With parts of the body or personal possessions (clothing, etc.)
3. Con partes del cuerpo o posesiones personales (ropa, etc.)

He has black hair.	El tiene pelo negro.
	(Ehl tee-eh-neh peh-loh neh-groh)
Mary has a broken foot.	María tiene el pie quebrado.
	(Mah-ree-ah tee-eh-neh ehl pee-eh keh-brah-doh)

4. With the time of day (*la hora*, the hour; *las horas*, the hours)
4. Con la hora del día (*la hora*, the hour; *las horas*, the hours).

It is one o'clock.	Es la una.
	(Ehs lah oo-nah)
I go to sleep at eleven.	Me duermo a las once.
	(Meh doo-ehr-moh ah lahs ohn-seh)

5. With the names of seasons.
5. Con las estaciones.

I like summer.	Me gusta el verano.
	(Meh goos-tah ehl beh-rah-noh)

6. With the days of the week, except after the verb **ser** *(to be)*.
6. Con los días de la semana, excepto después del verbo ser *(to be)*.

I go downtown (on) Tuesdays.	Los martes voy al centro.
	(Lohs mahr-tehs boy ahl sehn-troh)
Today is Monday.	Hoy es lunes.
	(Oh-ee ehs loo-nehs)

7. Before certain geographic areas.
7. Antes de ciertas areas geográficas.

Canada	el Canadá
	(ehl kah-nah-dah)
Argentina	la Argentina
	(lah ahr-hehn-tee-nah)

NEUTER ARTICLE *LO*

EL ARTÍCULO NEUTRO *LO*

1. The neuter article **lo** precedes an adjective used as a noun to express a quality or an abstract idea.
1. El artículo neutro *lo*, precede un adjetivo que se usa como nombre para expresar una cualidad o una idea abstracta.

I like red (that which is red).	Me gusta lo rojo.
	(Meh goos-tah loh roh-hoh)
I think the same as you.	Pienso lo mismo que usted.
	(Pee-ehn-soh loh mees-moh keh oos-tehd)

2. **Lo** + adjective or adverb + **que** = *how*.
2. *Lo* + el adjetivo o adverbio + *que* = *como*.

I see how good she is.
Ya veo lo buena que es.
(Yah beh-oh loh boo-eh-nah keh ehs)

Since the article *lo* is neuter, it has no plural form. Therefore, *lo* is used whether the adjective is masculine or feminine, singular or plural.

Como el artículo *lo* es neutro, no tiene forma plural. Así que, *lo* se usa aunque el adjetivo sea masculino o femenino.

OMISSION OF THE ARTICLES

OMISION DE LOS ARTICULOS

1. The definite articles are omitted:
1. Los artículos definitivos se omiten:
   A. Before nouns in apposition (that refer to the same noun)
   A. Antes de los nombres en aposición (que se refieren al mismo nombre)
      Austin, the capital of Texas, is at the center of the state.
      Austin, capital de Texas, está en el centro del estado.
   B. Before numerals expressing the numerical order of rulers.
   B. Antes de los números que se refieren a soberanos (monarcas).

Charles the Fifth
Carlos Quinto
(Kahr-lohs Keen-toh)
Mary the Second
María Segunda
(Mah-ree-ah Seh-goon-dah)

2. The indefinite article is omitted before predicate nouns denoting a class or group (social class, occupation, nationality, religion, etc.).
2. El artículo indefinido se omite antes de los nombres predicados que denotan una clase o grupo (clase social, ocupación, nacionalidad, religión, etc.).

He is a barber.
Es barbero.
(Ehs bahr-beh-roh)
I am Mexican.
Soy mexicana.
(Soh-ee meh-hee-kah-nah)
I want to be a nurse.
Quiero ser enfermera.
(Kee-eh-roh sehr ehn-fehr-meh-rah)

If the predicate noun is modified, the indefinite article is stated.
Si el predicado se modifica, el artículo indefinido se indica.

He is a hard-working barber.

Es un barbero muy trabajador.
(Ehs oon bahr-beh-roh moo-ee trah-bah-hah-dohr)

I want to be a good nurse.

Quiero ser una buena enfermera.
(Kee-eh-roh sehr oo-nah boo-eh-nah ehn-fehr-meh-rah)

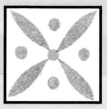

CHAPTER THIRTY-NINE
Adjectives and Pronouns

CAPITULO
TREINTA Y NUEVE
Adjetivos y Pronombres

Adjectives describe nouns and pronouns. In Spanish, adjectives are placed after the noun. They agree in number and gender with the noun they modify.

Los adjetivos describen nombres y pronombres. En español, los adjetivos se colocan después del nombre. Concuerdan en número y género con el nombre que modifican.

Adjectives ending in *o*:
Adjetivos que terminan en *o*:

Masculine singular:	The patient is happy.
	El paciente está contento.
	(Ehl pah-see-ehn-teh ehs-tah kohn-tehn-toh)
Feminine singular:	She is happy.
	Ella está contenta.
	(Eh-yah ehs-tah kohn-tehn-tah)
Masculine plural:	They are happy.
	Ellos están contentos.
	(Eh-yohs ehs-tahn kohn-tehn-tohs)
Feminine plural:	They are happy.
	Ellas están contentas.
	(Eh-yahs ehs-tahn kohn-tehn-tahs)

Adjectives ending in *e*:
Adjetivos que terminan en e:

Masculine singular:	He is sad.
	El está triste.
	(Ehl ehs-tah trees-teh)
Feminine singular:	She is sad.
	Ella está triste.
	(Eh-yah ehs-tah trees-teh)
Masculine plural:	They are sad.
	Ellos están tristes.
	(Eh-yohs ehs-tahn trees-tehs)
Feminine plural:	They are sad.
	Ellas están tristes.
	(Eh-yahs ehs-tahn trees-tehs)

Adjectives ending in a consonant:
Adjetivos que terminan en consonante:

Masculine singular:	The procedure is difficult.
	El procedimiento es difícil.
	(ehl proh-seh-dee-mee-ehn-toh ehs dee-fee-seel)
Feminine singular:	The measurement is difficult.
	La medida es difícil.
	(Lah meh-dee-dah ehs dee-fee-seel)
Masculine plural:	The exams are difficult.
	Los exámenes son difíciles.
	(Lohs ehx-ah-meh-nehs sohn dee-fee-see-lehs)
Feminine plural:	The measurements are difficult.
	Las medidas son difíciles.
	(Lahs meh-dee-dahs sohn dee-fee-see-lehs)

TABLE 39-1   Adjectives That Denote the Feminine or Masculine Gender
TABLA 39-1   Adjetivos que se Acomodan al género del pronombre

Adjective	Feminine	Masculine
this	esta *(ehs-tah)*	este *(ehs-teh)*
these	estas *(ehs-tahs)*	estos *ehs-tohs)*
that	esa *(eh-sah)*	ese *(eh-seh)*
those	esas *(eh-sahs)*	esos *(eh-sohs)*
that	aquella *(ah-keh-yah)*	aquel *(ah-kehl)*
those	aquellas *(ah-keh-yahs)*	aquellos *(ah-keh-yohs)*

Demonstrative adjectives precede the nouns they modify and agree with them in number and gender.

Los adjetivos demostrativos preceden los nombres que modifican y concuerdan con ellos en número y género.

| this book | este libro | *(ehs-teh lee-broh)* |
| these pens | estas plumas | *(ehs-tahs ploo-mahs)* |

Este *this* refers to what is near or directly concerns me.

Este *this* se refiere a lo que está cerca o que me concierne directamente.

Esos *those* refers to what is near or directly concerns you.

Esos *those* se refiere a lo que está cerca o que le concierne directamente.

Aquel *that* refers to what is remote to the speaker or the person addressed.

Aquel *that se refiere a lo que es remoto a la persona que habla (orador)o a la persona que se dirige.*

This pencil is red.	Este lápiz es rojo.
	(Ehs-teh lah-pees ehs roh-hoh)
John, give me that bone.	Juan, déme aquél hueso.
	(Hoo-ahn, deh-meh ah-kehl oo-eh-soh)

Some common limiting adjectives:

Algunos adjetivos comúnes que limitan:

more	mucho, más	*(moo-choh, mahs)*
little, few	poco	*(poh-koh)*
all, everything	todo	*(toh-doh)*
nothing	nada	*(nah-dah)*
one, a, an	un	*(oon)*
first	primero	*(pree-meh-roh)*
fourth	cuarto	*(koo-ahr-toh)*
good	bueno	*(boo-eh-noh)*
bad	malo	*(mah-loh)*
big (age)	grande	*(grahn-deh)*
small (age, it)	pequeño/chico	*(peh-keh-nyoh/chee-koh)*
less	menos	*(meh-nohs)*
better	mejor	*(meh-hohr)*

TABLE 39-2	Personal Pronouns
TABLA 39-2	Pronombres Personales

Singular		Plural	
I	yo *(yoh)*	we (masculine)	nosotros *(noh-soh-trohs)*
		we (feminine)	nosotras *(noh-soh-trahs)*
you (familiar)	tú *(too)*	you	vosotros/as *(boh-soh-trohs/ahs)*
you (formal)	usted *(oos-tehd)*	you	ustedes *(oos-teh-dehs)*
he	él *(ehl)*	they (masculine)	ellos *(eh-yohs)*
she	ella *(eh-yah)*	they (feminine)	ellas *(eh-yahs)*

POSSESSIVE PRONOUNS

PRONOMBRES POSESIVOS

	SINGULAR	PLURAL
mine	el mío, la mía *(ehl mee-oh, lah mee-ah)*	los míos, las mías *(lohs mee-ohs, lahs mee-ahs)*
yours	el tuyo, la tuya *(ehl too-yoh, lah too-yah)*	los tuyos, las tuyas *(lohs too-yohs, lahs too-yahs)*
his, hers, theirs	el suyo, la suya *(ehl soo-yoh, lah soo-yah)*	los suyos, las suyas *(lohs soo-yohs, lahs soo-yahs)*
ours	el nuestro, la nuestra *(ehl noo-ehs-troh, lah noo-ehs-trah)*	los nuestros, las nuestras *(lohs noo-ehs-trohs, lahs noo-ehs-trahs)*

Possessive pronouns are formed by the definite article + the long form of the possessive adjective.

Los pronombres posesivos se forman por el artículo definitivo + la forma larga del adjetivo posesivo.

My nose is prettier than yours.   Mi nariz es más bonita que la tuya.
(Mee nah-rees ehs mahs boh-nee-tah keh lah too-yah)

After the verb *ser*, the article preceding the possessive pronoun is generally omitted.

Después del verbo *ser*, el artículo que precede al pronombre posesivo se omite generalmente.

The bones are mine.	Los huesos son míos.
	(Lohs oo-eh-sohs soh mee-ohs)
That gown is yours.	Aquella bata es suya.
	(Ah-keh-yah bah-tah ehs soo-yah)
These books are mine.	Estos libros son míos.
	(Ehs-tohs lee-brohs sohn mee-ohs)

Possession is expressed by *de* + the possessor. This corresponds to *'s* or *s'* in English.

La posesión se indica por *de + el poseedor. Esto corresponde a 's o s' en inglés.*

his pens and yours	sus plumas y las de usted
	(soos ploo-mahs ee lahs deh oos-tehd)
Martin's pencil	el lápiz de Martín
	(ehl lah-pees deh Mahr-teen)
my book and Louisa's	mi libro y el de Luisa
	(mee lee-broh ee ehl deh Loo-ee-sah)
our patient	nuestro paciente
	(noo-ehs-troh pah-see-ehn-teh)
her rings	sus anillos
	(soos ah-nee-yohs)
a friend of theirs	un amigo de ellos
	(oon ah-mee-goh deh eh-yohs)

WHOSE?

¿DE QUIEN ES?

The interrogative pronoun *whose* is expressed in Spanish by **¿de quién es?**

El pronombre interrogativo *whose* se indica en Español como *¿de quién es?*

Whose pen is it?	¿De quién es la pluma?
	(Deh kee-ehn ehs lah ploo-mah)
It belongs to the doctor.	Es del doctor.
	(Ehs dehl dohk-tohr)
Whose card is it?	¿De quién es la tarjeta?
	(Deh kee-ehn ehs lah tahr-heh-tah)
Mr. García's.	Del señor García.
	(Dehl seh-nyohr Gahr-see-ah)
Whose x-rays are these?	¿De quién son estas radiografías?
	(Deh kee-ehn sohn ehs-tahs rah-dee-oh-grah-fee-ahs)

They are Mrs. Luna's.   Son de la señora Luna.
                                   (Sohn de lah seh-nyoh-rah Loo-nah)

SOME COMMON PREPOSITIONS

ALGUNAS PREPOSICIONES COMÚNES

to, at	a	*(ah)*
about	acerca de	*(ah-sehr-kah deh)*
around	alrededor de	*(ahl-reh-deh-dohr deh)*
in front of	enfrente de/	*(ehn-frehn-teh deh/*
	delante de	*deh-lahn-teh deh)*
within	dentro de	*(dehn-troh deh)*
beneath, under	debajo de	*(deh-bah-hoh deh)*
outside of	fuera de	*(foo-eh-rah deh)*
besides	además de	*(ah-deh-mahs deh)*
far	lejos de	*(leh-hohs deh)*
behind	detrás de	*(deh-trahs deh)*
near	cerca de	*(sehr-kah deh)*
since	desde	*(dehs-deh)*
before	antes de	*(ahn-tehs deh)*
after	después de	*(dehs-poo-ehs deh)*
during	durante	*(doo-rahn-teh)*
with	con	*(kohn)*
in, on	en	*(ehn)*
against	contra	*(kohn-trah)*
from, of	de	*(deh)*
among, between	entre	*(ehn-treh)*
for	para	*(pah-rah)*
toward	hacia	*(ah-see-ah)*
for, by, therefore	por	*(pohr)*
until	hasta	*(ahs-tah)*
according	según	*(seh-goon)*
over, above	sobre	*(soh-breh)*

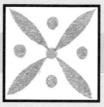

CHAPTER FORTY
Negatives, Affirmatives

CAPITULO CUARENTA
Negativos, Afirmativos

T he principal negative words and their affirmative opposites are:
Las principales palabras negativas y sus opuestas afirmativas son:

EXAMPLES

You do not know the plan.

I see no one here.

I have neither paper nor pencil.

He left without saying anything.

EJEMPLOS

Usted no sabe el plan.
(Oos-tehd noh sah-beh ehl plahn)

No veo a nadie aquí.
(Noh beh-oh ah nah-dee-eh ah-kee)

No tengo ni papel ni lápiz.
*(Noh tehn-goh nee pah-pehl nee
lah-pees)*

Salió sin decir nada.
(Sah-lee-oh seen deh-seer nah-dah)

BUT

PERO/SINO

Though both **pero** *(but, nevertheless)* and **sino** *(on the contrary)* are translated *but*, their use differs as follows: **Sino** is used only if the first clause of the sentence is negative and the second clause is in direct contrast to the first. **Pero** is used in all other cases where *but* is required.

TABLE 40-1	Negatives and Affirmatives
TABLA 40-1	Negativos y Afirmativos

Negative		Affirmative	
no, not	no *(noh)*	yes	sí *(see)*
no one, nobody	nadie *(nah-dee-eh)*	someone, somebody	alguien *(ahl-ghee-ehn)*
nothing	nada *(nah-dah)*	something	algo *(ahl-goh)*
never, not ever	nunca, jamás *(noon-kah, hah-mahs)*	always	siempre *(see-ehm-preh)*
neither	tampoco *(tahm-poh-koh)*	also	también *(tahm-bee-ehn)*
neither/nor	ni/ni *(nee/nee)*	either/or	o/o *(oh oh)*
not one, not any	ninguno *(neen-goo-noh)*	some, any	alguno *(ahl-goo-noh)*
without	sin *(seen)*	with	con *(kohn)*

Aunque *pero* y *sino* se traducen *but*, su uso se distingue como lo siguiente: *sino* se usa sólo si la primera cláusula de la oración es negativa y la segunda cláusula está en contraste directo con la primera. *Pero* se usa en todos los otros casos cuando se requiere.

He doesn't speak English, but Spanish.	No habla inglés, sino español. *(Noh ah-blah een-glehs, see-noh ehs-pah-nyohl)*
He is not wearing a green shirt, but a blue one.	No usa camisa verde, sino azul. *(Noh oo-sah kah-mee-sah behr-deh, see-noh ah-sool)*
I don't like to study, but (rather) to go to the theater.	No me gusta estudiar, sino ir al teatro. *(Noh meh goos-tah ehs-too-dee-ahr, see-noh eer ahl teh-ah-troh)*

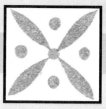

CHAPTER FORTY-ONE
Accents

CAPITULO
CUARENTA Y UNO
Acentos

The acute accent is the only mark of its kind in Spanish. It is a small oblique line (**á**) that is drawn from right to left and specifies a syllable that has a stronger sound when pronouncing it. Accents are used generally to distinguish words written alike and identical in form with other parts of speech, but with a different meaning. For example: **papá** (father), **papa** (vegetable); **café** (drink), **cafe** (color). Accents are sometimes omitted from capital letters.

El acento es la mayor intensidad con que se marca determinada sílaba al pronunciar una palabra. Es una rayita oblicua (á) que se escribe de derecha a izquierda y se coloca en ciertos casos sobre la vocal de la sílaba en que se carga la pronunciación. En español es muy necesario acentuar las palabras para darles el significado correcto que llevan. Por ejemplo: papá (padre), papa (vegetal); café (bebida), cafe (color).

I love	amo	*(ah-moh)*
he loved	él amó	*(ehl ah-moh)*
the owner	el dueño/amo	*(ehl doo-eh-nyoh/ah-moh)*
road	el camino	*(ehl kah-mee-noh)*
he walked	él caminó	*(ehl kah-mee-noh)*
copper	cobre	*(koh-breh)*
I charged	yo cobré	*(yoh koh-breh)*
volumes	volúmenes	*(boh-loo-meh-nehs)*
never	jamás	*(hah-mahs)*
pencil	lápiz	*(lah-pees)*

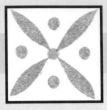

CHAPTER FORTY-TWO
Cognates

CAPITULO CUARENTA Y DOS
Cognados

Similar terms are those in which words are written and/or pronounced almost like others in a different language. These similar terms have very small variations in their spelling. In this chapter, we will mention only those terms useful to the medical practice.

Los términos similares son aquellos en los cuales las palabras se escriben y se pronuncian casi igual en ambos idiomas. Estos términos tienen variaciones muy pequeñas en ortografía. En este capítulo mencionaremos términos útiles en la práctica de la medicina.

abdomen	abdomen	*(ahb-doh-mehn)*
accident	accidente	*(ahk-see-dehn-teh)*
acetic	acético	*(ah-seh-tee-koh)*
acid	ácido	*(ah-see-doh)*
acne	acné	*(ahk-neh)*
acoustic	acústico	*(ah-koos-tee-koh)*
adenoid	adenoide	*(ah-deh-noh-ee-deh)*
adrenalism	adrenalismo	*(ah-dreh-nah-lees-moh)*
air	aire	*(ah-ee-reh)*
alcohol	alcohol	*(ahl-kohl)*
alcoholic	alcohólico	*(ahl-koh-lee-koh)*
allergy	alergia	*(ah-lehr-hee-ah)*
amebic	amébico	*(ah-meh-bee-koh)*
amygdala	amígdala	*(ah-meeg-dah-lah)*
analyze	analizar	*(ah-nah-lee-sahr)*
anemia	anemia	*(ah-neh-mee-ah)*

anesthesia	anestesia	(ah-nehs-teh-see-ah)
angioma	angioma	(ahn-hee-oh-mah)
angle	ángulo	(ahn-goo-loh)
antibiotic	antibiótico	(ahn-tee-bee-oh-tee-koh)
anticoagulant	anticoagulante	(ahn-tee-koo-ah-goo-lahn-teh)
asthma	asma	(ahs-mah)
bacteria	bacteria	(bahk-teh-ree-ah)
barbaric	bárbaro	(bahr-bah-roh)
bradycardia	bradicardia	(brah-dee-kahr-dee-ah)
cafe (coffee)	café	(kah-feh)
caffeine	cafeína	(kah-feh-ee-nah)
callus	callo	(kah-yoh)
calm	calma	(kahl-mah)
cancer	cáncer	(kahn-sehr)
cardiac	cardíaco	(kahr-dee-ah-koh)
caries	caries	(kah-ree-ehs)
carotid	carótida	(kah-roh-tee-dah)
cause	causa	(kah-oo-sah)
cavity	cavidad	(kah-bee-dahd)
chancre	chancro	(chahn-kroh)
chemotherapy	quimioterapia	(kee-mee-oh-teh-rah-pee-ah)
chocolate	chocolate	(choh-koh-lah-teh)
claustrophobia	claustrofobia	(klah-oos-troh-foh-bee-ah)
coagulation	coagulación	(koh-ah-goo-lah-see-ohn)
color	color	(koh-lohr)
coma	coma	(koh-mah)
comatose	comatoso	(koh-mah-toh-soh)
common	común	(koh-moon)
communication	comunicación	(koh-moo-nee-kah-see-ohn)
compromise	compromiso	(kohm-proh-mee-soh)
consultant	consultante	(kohn-sool-tahn-teh)
continued	continuado	(kohn-tee-noo-ah-doh)
control	control	(kohn-trohl)
cortisone	cortisona	(kohr-tee-soh-nah)
deficiency	deficiencia	(deh-fee-see-ehn-see-ah)
dehydration	deshidratación	(deh-see-drah-tah-see-ohn)
delirious	delirio	(deh-lee-ree-oh)
demented	demente	(deh-mehn-teh)
dental	dental	(dehn-tahl)
dentifrice	dentífrico	(dehn-tree-free-koh)
ecchymosis	equimosis	(eh-kee-moh-sees)
eczema	eczema	(ehk-seh-mah)
embolism	embolismo	(ehm-boh-lees-moh)
emetic	emético	(ehm-eh-tee-koh)
employ	emplear	(ehm-pleh-ahr)
English	inglés	(een-glehs)

epilepsy	epilepsia	*(eh-peel-ehp-see-ah)*
error	error	*(eh-rohr)*
exercise	ejercicio	*(eh-hehr-see-see-oh)*
explain	explicar	*(ehx-plee-kahr)*
extraction	extracción	*(ehx-trahk-see-ohn)*
exudate	exudado	*(ehx-oo-dah-doh)*
facial	facial	*(fah-see-ahl)*
fail	fallar	*(fah-yahr)*
false	falso	*(fahl-soh)*
family	familia	*(fah-mee-lee-ah)*
fatal	fatal	*(fah-tahl)*
fever	fiebre	*(fee-eh-breh)*
fibroid	fibroide	*(fee-broh-ee-deh)*
fistula	fístula	*(fees-too-lah)*
form	forma	*(fohr-mah)*
fremitus	frémito	*(freh-mee-toh)*
fresh	fresco	*(frehs-koh)*
frontal	frontal	*(frohn-tahl)*
function	función	*(foon-see-ohn)*
fundamental	fundamental	*(foon-dah-mehn-tahl)*
gastroenteritis	gastroenteritis	*(gahs-troh-ehn-teh-ree-tees)*
generic	genérico	*(heh-neh-ree-koh)*
genial	genial	*(heh-nee-ahl)*
glaucoma	glaucoma	*(glah-oo-koh-mah)*
globule	glóbulo	*(gloh-boo-loh)*
grave	grave	*(grah-beh)*
gynecologist	ginecólogo	*(hee-neh-koh-loh-goh)*
hematoma	hematoma	*(eh-mah-toh-mah)*
hemolysis	hemólisis	*(eh-moh-lee-sees)*
hepatitis	hepatitis	*(eh-pah-tee-tees)*
history	historia	*(ees-toh-ree-ah)*
hygienist	higienista	*(ee-hee-eh-nees-tah)*
ignore	ignorar	*(eeg-noh-rahr)*
impression	impresión	*(eem-preh-see-ohn)*
independence	independencia	*(een-deh-pehn-dehn-see-ah)*
indigestion	indigestión	*(een-dee-hehs-tee-ohn)*
infancy	infancia	*(een-fahn-see-ah)*
infection	infección	*(een-fehk-see-ohn)*
inflammation	inflamación	*(een-flah-mah-see-ohn)*
injection	inyección	*(een-yehk-see-ohn)*
insect	insecto	*(een-sehk-toh)*
instrument	instrumento	*(een-stroo-mehn-toh)*
insulin	insulina	*(een-soo-lee-nah)*
intimate	íntimo	*(een-tee-moh)*
jugular	yugular	*(yoo-goo-lahr)*
just	justo	*(hoos-toh)*

juvenile	juvenil	*(hoo-beh-neel)*
kleptomania	cleptomanía	*(klehp-toh-mah-nee-ah)*
laboratory	laboratorio	*(lah-boh-rah-toh-ree-oh)*
lancet	lanceta	*(lahn-seh-tah)*
laparoscopy	laparoscopía	*(lah-pah-rohs-koh-pee-ah)*
ligament	ligamento	*(lee-gah-mehn-toh)*
linen	lino	*(lee-noh)*
lingual	lingual	*(leen-goo-ahl)*
lithium	litio	*(lee-tee-oh)*
lupus	lupus	*(loo-poos)*
manual	manual	*(mah-noo-ahl)*
material	material	*(mah-teh-ree-ahl)*
maternal	maternal	*(mah-tehr-nahl)*
mathematics	matemáticas	*(mah-teh-mah-tee-kahs)*
medicine	medicina	*(meh-dee-see-nah)*
medication	medicamento	*(meh-dee-kah-mehn-toh)*
medulla	médula	*(meh-doo-lah)*
memory	memoria	*(meh-moh-ree-ah)*
meningitis	meningitis	*(meh-neen-hee-tees)*
minimum	mínimo	*(mee-nee-moh)*
model	modelo	*(moh-deh-loh)*
modern	moderno	*(moh-dehr-noh)*
molar	muela	*(moo-eh-lah)*
moral	moral	*(moh-rahl)*
nasal	nasal	*(nah-sahl)*
nausea	náusea	*(nah-oo-seh-ah)*
neonatal	neonatal	*(neh-oh-nah-tahl)*
nervous	nervioso	*(nehr-bee-oh-soh)*
neurotic	neurótico	*(neh-oo-roh-tee-koh)*
neutral	neutral	*(neh-oo-trahl)*
normal	normal	*(nohr-mahl)*
note	nota	*(noh-tah)*
Novocain	Novocaína	*(Noh-boh-kah-ee-nah)*
nutrition	nutrición	*(noo-tree-see-ohn)*
obsession	obsesión	*(ohb-seh-see-ohn)*
obstruction	obstrucción	*(ohb-strook-see-ohn)*
occipital	occipital	*(ohk-see-pee-tahl)*
occur	ocurrir	*(oh-koo-reer)*
office	oficina	*(oh-fee-see-nah)*
opinion	opinión	*(oh-pee-nee-ohn)*
optic	óptico	*(ohp-tee-koh)*
organ	órgano	*(ohr-gah-noh)*
ovary	ovario	*(oh-bah-ree-oh)*
oxygen	oxígeno	*(ohx-ee-heh-noh)*
palate	paladar	*(pahl-ah-dahr)*
palmar	palmar	*(pahl-mahr)*

palpation	palpación	*(pahl-pah-see-ohn)*
pancreas	páncreas	*(pahn-kreh-ahs)*
panic	pánico	*(pah-nee-koh)*
paralytic	paralítico	*(pah-rah-lee-tee-koh)*
pathogen	patogénico	*(pah-toh-heh-nee-koh)*
pathological	patológico	*(pah-toh-loh-hee-koh)*
pelvis	pelvis	*(pehl-bees)*
pharmacy	farmacia	*(fahr-mah-see-ah)*
philosophy	filosofía	*(fee-loh-soh-fee-ah)*
physique	físico	*(fee-see-koh)*
piece	pieza	*(pee-eh-sah)*
plan	plan	*(plahn)*
porcelain	porcelana	*(pohr-seh-lah-nah)*
practice	práctica	*(prahk-tee-kah)*
prepare	preparar	*(preh-pah-rahr)*
preventive	preventivo	*(preh-behn-tee-boh)*
probable	probable	*(proh-bah-bleh)*
problem	problema	*(proh-bleh-mah)*
pruritic	prurítico	*(proo-ree-tee-koh)*
pubic	púbico	*(poo-bee-koh)*
pulse	pulso	*(pool-soh)*
pure	puro	*(poo-roh)*
pyorrhea	piorrea	*(pee-oh-reh-ah)*
racial	racial	*(rah-see-ahl)*
radical	radical	*(rah-dee-kahl)*
radioactive	radioactivo	*(rah-dee-oh-ahk-tee-boh)*
rare	raro	*(rah-roh)*
rectal	rectal	*(rehk-tahl)*
repel	repeler	*(reh-peh-lehr)*
residue	residuo	*(reh-see-doo-oh)*
resin	resina	*(reh-see-nah)*
respect	respeto	*(rehs-peh-toh)*
rheumatic	reumático	*(reh-oo-mah-tee-koh)*
roseola	roseola	*(roh-seh-oh-lah)*
rubella	rubella	*(roo-beh-lah)*
rubeola	rubéola	*(roo-beh-oh-lah)*
saliva	saliva	*(sah-lee-bah)*
salt	sal	*(sahl)*
sanitary	sanitario	*(sah-nee-tah-ree-oh)*
science	ciencia	*(see-ehn-see-ah)*
scleral	escleral	*(ehs-kleh-rahl)*
sebaceous	sebásceo	*(seh-bah-seh-oh)*
secrete	secretar	*(seh-kreh-tahr)*
selection	selección	*(seh-lehk-see-ohn)*
serology	serología	*(seh-roh-loh-hee-ah)*
sex	sexo	*(sehx-oh)*

sexual	sexual	*(sehx-oo-ahl)*
situation	situación	*(see-too-ah-see-ohn)*
social	social	*(soh-see-ahl)*
solution	solución	*(soh-loo-see-ohn)*
solvent	solvente	*(sohl-behn-teh)*
somatic	somático	*(soh-mah-tee-koh)*
Spanish	español	*(ehs-pah-nyohl)*
spectrum	espectro	*(ehs-pehk-troh)*
spinal	espinal	*(ehs-pee-nahl)*
spirit	espíritu	*(ehs-pee-ree-too)*
stethoscope	estetoscopio	*(ehs-teh-tohs-koh-pee-oh)*
stupor	estupor	*(ehs-too-pohr)*
subaxillary	subaxilar	*(soob-ahx-ee-lahr)*
subnormal	subnormal	*(soob-nohr-mahl)*
substernal	subesternal	*(soob-ehs-tehr-nahl)*
suffer	sufrir	*(soo-freer)*
syncope	síncope	*(seen-koh-peh)*
systole	sístole	*(sees-toh-leh)*
tea	té	*(teh)*
technician	técnico	*(tehk-nee-koh)*
technique	tecnica	*(tehk-nee-kah)*
temporal	temporal	*(tehm-poh-rahl)*
tension	tensión	*(tehn-see-ohn)*
tetanus	tétanos	*(teh-tah-nohs)*
thermometer	termómetro	*(tehr-moh-meh-troh)*
tolerant	tolerante	*(toh-leh-rahn-teh)*
torso	torso	*(tohr-soh)*
treatment	tratamiento	*(trah-tah-mee-ehn-toh)*
tube	tubo	*(too-boh)*
tumor	tumor	*(too-mohr)*
ulcer	úlcera	*(ool-seh-rah)*
union	unión	*(oo-nee-ohn)*
universal	universal	*(oo-nee-behr-sahl)*
urea	urea	*(oo-reh-ah)*
uremia	uremia	*(oo-reh-mee-ah)*
ureteritis	uretritis	*(oo-reh-tree-tees)*
urticaria	urticaria	*(oor-tee-kah-ree-ah)*
use	usar	*(oo-sahr)*
uterus	útero	*(oo-teh-roh)*
uvula	úvula	*(oo-boo-lah)*
vaginal	vaginal	*(bah-hee-nahl)*
vagus	vago	*(bah-goh)*
valve	válvula	*(bahl-boo-lah)*
vapor	vapor	*(bah-pohr)*
varicocele	varicocele	*(bah-ree-koh-seh-leh)*
vein	vena	*(beh-nah)*

venereal	venéreo	*(beh-neh-reh-oh)*
vertebrate	vertebrado	*(behr-teh-brah-doh)*
vertigo	vértigo	*(behr-tee-goh)*
vestibule	vestíbulo	*(behs-tee-boo-loh)*
veterinary	veterinaria	*(beh-teh-ree-nah-ree-ah)*
vinegar	vinagre	*(bee-nah-greh)*
visible	visible	*(bee-see-bleh)*
vision	visión	*(bee-see-ohn)*
vital	vital	*(bee-tahl)*
volume	volumen	*(boh-loo-mehn)*
vomit	vómito	*(boh-mee-toh)*
x-rays	rayos X	*(rah-yohs eh-kiss)*
xiphoid	xifoide	*(see-foh-ee-deh)*
yogurt	yogurt	*(yoh-goohrt)*
zone	zona	*(soh-nah)*
zoology	zoología	*(soh-oh-loh-hee-ah)*
zygomatic	cigomático	*(see-goh-mah-tee-koh)*

Unit 7

Cultural Considerations

Unidad 7

Consideraciones Culturales

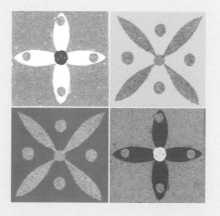

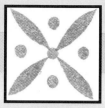

CHAPTER FORTY-THREE
A Cultural Perspective

CAPITULO
CUARENTA Y TRES
Una Perspectiva Cultural

Hispanic is a term often used to identify people who speak Spanish and who have Cuban, Central or South American, Mexican, or Puerto Rican backgrounds. Currently, Mexican Americans and Puerto Ricans are the two largest Hispanic groups in the United States. The movement of Hispanics into the United States seems to have occurred in phases. In 1910 many Mexicans entered the United States with permanent visas. In the early 1940s, the "Bracero" program (source of cheap agricultural labor) increased the Mexican population in the United States. During the 1950s Puerto Ricans were recruited to work as laborers in the United States. In the 1960s many Cubans and Latin Americans migrated to the United States in an attempt to better their social and economic status. A second influx of Cubans occurred in the early 1970s when entire families were ousted or chose to leave communist Cuba. Living conditions in Mexico and in South and Central America have fluctuated considerably over the years, forcing many people to immigrate or to settle illegally in the United States year after year. Although one can find Hispanics throughout the United States, the largest groups are in Arizona, California, Colorado, Florida, New Mexico, New York, and Texas.

As a group, Hispanics have certain similarities. They are young (median age ranges from 17 to 28 years), their median level of education ranges from 9 to 12 years, they are mostly employed in blue-collar jobs (well over 50%), and their median annual income is about $35,050. If one relates the socioeconomic conditions of a group to their level of health, then one can agree that Hispanics (with the preceding statistics), in general, are at risk for health problems. This risk doubles when Hispanics are not able to communicate with health care providers due to language barriers. The use of interpreters is not uncommon. In major university hospitals, where Hispanic patient populations are large, bilingual staff members often act as interpreters. Very often, hospitals refuse to hire interpreters that would facilitate communication; but instead, housekeepers, orderlies, physical plant, or transportation employees are burdened with this additional task. The medical staff who are not able to communicate in Spanish are at a disadvantage because they cannot verify whether the information that the patient is receiving is being translated adequately.

Hispanics have lived in the United States for decades. Many members of the third and fourth generations may not have retained Spanish as their primary language. However, in large cities where Hispanics concentrate, one commonality is evident: the use of Spanish, especially among teenagers and the elderly, is still practiced. Perhaps the current use of Spanish among the young relates to a new influx of Hispanic immigrants.

Hispanics tend to cluster, as do other cultural groups who share similar ethnicity, socioeconomic level, or belief systems. Because Hispanics value camaraderie and rely on familial support systems, they frequently gather in large numbers when one of the members is sick in the hospital. This is often annoying to staff who have to complete myriad of documents, deal with multiple services, and do not understand why so many people insist on visiting the patient even when the crisis is over. Determining the severity of the condition of the patient, reviewing the hospital's policies and procedures, and identifying the benefits/liabilities of having family members present, may help to alleviate the medical staff's confusion caused by the many visitors.

The concept of health varies in many cultures. For most Hispanics being healthy means being free from pain. It also means being able to perform all daily activities. Many think that health is a gift from God and that there is very little that one can do to avoid illness. In all cultures, behavior is learned; and as it is shared through the years, it tends to change and new behaviors are added. For some Hispanics, being sick is viewed as a punishment. Penance may include going to confession, making a long pilgrimage to a church, wearing a habit for a prescribed number of days, or keeping a *promesa/mandas (promise)* made to a patron saint. Some people kneel and "walk" on their knees several blocks to church, thus helping the illness disappear.

Music plays an important role in Hispanic lives. One often hears popular ballads while traveling through Hispanic communities. It is not unusual for hospitalized patients to ask to see a favorite Spanish program. Again, this is not only observed in the elder population, but also in the younger population (teenagers).

A Cultural Perspective

Catholicism is predominant in many Hispanic groups. However, other religions such as Baptist, Jehovah's Witness, and Methodist claim to have large numbers of Hispanic members. It is not unusual to see that some patients may take candles (*veladoras*) or their favorite religious medals to the hospital. Understanding the importance of religion (for any ethnic group) will facilitate the care and treatment of the patient.

Vibrant colors in clothes, jewelry, and make-up are trademarks of Hispanics. These, along with what appear to be loud intonations, rapid speech, and hand movements, often confuse medical staff who may not be aware of Hispanic cultural characteristics. It is extremely important to assess the patient's cultural background before diagnosing the unusual behavior or mannerisms.

Hospital food, traditionally, would not win any awards. Besides not being hot (temperature) it is often too bland (not enough condiments/spices) for Hispanic (and many other) tastes.

It is important to communicate the availability of foods to the patient. It is also helpful to assist in the decision-making process when selecting a menu. Often the patient's religion, ethnicity, age, and illness make it difficult to choose a menu.

Acculturation to a different group is often difficult. While parents may resent having to change, young members of an ethnic group may embrace the new groups' ideologies and way of living. This often causes stress within the family and outside the family. Careful assessment must be made by medical staff who may not be aware of the degree of acculturation of Hispanic patients. This is a great opportunity to provide anticipatory guidance and teaching related to assimilation to a new group.

REFERENCES

Berger PL, Huntington SP: *Many Globalizations: Cultural Diversity in the Contemporary World*. Cambridge, UK, 2002, Oxford University Press.

Clark MJ: *Nursing in the Community*, ed 3, Stamford, CT, 1999, Appleton & Lange.

Friedman MM: *Family Nursing: Theory and Practice*, ed 4, Norwalk, CT, 1998, Appleton & Lange.

Giger JN, Davidhizar RE: *Transcultural Nursing: Assessment and Intervention*. St. Louis, 1999, Mosby.

Hitchcock JE, Schubert PE, Thomas SA: *Community Health Nursing*. Albany, 1999, Del Mar Publishers.

Hooper-Greenhill E, editor: *Cultural Diversity*. Leicester, UK, 2001, Leicester University.

Ignatavicius DD, Workman ML, editors: *Medical Surgical Nursing: Critical Thinking for Collaborative Care*, ed 4, Philadelphia, 2001, Saunders.

Leininger M, McFarland M, McFarland MR: *Transcultural Nursing*, ed 3, New York, 2002, McGraw-Hill.

Maffi L, editor: *On Biocultural Diversity*, Washington, DC, 2001, Smithsonian Institution Press.

O'Loughlin J: Understanding the role of ethnicity in chronic disease: A challenge for the new millennium, *JAMC* 27(7):161–162, 1999.

Purnell LD, Paulanka BJ: *Transcultural Health Care*, Philadelphia, 1998, F.A. Davis Company.

San Antonio Express News. Curanderismo Still Has a Place in Many Homes. September 25, 2000, p.3D.

Spector RE: *Cultural Diversity in Health and Illness*, ed 5, Stamford, CT, 1999, Appleton & Lange.

Stewart M: Nurses need to strengthen cultural competence for the next century to ensure quality patient care, *American Nurse* 30(1):26–27, 1998.

United States Department of Health and Human Services: *Health Status of Minorities and Low-income Groups*, ed 3, Washington, DC, 1991, U.S. Government Printing Office.

U.S. Census Bureau: *Census Data*. Washington, DC, 2000, U.S. Government Printing Office.

Williams SR: *Essentials of Nutrition and Diet Therapy*, ed 7, St. Louis, 1999, Mosby.

Wurzbach ME: *Community Health Education and Promotion*. Gaithersburg, MD, 2002, Aspen Publishers.

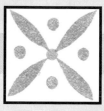

CHAPTER FORTY-FOUR
Home Cures and Popular Beliefs

CAPITULO CUARENTA Y CUATRO
Remedios Caseros y Creencias Populares

Data about cultures have been collected by anthropologists, nursing scientists, sociologists, psychologists, and others with interest in studying behaviors exhibited by different ethnic groups. Since behaviors are learned from generation to generation, it is beneficial to understand a patient's cultural background in order to understand his or her behavior.

In times of crisis or physical distress a patient may revert to treatment modalities used during childhood. During the initial interview, it is not uncommon to find that Hispanic patients favor a variety of home treatment modalities even when complying with Western medical regimes. It is imperative that the health care provider be nonjudgmental regarding these differences in beliefs and practices because it is the patient's perception of the illness that governs his or her behavior. Failure to assess the use of treatment modalities may result in frustration both for the patient and for the health care provider. It is also important not to stereotype patients even within a specific culture. Ideally, each patient must be viewed as a unique individual with care plans that incorporate his or her beliefs and practices.

For years, medicinal plants have been used throughout the world. According to Dr. Hero Gali (1985) there are more than 20,000 plants being used for medicinal purposes in Mexico. It is not difficult to find *hierberías* in open market places where vendors are allowed to recommend dried herbs that have been successful in alleviating certain ailments. Along the Texas-Mexico border, in rural areas, and in larger cities where a high concentration of Mexican Americans is found, many (especially the older generations) still tend to shop at *hierberías* and have specific prescriptions for their ailments. Popular among Hispanics is the use of herbal teas. Chamomile *(manzanilla)*, mint *(hierba buena)*, eucalyptus *(eucalipto)* ginger *(jengibre)*, and vanilla *(vainilla)*, and olive *(olivo)* are often used for common ailments such as colic, colds, cough, and indigestion.

Some folk medicine beliefs and practices can be traced ancient Greece. These beliefs were elaborated on by the Arabs and brought to Spain by the Moslems. Eventually, those beliefs were transmitted to America at the time of the Spanish conquest of Mexico. The combination of Spanish-Catholic tradition in Mexico with the Indian heritage (Aztecs, Mayans, etc.) yields the practice of *curanderismo* as it is observed today.

Expensive and time-consuming treatment is avoided by the lower socioeconomic groups when they visit a *curandero*. The *curandero* successfully integrates concepts and practices from diverse sources. He combines psycho-therapeutic skills and ritualistic herbal remedies. Many of the *curandero's* tools are religious in nature. In his "office" he usually has a large number of crosses and pictures of saints. He centers his thinking about illness on Christ and encourages patients to feel that they are doing what Christ did: suffer on earth. The *curandero* is usually sought for minor illnesses and chronic untreatable conditions that are feared to be supernatural. He is also seen for febrile conditions in children: convulsions, apathy, and disruptive behavior. Most *curanderos* do not charge for their services but they accept donations. The practitioners of *curanderismo* offer no barriers to care and have no waiting lists. This makes it attractive to many patients who do not have insurance or who find the health care system inaccessible. Other Hispanic groups rely on health care providers similar to the *curandero*. *Sobadoras* (female healers) are very popular in Puerto Rico. They use oils *(aceite de culebra, aceite de olivo)* in their treatment of patients. The *sobadoras* combine their listening skills with massage skills to assist the patient.

Acculturation and assimilation of persons of Hispanic origin has been slowed by various social mechanisms of the larger society that tend to keep massive numbers of people separate (in vast housing projects) and by a tendency on their part to separate themselves from the larger community by living in *barrios*. This isolation is not unusual. People tend to group because they find commonalities, acceptance, and comfort within the group. This sociocultural isolation results in the preservation of many folk beliefs of Spanish origin.

Prominent among health disease concepts are *mal de ojo (evil eye)*, *empacho (surfeit/indulgence)*, and *susto (fright)*.

Mal de ojo is an illness to which children and adults are susceptible. When a person with stronger vision looks at another admiringly, but does not touch him, he/she gives the person *mal de ojo*. Symptoms of fever, headache, restlessness, crying, and vomiting are most commonly reported. When the stronger vision person actually touches the other one the symptoms disappear. When the person is not available to touch the other, the treatment of choice is a *sweeping*. To sweep *(barrer)* means both to pass an unbroken raw egg over the body without touching, or actually rub the body with the egg. Prayers are recited during the sweeping. After the sweeping, to extract the fever from the patient's body and transmit it to the egg, the egg is broken and placed in a bowl of water. The bowl is placed under the head of the patient's bed. The egg is said to absorb the fever and, by morning, it should be "cooked." The cooked egg is a sign that the patient had *ojo.*

Empacho is caused by a bolus of poorly digested or uncooked food sticking to the wall of the stomach. This is a disease primarily seen in children and attributed to overeating foods such as bread and bananas. Most common symptoms are lack of appetite, stomachache, diarrhea, and vomiting. Other reported symptoms include fever, crying, and restlessness in children. The treatment includes rubbing the stomach and rubbing and pinching the back. In order to dislodge the bolus, grasp a fold of skin on the back, pull it up, and release it. This procedure is done with both hands at least three times before breakfast. The patient is then administered a tea made with *estafiate* (larkspur) or *manzanilla* (chamomile). It is important to determine how long the child has been ill and what procedures have been performed. There could be intestinal blockage that may lead to toxic megacolon if medical attention is not sought.

Susto is the result of a traumatic experience that may be anything from a simple scare at night (lightning, loud noises) to witnessing an accident. Children are more susceptible than adults, but groups of individuals may develop symptoms at the same time. The most common symptom of *susto* is sleeping. Also, anorexia, insomnia, hallucinations, or weakness often accompany this condition. Treatment of *susto* involves sweeping. The sweeping of the body is generally done by the healer (usually a grandmother) with orange or lemon tree branches or with palm leaves while reciting or chanting prayers. An herbal tea is usually administered after the sweeping.

Hispanics tend to use the "hot and cold" theory of disease. This theory is often used to explain the cause of an ailment and to choose a form of treatment. When a person has a "hot" disease he or she may refuse to eat hot foods, medicines, or hot teas because he or she may think that the condition will worsen. Cold treatments and cold beverages are assumed to be beneficial in this case. On the other hand, when a person has a "cold" disease, he or she may ingest hot teas to alleviate his or her symptoms. Hot and cold diseases are often labeled differently by different cultural groups (Hispanic, Chinese, etc.). It is pertinent to ask a patient, during the history-taking phase of the visit, if he or she has determined to what category a certain disease belongs.

There is a widespread fatalistic attitude among many Hispanics, specifically those in the low-income, low-education segments. Because of lack of education related to health promotion and health prevention, many Hispanics leave their health status "up to God." Many also believe that the hospital is the place where one goes to die. Mr. T., one of our diabetic patients, believed that his son was "murdered" by doctors who gave him too much medicine and thus refused to go to the hospital when he needed help.

Many Hispanics may secure health information and treatment from many sources including relatives, magazines, radio, religion, and tradition. Given a choice, they often consult medical doctors but they may be ingesting their own home remedies. It is appropriate to ask what treatment modalities they have been using prior to the visit. It is important to respect cultural and value differences, and when possible, attempt to incorporate these treatments in the plan of care. Perhaps, if this is done, patient compliance with medical treatment will increase.

REFERENCES

Clark MJ: *Nursing in the Community*, ed 3, Stamford, CT, 1999, Appleton & Lange.

Ellis JR, Hartley CL: *Nursing in Today's World*, ed 4, New York, 1992, Lippincott.

Friedman MM: *Family Nursing: Theory and Practice*, ed 4, East Norwalk, CT, 1998, Appleton & Lange.

Gali H: *Las Hierbas del Indio*. Mexico City, Mexico, 1985, Gomez Gomez Hnos.

Giger JN, Davidhizar RE: *Transcultural Nursing: Assessment and Intervention*, ed 4, St. Louis, 1999, Mosby.

Huff RM, Kline MV: *Promoting Health in Multicultural Populations*, Thousand Oaks, CA, 1999, Sage Publications.

Leininger M, McFarland M, McFarland RM: *Transcultural Nursing*, ed 3, New York, 2002, McGraw-Hill.

Purnell LD, Paulanka BJ: *Transcultural Health Care*, Philadelphia, 1998, F.A. Davis Company.

San Antonio Express News: Curanderismo Still Has a Place in Many Homes. September 25, 2000, p. 3D.

Spector RE: *Cultural Diversity in Health and Illness*, ed 5, Norwalk, CT, 1999, Appleton & Lange.

Torres E: *Green Medicine*, Kingsville, Texas, 1989a, Nieves Press.

Torres E: *The Folk Healer*, Kingsville, Texas, 1989b, Nieves Press.

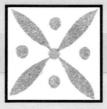

Phrase and Sentence Index

Índice de Frases y Oraciones

A bowel movement.
Hacer del baño.
(Ah-sehr dehl bah-nyoh)

A friend of theirs.
Un amigo de ellos.
(Oon ah-mee-goh deh eh-yohs)

A nurse will see you.
Una enfermera la atenderá.
(Oon-nah ehn-fehr-meh-rah lah ah-tehn-deh-rah)

A pharmacist assists with patient education.
Un farmacéutico asiste con la educación del paciente.
(Oon fahr-mah-seh-oo-tee-koh ah-sees-teh kohn lah eh-doo-kah-see-ohn dehl pah-see-ehn-teh)

A sore that does not heal.
Un grano que no se cura.
(Oon grah-noh keh noh seh koo-rah)

A standard schedule is used.
Se usa un horario estándar.
(Seh oo-sah oon oh-rah-ree-oh ehs-tahn-dahr)

A virus known as HIV.
El virus causal del SIDA se conoce como VIH.
(Ehl bee-roos kah-oo-sahl dehl see-dah seh koh-noh-seh coh-moh bee-ee-ah-cheh)

About 99 degrees today.
Cerca de noventa y nueve grados hoy.
(Sehr-kah deh noh-behn-tah ee noo-eh-beh grah-dohs oh-ee)

About your baby.
En cuanto a su bebé.
(Ehn koo-ahn-toh ah soo beh-beh)

Absence of insulin in the body is called insulin-dependent DM.
A la ausencia de insulina se le llama diabetes insulino-dependiente.
(Ah lah ah-oo-sehn-see-ah deh een-soo-lee-nah seh leh yah-mah dee-ah-beh-tehs een-soo-lee-noh-deh-pehn-dee-ehn-teh)

According to. . .
De acuerdo con. . .
(Deh ah-koo-ehr-doh kohn)

Activities are part of the plan while you are here.
Las actividades son parte del plan de su tratamiento mientras esté aquí.
(Lahs ahk-tee-bee-dah-dehs sohn pahr-teh dehl plahn deh soo trah-tah-mee-ehn-toh mee-ehn-trahs ehs-teh ah-kee)

Administer intravenous fluids and blood.
Administre sueros intravenosos y sangre.
(Ahd-mee-nees-treh soo-eh-rohs een-trah-beh-noh-sos ee sahn-greh)

315

After meals.
Después de las comidas.
(Dehs-poo-ehs deh lahs koh-mee-dahs)

After the bloodwork, you may have
your breakfast.
Después de tomar la muestra, puede
desayunar.
*(Dehs-poo-ehs deh toh-mahr lah moo-
ehs-trah, poo-eh-deh deh-sah-yoo-
nahr)*

After you finish brushing, we will
practice flossing.
Después de terminar de cepillar
practicaremos usando el hilo
dental.
*(Dehs-poo-ehs deh tehr-mee-nahr deh
seh-pee-yahr prahk-tee-kah-reh-mohs
oo-sahn-doh ehl ee-loh dehn-tahl)*

Again.
Otra vez.
(Oh-trah behs)

AIDS has a high fatality rate
approaching 100%.
El SIDA tiene una tasa cercana al 100
por ciento de mortalidad.
*(Ehl see-dah tee-eh-neh oo-nah tah-
sah sehr-kah-nah ahl see-ehn pohr
see-ehn-toh deh mohr-tah-lee-dahd)*

All of a sudden. . .
De golpe. . .
(Deh gohl-peh)

Allow time for ventilation of feelings.
Permita tiempo para ventilar
sentimientos.
*(Pehr-mee-tah tee-ehm-poh pah-rah
behn-tee-lahr sehn-tee-mee-ehn-tohs)*

All physicians furnishing services to me.
Todos los médicos presten sevicios.
*(Toh-dohs lohs meh-dee-kohs prehs-
tehn sehr-bee-see-ohs)*

Almost always the technician comes at
six in the morning.
Casi siempre el técnico viene a las
seis de la mañana.
*(Kah-see see-ehm-preh ehl tehk-nee-
koh bee-eh-neh ah lahs seh-ees deh
lah mah-nyah-nah)*

Also, I have a headache.
También, tengo dolor de cabeza.
*(Tahm-bee-ehn, tehn-goh doh-lohr deh
kah-beh-sah)*

Also, make an appointment for
Wednesday.
También, pida cita para el
miércoles.
*(Tahm-bee-ehn, pee-dah see-tah pah-
rah ehl mee-ehr-koh-lehs)*

Always!
¡Siempre!
(See-ehm-preh)

Answer "yes" or "no."
Conteste "sí" o "no."
(Kohn-tehs-teh "see" oh "noh")

Any blood disorders such as anemia or
leukemia?
¿Problemas de sangre como anemia
o leucemia?
*(Proh-bleh-mahs deh sahn-greh koh-
moh ah-neh-mee-ah oh loo-seh-mee-
ah)*

Any questions?
¿Alguna pregunta?
(Ahl-goo-nah preh-goon-tah)

Anything else?
¿Alguna otra cosa?
(Ahl-goo-nah oh-trah koh-sah)

Are there elevators?
¿Hay elevadores?
(Ah-ee eh-leh-bah-doh-rehs)

Are there ramps?
¿Hay rampas?
(Ah-ee ram-pahs)

Are you a housewife?
¿Es ama de casa?
(Ehs ah-mah deh kah-sah)

Are you a smoker?
¿Es fumador?
(Ehs foo-mah-dohr)

Are you a widow/widower?
¿Es usted viudo(a)?
(Ehs oos-tehd bee-oo-doh[-dah])

Are you allergic to anything?
¿Es alérgico a alguna cosa?
(Ehs ah-lehr-hee-koh ah ahl-goo-nah
koh-sah)

Are you allergic to drugs?
Es alérgico a drogas?
(Ehs ah-lehr-hee-koh ah droh-gahs)

Are you allergic to foods?
¿Es alérgico a comidas?
(Ehs ah-lehr-hee-koh ah koh-mee-
dahs)

Are you allergic to penicillin or other
medications?
¿Tiene alergias a la penicilina u otros
medicamentos?
(Tee-eh-neh ah-lehr-hee-ahs ah lah
peh-nee-see-lee-nah oo oh-trohs
meh-dee-kah-mehn-tohs)

Are you allergic to plants?
¿Es alérgico a plantas?
(Ehs ah-lehr-hee-koh ah plahn-
tahs)

Are you bleeding?
¿Está sangrando?
(Ehs-tah sahn-grahn-doh)

Are you cold?
¿Tiene frío?
(Tee-eh-neh free-oh)

Are you comfortable?
¿Está cómoda?
(Ehs-tah koh-moh-dah)

Are you constipated?
¿Está estreñido?
(Ehs-tah ehs-treh-nyee-doh)

Are you diabetic?
¿Es diabética?
(Ehs dee-ah-beh-tee-kah)

Are you divorced?
¿Es usted divorciado(a)?
(Ehs oos-tehd dee-bohr-see-ah-doh[-
dah])

Are you dizzy?
¿Tiene mareos?
(Tee-eh-neh mah-reh-ohs)

Are you employed?
¿Trabaja usted?
(Trah-bah-hah oos-tehd)

Are you feeling a contraction?
¿Está sintiendo una contracción?
(Ehs-tah seen-tee-ehn-doh oo-nah
kohn-trahk-see-ohn)

Are you from this area?
¿Es usted de esta área?
(Ehs uhs-tehd deh ehs-tah ah-reh-
ah)

Are you having problems breathing?
¿Tiene problemas al respirar?
(Tee-eh-nch proh-bleh-mahs ahl
rehs-pee-rahr)

Are you hot?
¿Tiene calor?
(Tee-eh-neh kah-lohr)

Are you hungry?
¿Tiene hambre?
(Tee-eh-neh ahm-breh)

Are you hurting?
¿Tiene dolor?
(Tee-eh-neh doh-lohr)

Are you in a hurry?
¿Estás de prisa?
(Ehs-tahs deh pree-sah)

Are you mad?
¿Está enojado?
(Ehs-tah eh-noh-hah-doh)

Are you married/single?
¿Está casada/soltera?
(Ehs-tah kah-sah-dah/sohl-tch-rah)

Are you nauseated?
¿Tiene náuseas?
(Tee-eh-neh nah-oo-seh-ahs)

Are you okay?
¿Está bien/Se siente bien?
(Ehs-tah bee-ehn/Seh see-ehn-teh
bee-ehn)

Are you on vacation?
¿Está de vacaciones?
(Ehs-tah deh bah-kah-see-ohn-ehs)

Are you pregnant?
¿Está embarazada?
(Ehs-tah ehm-bah-rah-sah-dah)

Are you related?
¿Es pariente?
(Ehs pah-ree-ehn-teh)

Are you single?
Es usted soltero(a)?
(Ehs oos-tehd sohl-teh-roh[-rah])

Are you sleepy?
¿Tiene sueño?
(Tee-eh-neh soo-eh-nyoh)

Are you taking anticoagulants?
¿Está tomando anticoagulantes?
(Ehs-tah toh-mahn-doh ahn-tee-koo-ah-goo-lahn-tehs)

Are you taking antidepressants?
¿Está tomando antidepresivos?
(Ehs-tah toh-mahn-doh ahn-tee-deh-preh-see-bohs)

Are you taking any medications?
¿Está tomando algunas medicinas?
(Ehs-tah toh-mahn-doh ahl-goo-nahs meh-dee-see-nahs)

Are you taking nitroglycerin?
¿Está tomando nitroglicerina?
(Ehs-tah toh-mahn-doh nee-troh-glee-seh-ree-nah)

Are you taking steroids?
¿Está tomando esteroides?
(Ehs-tah toh-mahn-doh ehs-teh-roh-ee-dehs)

Are you taking your medicines?
¿Está tomando sus medicinas?
(Ehs-tah toh-mahn-doh soos meh-dee-see-nahs)

Are you the patient?
Es usted el/la paciente?
(Ehs oos-tehd ehl/lah pah-see-ehn-teh)

Are you thirsty?
¿Tiene sed?
(Tee-eh-neh sehd)

Are you under a doctor's care?
¿Está bajo el cuidado de un doctor?
(Ehs-tah bah-hoh ehl koo-ee-dah-doh deh oon dohk-tohr)

Are you working also?
¿Trabaja también?
(Trah-bah-hah tahm-bee-ehn)

Are your teeth sensitive to cold?
¿Tiene sensibilidad al tomar frío?
(Tee-eh-neh sehn-see-bee-lee-dahd ahl toh-mahr free-oh)

As soon as you can, go to your doctor.
En cuanto pueda, acuda a su medico.
(Ehn koo-ahn-toh poo-eh-dah, ah-koo-dah ah soo meh-dee-koh)

Ask about rehabilitation.
Pregunte sobre la rehabilitación.
(Preh-goon-teh soh-breh lah reh-ah-bee-lee-tah-see-ohn)

Ask for unit Six A.
Pregunte por la unidad Seis A.
(Preh-goon-teh pohr lah oo-nee-dahd Seh-ees Ah)

Ask if you will use devices, prosthesis, or crutches.
Pregunte si va a usar aparatos, prótesis o muletas.
(Preh-goon-teh see bah ah oo-sahr ah-pah-rah-tohs, oh moo-leh-tahs)

Ask the receptionist for a number.
Pídale un número a la recepcionista.
(Pee-dah-leh oon noo-meh-roh ah lah reh-sehp-see-ohn-ees-tah)

Assess circulatory status, color, capillary refill, coolness.
Evalúe el estado circulatorio, color, relleno capilar, piel fría.
(Eh-bah-loo-eh ehl ehs-tah-doh seer-koo-lah-toh-ree-oh: koh-lohr, reh-yeh-noh kah-pee-lahr, pee-ehl free-ah)

Assess hemodynamic status.
Evalúe el estado hemodinámico.
(Eh-bah-loo-eh ehl ehs-tah-doh ee-moh-dee-nah-mee-koh)

Assure that family is informed of patient care.
Asegure que la familia esté informada sobre el cuidado del paciente.
(Ah-seh-goo-reh keh lah fah-mee-lee-ah ehs-teh een-fohr-mah-dah soh-breh ehl koo-ee-dah-doh dehl pah-see-ehn-teh)

At bedtime.
Al acostarse/hora de dormir.
(Ahl ah-kohs-tahr-seh/oh-rah deh dohr-meer)

At least thirty minutes!
¡Al menos treinta minutos!
(Ahl meh-nohs treh-een-tah mee-noo-tohs)

At the same time, we take the x-rays.
Al mismo tiempo, tomamos los rayos X.
(Ahl mees-moh tee-ehm-poh, toh-mah-mohs lohs rah-yohs eh-kiss)

At what hospital have you been treated?
¿En qué hospital lo han tratado?
(Ehn keh ohs-pee-tahl loh ahn trah-tah-doh)

At what time do they close?
¿A qué hora cierran?
(Ah keh oh-rah see-eh-rahn)

At what time do you get up?
¿A qué hora se levanta?
(Ah keh oh-rah seh leh-bahn-tah)

At what time do you go to bed?
¿A qué hora se acuesta?
(Ah keh oh-rah seh ah-koo-ehs-tah)

At what time do you go to sleep?
¿A qué hora te acuestas a dormir?
(Ah keh oh-rah teh ah-koo-ehs-tahs ah dohr-meer)

At what time?
¿A qué hora?
(Ah keh oh-rah)

Avoid scratching or cutting your skin.
Evite rasguños o heridas en la piel.
(Eh-bee-teh rahs-goo-nyohs oh eh-ree-dahs ehn lah pee-ehl)

Avoid sunlight.
Evite asolearse/los rayos del sol.
(Eh-bee-teh ah-soh-leh-ahr-seh/lohs rah-yohs dehl sohl)

Back pain?
¿Dolor de espalda?
(Doh-lohr deh ehs-pahl-dah)

Backward.
Atrás.
(Ah-trahs)

Bad breath?
¿Mal aliento?
(Mahl ah-lee-ehn-toh)

Bathe him every day.
Báñelo diariamente.
(Bah-nyeh-loh dee-ah-ree-ah-mehn-teh)

Be patient!
¡Tenga paciencia!
(Tehn-gah pah-see-ehn-see-ah)

Be still!
¡Quieto!
(Kee-eh-toh)

Be sure not eat or drink anything after nine PM.
No tome nada después de las nueve de la noche.
(Noh toh-meh nah-dah dehs-poo-ehs deh lahs noo-eh-beh deh lah noh-cheh)

Before he sits up in bed, lower the bed.
Antes de que él se levante, baje la cama.
(Ahn-tehs deh keh ehl seh leh-bahn-teh, bah-heh lah kah-mah)

Before/after meals.
Antes/después de las comidas.
(Ahn-tehs/dehs-poo-ehs deh lahs koh-mee-dahs)

Bend it.
Dóblala.
(Doh-blah-lah)

Bend over.
Agáchese.
(Ah-gah-cheh-seh)

Bend the wrist.
Dobla la muñeca.
(Doh-blah lah moo-nyeh-kah)

Bend the elbow.
Doble el codo.
(Doh-bleh ehl koh-doh)

Bend your hip.
Dobla su cadera.
(Doh-blah soo kah-deh-rah)

Bend your knee!
¡Doble su rodilla!
(Doh-bleh soo roh-dee-yah)

Bend your shoulder.
Dobla tu hombro.
(Doh-blah too ohm-broh)

Bend your toes.
Dobla tus dedos.
(Doh-blah toos deh-dohs)

Bend!
¡Doble!
(Doh-bleh)

Besides your cholesterol, are there any
   other medical problems?
¿Además de su colesterol, tiene otros
   problemas médicos?
(Ah-deh-mahs deh soo koh-lehs-teh-
   rohl, tee-eh-neh oh-trohs proh-bleh-
   mahs meh-dee-kohs)

Bite!
¡Muerda!
(Moo-ehr-dah)

Blink if you understand me.
Parpadee si me entiende.
(Pahr-pah-dee-eh see meh ehn-tee-ehn-
   deh)

Boil the water he drinks.
Hierva el agua que toma.
(Ee-ehr-bah ehl ah-goo-ah keh toh-
   mah)

Breast feed or give a bottle every three
   hours.
Déle pecho o biberón cada tres
   horas.
(Deh-leh peh-choh oh bee-beh-rohn
   kah-dah trehs oh-rahs)

Breathe!
¡Respire!
(Rehs-pee-reh)

Breathe out!
¡Saque el aire/Exhale!
(Sah-keh ehl ah-ee-reh/Ehx-ah-leh)

Breathe deep; let it out slowly.
Respira hondo; déjalo ir despacio.
(Rehs-pee-rah oon-doh; deh-hah-loh
   eer dehs-pah-see-oh)

Breathe deeply!
¡Respire hondo/profundo!
(Rehs-pee-reh ohn-doh/proh-foon-doh)

Breathe regularly.
Respire regular/normal.
(Rehs-pee-reh reh-goo-lahr/nohr-mahl)

Breathe through the mouth.
Respire por la boca.
(Rehs-pee-reh pohr lah boh-kah)

Breathe, deep!
¡Respire, hondo/profundo!
(Rehs-pee-reh oon-doh/proh-foon-doh)

Brush your teeth!
¡Cepíllese los dientes!
(Seh-pee-yeh-seh lohs dee-ehn-tehs)

But I don't have a pencil.
Pero no tengo un lápiz.
(Peh-roh noh tehn-goh oon lah-pees)

But we will give you something to
   drink.
Pero le daremos algo que tomar.
(Peh-roh leh dah-reh-mohs ahl-goh
   keh toh-mahr)

Buzzing in ears. . .
Zumbido en los oídos. . .
(Soom-bee-doh ehn lohs oh-ee-dohs)

Call!
¡Llame!
(Yah-meh)

Call for. . .
Llamar. . .
(Yah-mahr)

Call if you need help.
Llame sí necesita ayuda.
(Yah-meh see neh-seh-see-tah ah-yoo-dah)

Call your friends.
Llame a sus amigos.
(Yah-meh ah soos ah-mee-gohs)

Call your physician.
Llame a su médico.
(Yah-meh ah soo meh-dee-koh)

Can casual contact cause AIDS?
¿Los contactos eventuales pueden causar SIDA?
(Lohs kohn-tahk-tohs eh-behn-too-ah-lehs poo-eh-dehn kah-oo-sahr see-dah)

Can I be poisoned by the radiation?
¿Puedo ser dañada por la radiación?
(Poo-eh-doh sehr dah-nyah-dah pohr lah rah-dee-ah-see-ohn)

Can I join you?
¿Te puedo acompañar?
(Teh poo-eh-doh ah-kohm-pah-nyahr)

Can you breathe?
¿Puede respirar?
(Poo-eh-deh rehs-pee-rahr)

Can you do house chores?
¿Puede hacer quehacer?
(Poo-eh-deh ah-sehr keh-ah-sehr)

Can you feed yourself?
¿Puede alimentarse?
(Poo-eh-deh ah-lee-mehn-tahr-seh)

Can you feel?
¿Puede sentir?
(Poo-eh-deh sehn-teer)

Can you feel this?
¿Siente esto?
(See-ehn-teh ehs-toh)

Can you get out of bed?
¿Puede salir de la cama?
(Poo-eh-deh sah-leer deh lah kah-mah)

Can you give me directions?
¿Me puede dar direcciones?
(Meh poo-eh-deh dahr dee-rek-see-ohn-ehs)

Can you go with me?
¿Puede ir conmigo?
(Poo-eh-deh eer kohn-mee-goh)

Can you hear me?
¿Puede oírme?
(Poo-eh-deh oh-eer-meh)

Can you move in bed?
¿Puede moverse en la cama?
(Poo-eh-deh moh-behr-seh ehn lah kah-mah)

Can you read?
¿Puede leer?
(Poo-eh-deh leh-ehr)

Can you see the blackboard well?
¿Puedes ver bien el pizarrón?
(Poo-eh-dehs behr bee-ehn ehl pee-sah-rohn)

Can you see the fire extinguisher?
¿Ve el extinguidor de fuego?
(Beh ehl ehx-teen-ghee-dohr deh foo-eh-goh)

Can you see the places that are stained?
Puede ver los lugares que están dañados?
(Poo-eh-deh behr lohs loo-gah-rehs keh ehs-tahn dah-nyah-dohs)

Can you sit up?
¿Puede sentarse?
(Poo-eh-deh sehn-tahr-seh)

Can you take off work?
¿Puede faltar al trabajo?
(Poo-eh-deh fahl-tahr ahl trah-bah-hoh)

Can you take vacation?
¿Puede tomar vacaciones?
(Poo-eh-deh toh-mahr bah-kah-see-ohn-ehs)

Can you talk?
¿Puede hablar?
(Poo-eh-deh ah-blahr)

Can you tell me what kind of diet you have?
¿Puede decirme que dieta tiene?
(Poo-eh-deh deh-seer-meh keh dee-eh-tah tee-eh-neh)

Can you write the name?
¿Puede escribir el nombre?
(Poo-eh-deh ehs-kree-beer ehl nohm-breh)

Can you write?
¿Puede escribir?
(Poo-eh-deh ehs-kree-beer)

Car accidents?
¿Accidentes de auto?
(Ahk-see-dehn-tehs deh ah-oo-toh)

Change in bowel or bladder habits.
Cambio en el hábito de la orina o el excremento.
(Kahm-bee-oh ehn ehl ah-bee-toh deh lah oh-ree-nah oh ehl ehx-kreh-mehn-toh)

Change in wart or mole.
Cambio en lunar o verruga.
(Kahm-bee-oh ehn loo-nahr oh beh-ruh-ah)

Change into this gown.
Póngase está bata.
(Pohn-gah-seh ehs-tah bah-tah)

Choose!
¡Escoja!
(Ehs-koh-hah)

Clean your breasts thoroughly.
Lave muy bien sus senos/pechos.
(Lah-beh moo-eeh bee-ehn soohs seh-nohs/peh-chohs)

Clean your nipples before you breast feed.
Lave sus pezones antes de dar pecho.
(Lah-beh soos peh-sohn-ehs ahn-tehs deh dahr peh-choh)

Close it.
Ciérrala(lo).
(See-eh-rah-lah[-loh])

Close your books, please.
Cierren sus libros, por favor.
(See-eh-rehn soos lee-brohs, pohr fah-bohr)

Close your eyes!
¡Cierre los ojos!
(See-eh-reh lohs oh-hohs)

Close your mouth!
¡Cierre la boca!
(See-eh-reh lah boh-kah)

Come in.
Pase/Entre Usted.
(Pah-seh/ehn-treh oos-tehd)

Complications.
Complicaciones.
(Kohm-plee-kah-see-oh-nehs)

Cough deeply.
Tosa más fuerte.
(Toh-sah mahs foo-ehr-teh)

Cough harder!
¡Tose más fuerte!
(Toh-seh mahs foo-ehr-teh)

Cough!
¡Tosa!
(Toh-sah)

Cross your arms.
Cruza tus brazos.
(Kroo-sah toos brah-sohs)

Cross your legs.
Cruza tus piernas.
(Kroo-sah toos pee-ehr-nahs)

Curve the floss into a "C."
Ponga el hilo en forma de "C."
(Pohn-gah ehl ee-loh ehn fohr-mah deh seh)

Daily.
Diariamente/Una por día/Cada día.
(Dee-ah-ree-ah-mehn-teh/Oo-nah pohr dee-ah/Kah-dah dee-ah)

Date.
Fecha.
(Feh-chah)

Deal with. . .
Tratar. . .
(Trah-tahr)

Describe different types of amputations.
Describa los diferentes tipos de amputaciones.
(Dehs-kree-bah lohs dee-feh-rehn-tehs tee-pohs deh ahm-poo-tah-see-oh-nehs)

Diabetes mellitus is characterized by
the body's inability to utilize
glucose.
La diabetes mellitus se caracteriza
por la incapacidad del cuerpo para
utilizar glucosa.
*(Lah dee-ah-beh-tehs meh-lee-toos seh
kah-rahk-teh-ree-sah pohr lah een-
kah-pah-see-dahd dehl koo-ehr-poh
puh-rah oo-tee-lee-sahr gloo-koh-sah)*

Diagnostic tests and procedures.
Pruebas de diagnóstico y
procedimientos.
*(Proo-eh-bahs deh dee-ahg-nohs-tee-
koh ee proh-seh-dee-mee-ehn-tohs)*

Dial nine, wait for the tone, then dial
the number you want to call.
Marque el nueve, espere el tono,
luego marque el número que
quiera llamar.
*(Mahr-keh ehl noo-eh-beh, ehs-peh-reh
ehl toh-noh, loo-eh-goh mahr-keh
ehl noo-meh-roh keh kee-eh-rah
yah-mahr)*

Did anyone treat you prior to our
arrival?
¿Lo trató alguien antes de nuestra
llegada?
*(Loh trah-toh ahl-ghee-ehn ahn-tehs
deh noo-ehs-trah yeh-gah-dah)*

Did the doctor explained the
procedure to you?
¿Le explicó el médico el
procedimiento?
*(Leh ehx-plee-koh ehl meh-dee-koh ehl
proh-seh-dee-mee-ehn-toh)*

Did you arrive in a wheelchair?
¿Llegó en silla de ruedas?
(Yeh-goh ehn see-yah deh roo-eh-dahs)

Did you bring a hearing aid?
¿Trajo un aparato para oír?
*(Trah-hoh oon ah-pah-rah-toh pah-
rah oh-eer)*

Did you bring an artificial eye?
¿Trajo un ojo artificial?
*(Trah-hoh oon oh-hoh ahr-tee-fee-see-
ahl)*

Did you bring contact lenses?
¿Trajo lentes de contacto?
*(Trah-hoh lehn-tehs deh kohn-tahk-
toh)*

Did you bring dentures?
¿Trajo una dentadura postiza?
*(Trah-hoh oon-ah dehn-tah-doo-rah
pohs-tee sah)*

Did you bring glasses?
¿Trajo anteojos/lentes?
(Trah-hoh ahn-teh-oh-hohs/lehn-tehs)

Did you bring jewelry/cash?
¿Trajo joyeria/dinero?
*(Trah-hoh hoh-yeh-ree-ah/
dee-neh-roh)*

Did you bring valuables?
¿Trajo algo de valor?
(Trah-hoh ahl-goh deh bah-lohr)

Did you call anyone?
¿Llamó a alguien?
(Yah-moh ah ahl-ghee-ehn)

Did you come by car?
¿Vino en carro?
(Bee-noh ehn kah-roh)

Did you faint?
¿Se desmayó?
(Seh dehs-mah-yoh)

Did you fall?
¿Se cayó?
(Seh kah-yoh)

Did you feel warm water run out of
your vagina?
¿Sintió que salió agua tibia de su
vagina?
*(Seen-tee-oh keh sah-lee-oh
ah-goo-ah tee-bee-ah deh soo
bah-hee-nah)*

Did you have a bowel movement?
¿Hizo del baño/caca/evacuó?
*(Ee-soh dehl bah-nyoh/kah-kah/eh-
bah-koo-oh)*

Did you have a miscarriage?
¿Tuvo un niño nacido muerto?
*(Too-boh oon nee-nyoh nah-see-doh
moo-ehr-toh)*

Did you have an ectopic (tubal) pregnancy?
¿Tuvo un embarazo fuera de la matriz o en las trompas?
(Too-boh oon ehm-bah-rah-soh foo-eh-rah deh lah mah-trees oh ehn lahs trohm-pahs)

Did you hit the windshield/steering wheel?
¿Se pegó contra el parabrisas/volante?
(Seh peh-goh kohn-trah ehl pah-rah-bree-sahs/boh-lahn-teh)

Did you loose consciousness?
¿Perdió el conocimiento/Se desmayó?
(Pehr-dee-oh ehl koh-noh-see-mee-ehn-toh/Seh dehs-mah-yoh)

Did you see blood in the urine?
¿Vio sangre en la orina?
(Bee-oh sahn-greh ehn lah oh-ree-nah)

Did you see how the accident happen?
¿Vio cómo pasó el accidente?
(Bee-oh koh-moh pah-soh ehl ahk-see-dehn-teh)

Did you sleep well?
¿Durmió bien?
(Door-mee-oh bee-ehn)

Did you take drugs or alcohol in the last three hours?
¿Tomó drogas o alcohol en las últimas tres horas?
(Toh-moh droh-gahs oh ahl-kohl ehn lahs ool-tee-mahs trehs oh-rahs)

Did you take medications today? When?
¿Tomó sus medicinas hoy? ¿Cuándo?
(Toh-moh soos meh-dee-see-nahs oh-ee) (Koo-ahn-do)

Did you walk?
¿Caminó?
(Kah-mee-noh)

Did you take your medicines this morning?
¿Tomó las medicinas esta mañana?
(Toh-moh lahs meh-dee-see-nahs ehs-tah mah-nyah-nah?

Difficulty in swallowing. . .
Dificultad al tragar. . .
(Dee-fee-kool-tahd ahl trah-gahr)

Diminished amounts of insulin to meet requirements is called non-insulin-dependent DM.
A la disminución de insulina requerida se le llama diabetes no-insulino-dependiente.
(Ah lah dees-mee-noo-see-ohn deh een-soo-lee-nah reh-keh-ree-dah seh leh yah-mah dee-ah-beh-tehs noh-een-soo-lee-noh-deh-pehn-dee-ehn-teh)

Discuss medical and surgical management of the amputated patient.
Discuta el manejo médico y quirúrgico del paciente amputado.
(Dees-koo-tah ehl mah-neh-hoh meh-dee-koh ee kee-roor-hee-koh dehl pah-see-ehn-teh ahm-poo-tah-doh)

Do all go to school?
¿Todos van a la escuela?
(Toh-dohs bahn ah lah ehs-koo-eh-lah)

Do any of your children have asthma?
¿Algunos de sus niños tienen ahs-mah?
(Ahl-goo-nohs deh soos nee-nyohs tee-eh-nehn asma)

Do any of your children have bad coordination?
¿Algunos de sus niños tienen mala coordinacion?
(Ahl-goo-nohs deh soos nee-nyohs tee-eh-nehn mah-lah kohr-dee-nah-see-ohn)

Do any of your children have chickenpox?
¿Algunos de sus niños tienen viruelas?
(Ahl-goo-nohs deh soos nee-nyohs tee-eh-nehn bee-roo-eh-lahs)

Do any of your children have cold?
¿Algunos de sus niños tienen
resfriado?
(Ahl-goo-nohs deh soos nee-nyohs tee-eh-nehn rehs-free-ah-doh)

Do any of your children have
convulsions?
¿Algunos de sus niños tienen
convulsiones?
(Ahl-goo-nohs deh soos nee-nyohs tee-eh-nehn kohn-bool-see-ohn-ehs)

Do any of your children have delayed
speech?
¿Algunos de sus niños tienen tardío
el lenguaje?
(Ahl-goo-nohs deh soos nee-nyohs tee-eh-nehn tahr-dee-oh ehl lehn-goo-ah-heh)

Do any of your children have
diphtheria?
¿Algunos de sus niños tienen difteria?
(Ahl-goo-nohs deh soos nee-nyohs tee-eh-nehn deef-teh-ree-ah)

Do any of your children have hearing
defects?
¿Algunos de sus niños tienen
defectos del oído?
(Ahl-goo-nohs deh soos nee-nyohs tee-eh-nehn deh-fehk-tohs dehl oh-ee-doh)

Do any of your children have measles?
¿Algunos de sus niños tienen
sarampión?
(Ahl-goo-nohs deh soos nee-nyohs tee-eh-nehn sah-rahm-pee-ohn)

Do any of your children have mumps?
¿Algunos de sus niños tienen
paperas?
(Ahl-goo-nohs deh soos nee-nyohs tee-eh-nehn pah-peh-rahs)

Do any of your children have nausea
and vomiting?
¿Algunos de sus niños tienen náusea
y vómitos?
(Ahl-goo-nohs deh soos nee-nyohs tee-eh-nehn nah-oo-seh-ah ee boh-mee-tohs)

Do any of your children have
pneumonia?
¿Algunos de sus niños tienen
pulmonía?
(Ahl-goo-nohs deh soos nee-nyohs tee-eh-nehn pool-moh-nee-ah)

Do any of your children have visual
defects?
¿Algunos de sus niños tienen
defectos de la vista?
(Ahl-goo-nohs deh soos nee-nyohs tee-eh-nehn deh-fehk-tohs deh lah bees-tah)

Do each movement ten times.
Haga cada movimiento diez veces.
(Ah-gah kah-dah moh-bee-mee-ehn-toh dee-ehs beh-sehs)

Do I have time?
¿Tengo tiempo?
(Tehn-goh tee-ehm-poh)

Do not assume others don't
understand what you are feeling.
No presuma que otros no entienden
lo que está sintiendo.
(Noh preh-soo-mah keh oh-trohs noh ehn-tee-ehn-dehn loh keh ehs-tah seen-tee-ehn-doh)

Do not bend your leg!
¡No doble la pierna!
(Noh doh-bleh lah pee-ehr-nah)

Do not deny your feelings.
No niege sus sentimientos.
(Noh nee-eh-geh soos sehn-tee-mee-ehn-tohs)

Do not drink alcohol with this
medication.
No tome alcohol con está medicina.
(Noh toh-meh ahl-kol kohn ehs-tah meh-dee-see-nah)

Do not drive!
¡No maneje/conduzca!
(Noh mah-neh-heh/kohn-doos-kah)

Do not eat or drink anything for thirty
minutes.
No coma o beba nada por treinta
minutos.
*(Noh koh-mah oh beh-bah nah-dah
pohr treh-een-tah mee-noo-tohs)*

Do not get up!
¡No se levante!
(Noh seh leh-bahn-teh)

Do not hold on to the wall.
No se agarre de la pared.
*(Noh seh ah-gah-reh deh lah pah-
rehd)*

Do not isolate yourself.
No se aparte.
(Noh seh ah-pahr-teh)

Do not lift more than ten pounds of
weight.
No levante más de diez libras de
peso.
*(Noh leh-bahn-teh mahs deh dee-ehs
lee-brahs deh peh-soh)*

Do not move the patient!
¡No mueva al paciente!
(Noh moo-eh-bah ahl pah-see-ehn-teh)

Do not move!
¡No se mueva!
(Noh seh moo-eh-bah)

Do not operate machinery!
¡No maneje/opere una
máquina/maquinaria!
*(Noh mah-neh-heh/oh-peh-reh
oo-nah mah-kee-nah/mah-kee-nah-
ree-ah)*

Do not put on plastic panties.
No le ponga calzones de plástico.
*(Noh leh pohn-gah kahl-sohn-ehs deh
plahs-tee-koh)*

Do not smoke in the room where the
oxygen is being used.
No fume en el cuarto donde se usa el
oxígeno.
*(Noh foo-meh ehn ehl koo-ahr-toh
dohn-deh seh oo-sah ehl ohx-ee-heh-
noh)*

Do they have a bad coordination?
¿Tienen mala coordinación?
*(Tee-eh-nehn mah-lah kohr-dee-nah-
see-ohn)*

Do they have chickenpox?
¿Tienen varicela?
(Tee-eh-nehn bah-ree-seh-lah)

Do they have cold/flu?
¿Tienen resfriado/gripa?
*(Tee-eh-nehn rehs-free-ah-doh/gree-
pah)*

Do they have convulsions?
¿Tienen convulsiones?
(Tee-eh-nehn kohn-bool-see-ohn-ehs)

Do they have delayed speech?
¿Tienen tardío del lenguaje?
*(Tee-eh-nehn tahr-dee-oh dehl lehn-
goo-ah-heh)*

Do they have diphtheria?
¿Tienen difteria?
(Tee-eh-nehn deef-teh-ree-ah)

Do they have hearing defects?
¿Tienen defectos del oído?
*(Tee-eh-nehn deh-fehk-tohs dehl oh-ee-
doh)*

Do they have measles?
¿Tienen sarampión?
(Tee-eh-nehn sah-rahm-pee-ohn)

Do they have mumps?
¿Tienen paperas?
(Tee-eh-nehn pah-peh-rahs)

Do they have nausea and vomiting?
¿Tienen náusea y vómitos?
*(Tee-eh-nehn nah-oo-seh-ah ee boh-
mee-tohs)*

Do they have pneumonia?
¿Tienen pulmonía?
(Tee-eh-nehn pool-moh-nee-ah)

Do they have visual defects?
¿Tienen defectos de la vista?
*(Tee-eh-nehn deh-fehk-tohs deh lah
bees-tah)*

Do they live close to you?
¿Viven cerca de usted?
(Bee-behn sehr-kah deh oos-tehd)

Do not use flammable substances.
No use substancias flamables.
(Noh oo-seh soobs-tahn-see-ahs flah-mah-blehs)

Do you dribble urine?
¿Se orina sin sentir?
(Seh oh-ree-nah seehn sehn-teer)

Do you drink alcohol?
¿Toma bebidas alcohólicas?
(Toh-mah beh-bee-dahs ahl-koh-lee-kahs)

Do you drink coffee?
¿Toma café?
(Toh-mah kah-feh)

Do you eat breakfast/lunch?
¿Tomas desayuno/almuerzo?
(Toh-mahs deh-sah-yoo-noh/ahl-moo-ehr-soh)

Do you engage in protective sex?
¿Practica el sexo seguro?
(Prahk-tee-kah ehl sehx-oh seh-goo-roh)

Do you feed every three hours?
¿Le da de comer cada tres horas?
(Leh dah deh koh-mehr kah-dah trehs oh-rahs)

Do you feel all right?
¿Se siente bien?
(Seh see-ehn-teh bee-ehn)

Do you feel dizzy?
¿Se siente mareado?
(Seh see-ehn-teh mah-reh-ah-doh)

Do you feel nauseated?
¿Siente náuseas?
(Seh-ehn-teh nah-oo-seh-ahs)

Do you feel weak?
¿Se siente débil?
(Seh see-ehn-teh deh-beel)

Do you get distracted easily?
¿Te distraes fácilmente?
(Teh dees-trah-ehs fah-seel-mehn-teh)

Do you get headaches?
¿Tiene dolor de cabeza?
(Tee-eh-neh doh-lohr deh kah-beh-sah)

Do you get tired easily?
¿Se cansa con facilidad?
(Seh kahn-sah kohn fah-see-lee-dahd)

Do you have a doctor?
¿Tiene un doctor?
(Tee-eh-neh oon dohk-tohr)

Do you have a driver's license?
¿Tiene licencia de manejar?
(Tee-eh-neh lee-sehn-see-ah deh mah-neh-hahr)

Do you have a family doctor?
¿Tiene un doctor familiar?
(Tee-eh-neh oon dohk-tohr fah-mee-lee-ahr)

Do you have a hospital card?
¿Tiene usted tarjeta de hospital?
(Tee-eh-neh oos-tehd tahr-heh-tah deh ohs-pee-tahl)

Do you have a husband/wife?
¿Tiene esposo/esposa?
(Tee-eh-neh ehs-poh-soh/ehs-poh-sah)

Do you have a pacemaker?
¿Tiene marcapasos?
(Tee-eh-neh mahr-kah-pah-sohs)

Do you have pain?
¿Tiene dolor?
(Tee-eh-neh doh-lohr)

Do you have a phone?
¿Tiene teléfono?
(Tee-eh-nch teh-leh-foh-noh)

Do you have allergies, asthma, high blood pressure, cardiac problems, diabetes?
¿Tiene alergias, asma, alta presión, problemas cardíacos, diabetes?
(Tee-eh-neh ah-lehr-hee-ahs, ahs-mah, ahl-tah preh-see-ohn, proh-bleh-mahs kahr-dee-ah-kohs, dee-ah-beh-tehs)

Do you have allergies?
¿Tiene alergias?
(Tee-eh-neh ah-lehr-gee-ahs)

Do you have another car?
¿Tiene otro carro?
(Tee-eh-neh oh-troh kah-roh)

Do you have any children?
¿Tiene niños?
(Tee-eh-neh nee-nyohs)

Do you have any condition or disease not listed in this questionnaire?
Tiene problemas o condiciones de salud que no estén en este cuestionario?
(Tee-eh-neh proh-bleh-mahs oh kohn-dee-see-ohn-ehs deh sahl-ood keh noh ehs-tehn ehn ehs-teh koo-ehs-tee-oh-nah-ree-oh)

Do you have any further questions?
¿Tiene más preguntas que hacer?
(Tee-eh-neh mahs preh-goon-tahs keh ah-sehr)

Do you have any infectious disease now?
¿Tiene alguna enfermedad infecciosa ahora?
(Tee-eh-neh ahl-goo-nah ehn-fehr-meh-dahd een-fehk-see-oh-sah ah-oh-rah)

Do you have any questions?
¿Tiene preguntas?
(Tee-eh-neh preh-goon-tahs)

Do you have any symptoms: nausea, dizziness, other unusual feelings?
¿Tiene algún síntoma como: náuseas, vértigo, otra sensación rara?
(Tee-eh-neh ahl-goon seen-toh-mah koh-moh nah-oo-seh-ahs, behr-tee-goh, oh-trah sehn-sah-see-ohn rah-rah)

Do you have bad breath?
¿Tiene mal aliento?
(Tee-eh-neh mahl ah-lee-ehn-toh)

Do you have brothers/sisters?
¿Tiene hermanos/hermanas?
(Tee-eh-neh ehr-mah-nohs/ehr-mah-nahs)

Do you have cancer?
¿Tiene cáncer?
(Tee-eh-neh kahn-sehr)

Do you have car insurance?
¿Tiene seguro de carro?
(Tee-eh-neh seh-goo-roh deh kah-roh)

Do you have cardiac problems?
¿Tiene problemas cardíacos?
(Tee-eh-neh proh-bleh-mahs kahr-dee-ah-kohs)

Do you have chest pain?
¿Tiene dolor en el pecho?
(Tee-eh-neh doh-lohr ehn ehl peh-choh)

Do you have convulsions?
¿Tiene convulciones?
(Tee-eh-neh kohn-bool-see-oh-nehs)

Do you have diabetes?
¿Tiene diabetes?
(Tee-eh-neh dee-ah-beh-tehs)

Do you have diarrhea?
¿Tiene diarrea?
(Tee-eh-neh dee-ah-reh-ah)

Do you have dizzy spells?
¿Tiene mareos?
(Tee-eh-neh mah-reh-ohs)

Do you have health insurance?
¿Tiene seguro de salud?
(Tee-eh-neh seh-goo-roh deh sah-lood)

Do you have help at home?
¿Tiene ayuda en casa?
(Tee-eh-neh ah-yoo-dah ehn kah-sah)

Do you have her support in everything?
¿Tiene apoyo de ella en todo?
(Tee-eh-neh ah-poh-yoh deh eh-yah ehn toh-doh)

Do you have hesitancy (when urinating)?
¿Se corta el chorro de la orina?
(Seh kohr-tah ehl choh-roh deh lah oh-ree-nah)

Do you have high blood pressure?
¿Tiene la presión alta?
(Tee-eh-neh lah preh-see-ohn ahl-tah)

Do you have hospital insurance?
¿Tiene seguro de hospital?
(Tee-eh-neh seh-goo-roh deh ohs-pee-tahl)

Do you have insomnia?
¿Tiene insomnio?
(Tee-eh-neh een-sohm-nee-oh)

Do you have medical problems?
¿Tiene problemas médicos?
(Tee-eh-neh proh-bleh-mahs meh-dee-kohs)

Do you have Medicare?
¿Tiene Medicare?
(Tee-eh-neh meh-dee-kehr)

Do you have pain?
¿Tiene dolor?
(Tee-eh-neh doh-lohr)

Do you have problems with your teeth?
¿Tiene(s) problemas con los dientes?
(Tee-eh-neh[s] proh-bleh-mahs kohn lohs dee-ehn-tehs)

Do you have problems with starting to urinate?
¿Tiene dificultad para empezar a orinar?
(Tee-eh-neh dee-fee-kool-tahd pah-rah ehm-peh-sahr ah oh-ree-nahr)

Do you have problems you want the nurse to know?
¿Tiene problemas que quiere decirle a la enfermera?
(Tee-eh-neh proh-bleh-mahs keh kee-eh-reh deh-seer-leh ah lah ehn-fehr-meh-rah)

Do you have questions?
¿Tiene(s) preguntas/dudas?
(Tee-eh-neh[s] preh-goon-tahs/doo-dahs)

Do you have relatives with cardiac problems?
¿Tiene familiares con problemas cardíacos?
(Tee-eh-neh fah-mee-lee-ah-rehs kohn proh-bleh-mahs kahr-dee-ah-kohs)

Do you have relatives/friends?
¿Tiene parientes/amigos?
(Tee-eh-neh pah-ree-ehn-tehs/ah-mee-gohs)

Do you have renal problems?
¿Tiene problemas renales?
(Tee-eh-neh proh-bleh-mahs reh-nah-lehs)

Do you have respiratory problems?
¿Tiene problemas respiratorios?
(Tee-eh-neh proh-bleh-mahs rehs-pee-rah-toh-ree-ohs)

Do you have sexual relations?
¿Tiene relaciones sexuales?
(Tee-eh-neh reh-lah-see-oh-nehs sex-oo-ah-lehs)

Do you have special problems?
¿Tiene problemas especiales?
(Tee-eh-neh proh-bleh-mahs ehs-peh-see-ah-lehs)

Do you have time?
¿Tienes tiempo?
(Tee-eh-nehs tee-ehm-poh)

Do you have trouble making friends at work?
¿En su trabajo tiene dificultad para hacer amistades?
(Ehn soo trah-bah-hoh tee-eh-neh dee-fee-kool-tahd pah-rah ah-sehr ah-mees-tah-dehs)

Do you have tuberculosis?
¿Tiene tuberculosis?
(Tee-eh-neh too-behr-koo-loh-sees)

Do you have vision problems?
¿Tienes problemas con la visión?
(Tee-eh-nehs proh-bleh-mahs kohn lah bee-see-ohn)

Do you have your Medicare card?
¿Tiene usted su tarjeta de Medicare?
(Tee-eh-neh oos-tehd soo tahr-heh-tah deh meh-dee-kehr)

Do you know him/her?
¿Lo/la conoce?
(Loh/lah koh-noh-seh)

Do you know his/her phone number?
¿Sabe su teléfono?
(Sah-beh soo teh-leh-foh-noh)

Do you know how to return?
¿Sabe cómo regresar?
(Sah-beh koh-moh re-greh-sahr)

Do you know the day of the week?
¿Sabe el día de la semana?
(Sah-beh ehl dee-ah deh lah seh-mah-nah)

Do you know the day?
¿Qué día es hoy?
(Keh dee-ah ehs oh-ee)

Do you know the hospital name?
¿Sabe el nombre del hospital?
(Sah-beh ehl nohm-breh dehl ohs-pee-tahl)

Do you know the street name?
¿Sabe el nombre de la calle?
(Sah-beh ehl nohm-breh deh lah kah-yeh)

Do you know where you are?
¿Sabe dónde está?
(Sah-beh dohn-deh ehs-tah)

Do you know why?
¿Sabe por qué?
(Sah-beh pohr keh)

Do you know?
¿Sabe?
(Sah-beh)

Do you like going to school?
¿Te/le gusta ir a la escuela?
(Teh/leh goos-tah eer ah lah ehs-koo-eh-lah)

Do you like them hot/cold?
¿Le gustan calientes/fríos?
(Leh goos-tahn kah-lee-ehn-tehs/free-ohs)

Do you live by yourself?
¿Vive solo?
(Bee-beh soh-loh)

Do you live here?
¿Vive aquí?
(Bee-beh ah-kee)

Do you live with your husband?
¿Vive con su esposo?
(Bee-beh kohn soo ehs-poh-soh)

Do you miss school a lot?
¿Faltas mucho a la escuela?
(Fahl-tahs moo-choh ah lah ehs-koo-eh lah)

Do you need help with school work?
¿Necesitas ayuda con la tarea?
(Neh-seh-see-tahs ah-yoo-dah kohn lah tah-reh-ah)

Do you need help?
¿Necesita ayuda?
(Neh-seh-see-tah ah-yoo-dah)

Do you need ice?
¿Necesita hielo?
(Neh-seh-see-tah ee-eh-loh)

Do you need more pillows?
¿Necesita más almohadas?
(Neh-seh-see-tah mahs ahl-moh-ah-dahs)

Do you need the headboard up?
¿Necesita levantar la cabecera más alta?
(Neh-seh-see-tah leh-bahn-tahr lah kah-beh-seh-rah mahs ahl-tah)

Do you need to call a taxi?
¿Necesita llamar un taxi/carro de sitio?
(Neh-seh-see-tah yah-mahr oon tahx-ee/kah-roh deh see-tee-oh)

Do you need to see a dietitian?
¿Necesita ver a la dietista?
(Neh-seh-see-tah behr ah lah dee-eh-tees-tah)

Do you need to see a social worker?
¿Necesita ver a la trabajadora social?
(Neh-seh-see-tah behr ah lah trah-bah-hah-doh-rah soh-see-ahl)

Do you participate in homosexual relations?
¿Participa en relaciones homosexuales?
(Pahr-tee-see-pah ehn reh-lah-see-ohn-ehs oh-moh-sex-oo-ahl-ehs)

Do you play sports?
¿Juegas deportes?
(Joo-eh-gahs deh-pohr-tehs)

Do you remember me?
¿Se acuerda de mi?
(Seh ah-koo-ehr-dah deh mee)

Do you remember the street?
¿Recuerda la calle?
(Reh-koo-ehr-dah lah kah-yeh)

Do you sleep during the day?
¿Duerme durante el día?
(Doo-ehr-mch doo-rahn-teh ehl dee-ah)

Do you smoke or drink alcohol?
¿Fuma o toma alcohol?
(Foo-mah oh toh-mah ahl-kohl)

Do you smoke?
¿Fuma usted?
(Foo-mah oo-stehd)

Do you speak English?
¿Habla inglés?/Habla usted inglés?
(Ah-blah een-glehs/Ah-blah oos-tehd een glchs)

Do you speak Spanish?
¿Habla español?
(Ah-blah ehs-pah-nyohl)

Do you take a special diet?
¿Toma dieta especial?
(Toh-mah dee-eh-tah ehs-peh-see-ahl)

Do you take any drugs?
¿Toma drogas?
(Toh-mah droh-gahs)

Do you take any medicines?
¿Toma algunas medicinas?
(Toh-mah ahl-goo-nahs meh-dee-see-nahs)

Do you take any narcotics?
¿Toma narcóticos?
(Toh-mah nahr-koh-tee-kohs)

Do you take drugs from habit?
¿Tiene vicio de tomar drogas?
(Tee-eh-neh bee-see-oh deh toh-mahr droh-gahs)

Do you take medicines?
¿Toma medicinas?
(Toh-mah meh-dee-see-nahs)

Do you talk to your wife about your job?
¿Trata de hablar con su esposa acerca de su trabajo?
(Trah-tah deh ah-blahr kohn soo ehs-poh-sah ah-sehr-kah deh soo trah-bah-hoh)

Do you try to relax to forget your anxiety?
¿Procura distraerse para olvidar su ansiedad?
(Proh-koo-rah dees-trah-ehr-seh pah-rah ohl-bee-dahr soo ahn-see-eh-dahd)

Do you understand?
¿Comprende/Entiende?
(Kohm-prehn-deh/Ehn-tee-ehn-deh)

Do you use drugs/medicine?
¿Usa drogas/medicamento?
(Oo-sah droh-gahs/mch-dee-kah-mehn-toh)

Do you use sugar in the coffee?
¿Usa azúcar en el café?
(Oo-sah ah-soo-kahr ehn ehl kah-feh)

Do you wake up at night?
¿Te despiertas en la noche?
(Teh dehs-pee-ehr-tahs ehn lah noh-che)

Do you walk to school?
¿Camina(s) a la escuela?
(Kah-mee-nah[s] ah lah ehs-koo-eh-lah)

Do you want a cup of coffee?
¿Quiére una taza de cafe?
(Kee-eh-reh oo-nah tah-sah deh kah-feh)

Do you want a glass of juice?
¿Quiére un vaso de jugo?
(Kee-eh-reh oon bah-soh deh hoo-goh)

Do you want a glass of water?
¿Quiére un vaso de agua?
(Kee-eh-reh oon bah-soh deh ah-goo-ah)

Do you want something to drink?
¿Quiére algo de tomar/beber?
*(Kee-eh-reh ahl-goh deh toh-mahr/
beh-behr)*

Do you want something to eat?
¿Quiére algo de comer?
(Kee-eh-reh ahl-goh deh koh-mehr)

Do you want something to read?
¿Quiére algo de leer?
(Kee-eh-reh ahl-goh deh leh-ehr)

Do you want the bedpan?
¿Quiére el pato/el bacín?
*(kee-eh-reh ehl pah-toh/ehl
bah-seen)*

Do you want the toast with butter?
¿Quiére el pan tostado con
mantequilla?
*(Kee-eh-reh ehl pahn tohs-tah-doh
kohn mahn-teh-kee-yah)*

Do you want to go home?
¿Quiére ir a su casa?
(Kee-eh-reh eer ah soo kah-sah)

Do you want to see a priest?
¿Necesita ver al sacerdote?
*(Neh-seh-see-tah behr ahl sah-sehr-
doh-teh)*

Do you want to see our doctor?
¿Quiére ver a nuestro doctor?
*(Kee-eh-reh behr ah noo-ehs-troh
dohk-tohr)*

Do you want to take the stairs?
¿Quiére tomar la escalera?
*(Kee-eh-reh toh-mahr lah ehs-kah-leh-
rah)*

Do you want water?
¿Quiére agua?
(Kee-eh-reh ah-goo-ah)

Do you wear glasses?
¿Usa(s) anteojos/lentes?
(Oo-sah[s] ahn-teh-oh-hohs/lehn-tehs)

Do you wish a glass of juice?
¿Quiére un vaso con jugo?
*(Kee-eh-reh oon bah-soh kohn hoo-
goh)*

Do you wish a glass of water?
¿Quiére un vaso con agua?
*(Kee-eh-reh oon bah-soh kohn ah-goo-
ah)*

Do you wish to have a bowel
movement?
¿Quiére evacuar?
(Kee-eh-reh eh-bah-koo-ahr)

Do you wish to pass urine?
¿Quiére orinar?
(Kee-eh-reh oh-ree-nahr)

Do you wish/want something to eat?
¿Quiére algo de comer?
(Kee-eh-reh ahl-goh deh koh-mehr)

Do you wish/want to drink?
¿Quiére tomar/beber?
(Kee-eh-reh toh-mahr/beh-behr)

Do you wish/want to read?
¿Quiére leer?
(Kee-eh-reh leh-ehr)

Do you work everyday?
¿Trabaja todos los días?
(Trah-bah-hah toh-dohs lohs dee-ahs)

Do you work?
¿Trabaja usted?
(Trah-bah-hah oos-tehd)

Do your gums bleed?
¿Le sangran las encías?
(Leh sahn-grahn lahs ehn-see-ahs)

Doctor, I have had pain for the last
five hours.
Doctor, desde hace cinco horas tengo
dolor.
*(Dohk-tohr, dehs-deh ah-seh seen-koh
oh-rahs tehn-goh doh-lohr)*

Doctor, I think I am infected with
AIDS.
Doctor, pienso que estoy infectado
de SIDA.
*(Dohk-tohr, pee-ehn-so keh ehs-toh-ee
een-fek-tah-doh deh see-dah)*

Does he cough only at night?
¿Tose solo de noche?
(Toh-seh soh-loh deh noh-cheh)

Does he cry a lot?
¿Llora mucho?
(Yoh-rah moo-choh)

Does he go to school?
¿Va a la escuela?
(Bah ah lah ehs-koo-eh-lah)

Does he have any friends?
¿Tiene amigos?
(Tee-eh-neh ah-mee-gohs)

Does he have fever/diarrhea/colic?
¿Tiene fiebre/diarrea/cólico?
(Tee-eh-neh fee-eh-breh/dee-ah-reh-ah/koh-lee-koh)

Does he play outdoors?
¿Juega afuera de la casa?
(Joo-eh-gah ah-foo-eh-rah deh lah kah-sah)

Does he sleep well?
¿Duerme bien?
(Doo-ehr-meh bee-ehn)

Does he wet the bed?
¿Moja la cama?
(Moh-hah lah kah-mah)

Does he/she speak English?
¿El/ella habla inglés?
(Ehl/eh-yah ah-blah een-glehs)

Does it come and go?
¿Va y viene?
(Bah eeh bee-eh-neh)

Does it have undigested food?
¿Tiene restos de comida?
(Tee-eh-neh rehs-tohs deh koh-mee-dah)

Does it hurt to breathe?
¿Te duele al respirar?
(Teh doo-eh-leh ahl rehs-pee-rahr)

Does it hurt to cough?
¿Te duele al toser?
(Teh doo-eh-leh ahl toh-sehr)

Does it hurt when you chew very hard?
¿Le duele al masticar con fuerza?
(Leh doo-eh-leh ahl mahs-tee-kahr kohn foo-ehr-sah)

Does it hurts when I let go?
¿Duele cuando retiro la mano?
(Doo-eh-leh koo-ahn-doh reh-tee-roh lah mah-noh)

Does it hurts when I press?
¿Duele cuando presiono?
(Doo-eh-leh koo-ahn-doh preh-see-oh-noh)

Does it smell bad?
¿Huele mal?
(Oo-eh-leh mahl)

Does it still hurt?
¿Todavía le duele?
(Toh-dah-bee-ah leh doo-eh-leh)

Does the baby sleep all night?
¿Duerme el bebé toda la noche?
(Doo-ehr-meh ehl beh-beh toh-dah lah noh-cheh)

Does the cough produce vomit?
¿La tos le produce vómito?
(Lah tohs leh proh-doo-seh boh-mee-toh)

Does the pain get better if you stop and rest?
¿Se mejora el dolor si se detiene y descansa?
(Seh meh-hoh-rah ehl doh-lohr see seh deh-tee-eh-neh oh dehs kahn-sah)

Does the pain move from one place to another?
¿El dolor se mueve de un lugar a otro?
(Ehl doh-lohr seh moo-eh-beh deh oon loo-gahr ah oh-troh)

Does the school have complaints about him?
¿Tiene quejas de la escuela?
(Tee-eh-neh keh-hahs deh lah ehs-koo-eh-lah)

Does the vomit have blood?
¿Tiene sangre el vómito?
(Tee-eh-neh sahn-greh ehl boh-mee-toh)

Does the wind hurt your teeth?
¿Le molesta el aire?
(Leh moh-lehs-tah ehl ah-ee-reh)

Does this surgery require a blood transfusion?
¿Esta cirugía requiere transfusión de sangre?
(Ehs-tah see-roo-hee-ah reh-kee-eh-reh trahns-foo-see-ohn deh sahn-greh)

Don't lift more than five pounds.
No levante más de cinco libras.
(Noh leh-bahn-teh mahs deh seen-koh lee-brahs)

Don't move.
No se mueva.
(Noh seh moo-eh-bah)

Don't use intravenous drugs with contaminated needles; don't share needles or syringes.
No use drogas intravenosas con agujas contaminadas; no comparta agujas o jeringas.
(Noh oos-eh droh-gahs een-trah-beh-noh-sahs kohn ah-goo-hahs kohn-tah-mee-nah-dahs; noh kohm-pahr-tah ah-goo-hahs oh hehr-een-gahs)

Don't be afraid!
¡No tenga miedo!
(Noh tehn-gah mee-eh-doh)

Don't breathe!
¡No respire!
(Noh rehs-pee-reh)

Don't change clothes.
No se cambie de ropa.
(Noh seh kahm-bee-eh deh roh-pah)

Don't get constipated.
No se deje estreñir.
(Noh seh deh-heh ehs-treh-nyeer)

Don't get up!
¡No se levante!
(Noh seh leh-bahn-teh)

Don't hold on!
¡No se agarre!
(Noh seh ah-gahr-reh)

Don't hold the rail.
No agarre el barandal.
(Noh ah-gah-reh ehl bah-rahn-dahl)

Don't laugh!
¡No se ría!
(Noh seh ree-ah)

Don't let him put dirt in his mouth.
No deje que se meta tierra en la boca.
(Noh deh-heh keh seh meh-tah tee-eh-rah ehn lah boh-kah)

Don't let me bend it.
No me dejes que la doble.
(Noh meh deh-hehs keh lah doh-bleh)

Don't let me close them.
No me dejes cerrarlos.
(Noh meh deh-hehs seh-rahr-lohs)

Don't let me extend it.
No me dejes extenderlo.
(Noh meh deh-hehs ehx-tehn-dehr-loh)

Don't let the baby sleep more than three hours during the day.
No deje que el bebé duerma más de tres horas durante el día.
(Noh deh-heh keh ehl beh-beh doo-ehr-mah mahs deh trehs oh-rahs doo-rahn-teh ehl dee-ah)

Don't lie down!
¡No se acueste!
(Noh seh ah-koo-ehs-teh)

Don't move!
¡No se mueva!
(Noh seh moo-eh-bah)

Don't push!
¡No haga esfuerzo!
(Noh ah-gah ehs-foo-ehr-soh)

Don't sit!
¡No se siente!
(Noh seh see-ehn-teh)

Don't talk!
¡No hable!
(Noh ah-bleh)

Don't touch anything!
¡No toque nada!
(Noh toh-keh nah-dah)

Don't turn.
No voltee.
(Noh bohl-teh-eh)

Don't walk barefoot.
No camine descalzo.
(Noh kah-mee-neh dehs-kahl-soh)

Don't worry!
¡No se preocupe!
(Noh seh preh-oh-koo-peh)

Dress him with loose clothes.
Póngale ropa cómoda.
(Pohn-gah-leh roh-pah koh-moh-dah)

Dress the baby with few clothes.
Vista al bebé con poca ropa.
(Bees-tah ahl beh-beh kohn poh-kah roh-pah)

Drink a lot of water and juices.
Tome mucha agua y jugos.
(Toh-meh moo-chah ah-goo-ah ee hoo-gohs)

Drink!
¡Beba/tome!
(Beh-bah/toh-meh)

Drug carts are checked for quantity, number, and expiration dates on all items.
Los carros de drogas se checan/revisan para notar cantidad, número, y fecha de caducidad en todos los artículos.
(Lohs kah-rohs deh droh-gahs seh cheh-kahn/reh-bee-sahn pah-rah noh-tahr kahn-tee-dahd, noo-meh-roh, ee feh-chah deh kah-doo-see-dahd ehn toh-dohs lohs ahr-tee-koo-lohs)

Drugs are dispensed only upon the order of a physician.
Los medicamentos son distribuidos solamente por órdenes de un doctor.
(Lohs meh-dee-kah-mehn-tohs sohn dees-tree-boo-ee-dohs sohl-ah-mehn-teh pohr ohr-dehn-ehs deh oon dohk-tohr)

Eat!
¡Coma!
(Koh-mah)

Eat two to three servings of meat, fish or poultry.
Coma dos a tres porciones de carne, pescado o aves de corral.
(Koh-mah dohs ah trehs pohr-see-oh-nehs deh kahr-neh, pehs-kah-doh oh ah-behs deh ko-rahl)

Eat two to four servings of fruit.
Coma dos a cuatro porciones de fruta.
(Koh-mah dohs ah koo-ah-troh pohr-see-ohn-ehs deh froo-tah)

Eat three to five servings of vegetables.
Coma tres a cinco porciones de vegetales.
(Koh-mah trehs ah seen-koh pohr-see-oh-nehs deh beh-heh-tah-lehs)

Eat six to eleven servings of starches.
Coma seis a once porciones de almidones/féculas.
(Koh-mah seh-ees ah ohn-seh pohr-see-oh-nehs deh ahl-mee-doh-nehs/feh-koo-lahs)

Eat a 1500-calorie diet.
Lleve la dieta de mil quinientas calorías.
(Yeh-beh lah dee-eh-tah deh meel-kee-nee-ehn-tahs kah-loh-ree-ahs)

Eat and sleep well.
Aliméntese y duerma bien.
(Ah-lee-mehn-teh-seh ee doo-ehr-mah bee-ehn)

Eat soft foods.
Coma alimentos blandos.
(Koh-mah ah-lee-mehn-tohs blahn-dohs)

Eat wheat bread and cereals.
Coma pan de trigo y cereales.
(Koh-mah pahn deh tree-goh ee seh-reh-ah-lehs)

Elevate the limb to promote venous and lymphatic drainage.
Eleve el miembro para promover el desagüe venoso y linfático.
(Eh-leh-beh ehl mee-ehm-broh pah-rah proh-moh-behr ehl deh-sah-goo-eh beh-noh-soh ee leen-fah-tee-koh)

Eliminate multiple sexual partners.
Elimine múltiples compañeros sexuales.
(Eh-lee-mee-neh mool-tee-plehs kohm-pah-nyeh-rohs sehx-oo-ah-lehs)

Encourage relaxation exercises.
Estimule los ejercicios de relajamiento.
(Ehs-tee-moo-leh lohs eh-hehr-see-see-ohs deh reh-lah-hah-mee-ehn-toh)

Establish a contract so he does not harm himself.
Establece un contrato para que no se cause daño.
(Ehs-tah-bleh-seh oon kohn-trah-toh pah-rah keh noh seh kah-oo-seh dah-nyoh)

Every day spend time in exercise or a hobby.
Diariamente tome tiempo para hacer ejercicio o una actividad favorita.
(Dee-ah-ree-ah-mehn-teh toh-meh tee-ehm-poh pah-rah ah-sehr eh-hehr-see-see-oh oh oo-nah ahk-tee-bee-dahd fah-boh-ree-tah)

Every time you go to the bathroom to void, you must place the urine in the container.
Cada vez que vaya al baño a orinar, debe poner la orina en el recipiente.
(Kah-dah behs keh bah-yah ahl bah-nyoh ah oh-ree-nahr, deh-beh poh-nehr lah oh-ree-nah ehn ehl reh-see-pee-ehn-teh)

Everybody experiences some anxiety.
Todo el mundo pasa por cierta ansiedad.
(Toh-doh ehl moon-doh pah-sah pohr see-ehr-tah ahn-see-eh-dahd)

Everything sounds good.
Todo se oye bien.
(Toh-doh seh oh-yeh bee-ehn)

Everything will be alright.
Todo saldrá con exito.
(Toh-doh sahl-drah kohn ehx-ee-toh)

Excuse me!
¡Perdón/Excúseme/Con permiso!
(Pehr-dohn/Ehx-koo-seh-meh/Kohn pehr-mee-soh)

Exit to the right.
Salga a la derecha.
(Sahl-gah ah lah deh-reh-chah)

Expiration date.
Caducidad.
(Kah-doo-see-dahd)

Expired items on the unit are returned to the pharmacy.
Los artículos con fecha vencida se devuelven a la farmacia.
(Lohs ahr-tee-koo-lohs kohn feh-chah behn-see-dah seh boo-ehl-behn ah lah fahr-mah-see-ah)

Extend it.
Extiéndelo.
(Ehx-tee-ehn-deh-loh)

Extend your arm.
Extiende tu brazo.
(Ehx-tee-ehn-deh too brah-soh)

Extend your leg and foot.
Extiende tu pierna y pie.
(Ehx-tee-ehn-deh too pee-ehr-nah ee pee-eh)

Extend your wrist.
Extiende tu muñeca.
(Ehx-tee-ehn-deh too moo-nyeh-kah)

Family history of cancer?
¿Hay historia de cáncer en la familia?
(Ah-ee ees-toh-ree-ah deh kahn-sehr ehn lah fah-mee-lee-ah)

Fetus of infected mothers.
Fetos de madres contaminadas.
*(Feh-toohs deh mah-drehs kohn-tah-
mee-nah-dahs)*

Find out.
Descubrir.
(Dehs-koo-breer)

Flex it.
Dóblalo.
(Doh-blah-loh)

Flex the foot upward.
Dobla el pie hacia arriba.
*(Doh-blah ehl pee-eh ah-see-ah ah-ree-
bah)*

Flex your arm, don't let me extend it.
Dobla tu brazo, no me dejes
extenderlo.
*(Doh-blah too brah-soh, noh meh deh-
hehs ehx-tehn-dehr-loh)*

Flex your arm.
Dobla tu brazo.
(Doh-blah too brah-soh)

Flex your knee and turn it to the
middle.
Dobla tu rodilla y voltéala hacia
adentro.
*(Doh-blah too roh-dee-yah ee bohl-
teh-ah-lah ah-see-ah ah-dehn-
troh)*

Follow my finger.
Sigue mi dedo.
(See-geh mee deh-doh)

Follow the green line.
Siga la línea verde.
(See-gah lah lee-nee-ah behr-deh)

Follow the instructions carefully.
Siga las instrucciones con
cuidado.
*(See-gah lahs eens-trook-see-ohn-ehs
kohn koo-ee-dah-doh)*

Follow the red arrows.
Siga las flechas rojas.
(See-gah lahs fleh-chahs roh-hahs)

Foods you may not eat.
Comidas que no debe comer.
*(Koh-mee-dahs keh noh deh-beh koh-
mehr)*

For breakfast?
¿Para el desayuno?
(Pah-rah ehl deh-sah-yoo-noh)

For men: watch urinary problems,
evaluate yearly the size of the
prostate.
En hombres: vigile los problemas de
la orina, haga el examen de la
próstata cada año.
*(Ehn ohm-brehs: bee-hee-leh lohs
proh-bleh-mahs deh lah oh-ree-nah,
ah-gah ehl ehx-ah-mehn deh lah
prohs-tah-tah kah-dah ah-nyoh)*

For now, follow these
recommendations.
Por ahora, siga estas
recomendaciones.
*(Pohr ah-oh-rah see-gah ehs-tahs reh-
koh-mehn-dah-see-oh-nehs)*

For now, change into this gown.
Por ahora, póngase esta bata.
*(Pohr ah-oh-rah, pohn-gah-seh ehs-
tah bah-tah)*

For the birth control plan that you
wish to have.
Para el control de fertilidad que
desee.
*(Pah-rah ehl kohn-trohl deh fehr-tee-
lee-dahd keh deh-seh-eh)*

For what purpose?
¿Para qué?
(Pah-rah keh)

For what reason?
¿Cuál es la razón?
(Koo-ahl ehs lah rah-sohn)

For what?
¿Para qué?
(Pah-rah keh)

For whom?
¿Para quién?
(Pah-rah kee-ehn)

Forward!
¡Adelante!
(Ah-deh-lahn-teh)

Four times a day!
¡Cuatro veces al día!
(Koo-ah-troh beh-sehs ahl dee-ah)

Frequent blisters/ulcerations?
¿Ulceraciones frecuentes?
(Ool-seh-rah-see-oh-nehs freh-koo-ehn-tehs)

From here, turn to the left, then turn right.
De aquí, dé vuelta a la izquierda, luego voltee a la derecha.
(Deh ah-kee, deh boo-ehl-tah ah lah ees-kee-ehr-dah, loo-eh-goh bohl-teh-eh ah lah deh-reh-chah)

From time to time. . .
De vez en cuando. . .
(Deh behs ehn koo-ahn-doh)

From what height did he/she fall?
¿De qué altura cayó?
(Deh keh ahl-too-rah kah-yoh)

Get!
¡Consiga!
(Kohn-see-gah)

Get out!
¡Fuera!
(Foo-eh-rah)

Get up.
Levántese.
(Leh-bahn-teh-seh)

Give him/her the medicine every four hours.
Déle la medicina cada cuatro horas.
(Deh-leh lah meh-dee-see-nah kah-dah koo-ah-troh oh-rahs)

Give it to the clerk.
Déselo a la secretaria.
(Deh-seh-loh ah lah seh-kreh-tah-ree-ah)

Give the medicine every four hours.
Dé la medicina cada cuatro horas.
(Deh lah meh-dee-see-nah kah-dah koo-ah-troh oh-rahs)

Give the medicine with a dropper.
Dé la medicina con gotero.
(Deh lah meh-dee-see-nah kohn goh-teh-roh)

Give the patient a hand mirror and toothbrush.
Déle al paciente un espejo de mano y un cepillo de dientes.
(Deh-leh ahl pah-see-ehn-teh oon ehs-peh-hoh deh mah-noh ee oon seh-pee-yoh deh dee-ehn-tehs)

Go immediately to the hospital!
¡Vaya inmediatamente/enseguida al hospital!
(Bah-yah een-meh-dee-ah-tah-mehn-teh/ehn-seh-ghee-dah ahl ohs-pee-tahl)

Go on, please.
Continúe/Siga, por favor.
(Kohn-tee-noo-eh/See-gah, pohr fah-bohr)

Go through.
Atravesar/Cruzar.
(Ah-trah-beh-sahr/Kroo-sahr)

Go to the dentist every six months.
Vaya al dentista cada seis meses.
(Bah-yah ahl dehn-tees-tah kah-dah seh-ees meh-sehs)

Go to the glass doors.
Vaya a las puertas de vidrio.
(Bah-yah ah lahs poo-ehr-tahs deh bee-dree-oh)

Go to the hospital right away.
Acuda inmediatamente al hospital.
(Ah-koo-dah een-meh-dee-ah-tah-mehn-teh ahl ohs-pee-tahl)

Go to the ophthalmologist every year.
Vaya al oftalmólogo cada año.
(Bah-yah ahl ohf-tahl-moh-loh-goh kah-dah ah-nyoh)

Good afternoon, Miss Gonzalez.
Buenas tardes,señorita Gonzalez.
(Boo-eh-nahs tahr-dehs, seh-nyoh-ree-
tah Gohn-sah-lehs)

Good afternoon.
Buenas tardes.
(Boo-eh-nahs tahr-dehs)

Good evening/Good night!
¡Buenas noches!
(Boo-eh-nahs noh-chehs)

Good luck!
¡Buena suerte!
(Boo-eh-nah soo-ehr-teh)

Good morning doctor.
Buenos días, doctor.
(Boo-eh-nohs dee-ahs, dohk-tohr)

Good morning!
¡Buenos días!
(Boo-eh-nohs dee-ahs)

Good night.
Buenas noches.
(Boo-eh-nahs noh-chehs)

Good!
¡Bueno!
(Boo-eh-noh)

Good-bye!
¡Hasta luego!
(Ahs-tah loo-eh-goh)

Grab the spoon.
Coja la cuchara.
(Koh-hah lah koo-chah-rah)

Great!
¡Bien!
(Bee-ehn)

Has anything changed in your life?
¿Ha cambiado algo en su vida?
(Ah kahm-bee-ah-doh ahl-goh ehn soo
bee-dah)

Has the child been ill?
¿Ha estado enfermo el niño?
(Ah ehs-tah-doh ehn-fehr-moh ehl
nee-nyoh)

Has the pain gotten worse or gotten
better?
¿Se ha puesto el dolor peor o mejor?
(Seh ah poo-ehs-toh ehl doh-lohr peh-
ohr oh meh-hohr)

Has this happened before?
¿Pasó esto antes?
(Pah-soh ehs-toh ahn-tehs)

Has this happened to you before?
¿Le ha pasado esto antes?
(Leh ah pah-sah-doh ehs-toh ahn-
tehs)

Has this problem happened before?
¿Le ha pasado antes este problema?
(Leh ah pah-sah-doh ahn-tehs ehs-teh
proh-bleh-mah)

Have a good day!
¡Pase un buen día!
(Pah-seh oon boo-ehn dee-ah)

Have a yearly Pap smear.
Haga una prueba de papanicolau
cada año.
(Ah-gah oo-nah proo-eh-bah deh pah-
pah-nee-koh-lah-oo kah-dah ah-
nyoh)

Have someone help your husband to
stand up.
Asegure que alguien le ayude a su
esposo a levantarse.
(Ah-seh-goo-reh keh ahl-ghee-ehn leh
ah-yoo-deh ah soo ehs-poh-soh ah
leh-bahn-tahr-seh)

Have you been a patient before?
¿Ha sido paciente antes?
(Ah see-doh pah-see-ehn-teh ahn-tehs)

Have you been exposed to any
infectious diseases?
¿Ha estado expuesto a enfermedades
infecciosas?
(Ah ehs-tah-doh ex-poo-ehs-toh ah
ehn-fehr-meh-dah-dehs een-fek-see-
oh-sahs)

Have you been here before?
¿Ha estado aquí antes?
(Ah ehs-tah-doh ah-kee ahn-tehs)

Have you been sick?
¿Has estado enfermo(a)?
(Ahs ehs-tah-doh ehn-fehr-moh[mah])

Have you eaten?
¿Ha comido?
(Ah koh-mee-doh)

Have you ever been in this hospital?
¿Ha estado en este hospital?
(Ah ehs-tah-doh ehn ehs-teh ohs-pee-tahl)

Have you ever been to the emergency room?
¿Ha estado en el cuarto de emergencia/urgencias?
(Ah ehs-tah-doh ehn ehl koo-ahr-toh deh eh-mehr-hehn-see-ah/oor-hehn-see-ahs)

Have you ever had a heart attack or pains in your heart?
¿Ha tenido ataque al corazón o dolor en el pecho?
(Hah teh-nee-doh ah-tah-keh ahl koh-rah-sohn oh doh-lohr ehn ehl peh-cho)

Have you ever had allergic reaction to a local anesthetic?
¿Ha tenido alergia a la anestesia local?
(Ah teh-nee-doh ah-lehr-hee-ah ah lah ah-nehs-teh-see-ah loh-kahl)

Have you ever had cancer?
¿Ha tenido cáncer?
(Ah teh-nee-doh kahn-sehr)

Have you ever had chemotherapy treatment?
¿Ha tenido tratamiento de quimioterapia?
(Ah teh-nee-doh trah-tah-mee-ehn-toh deh kee-mee-oh-tehr-ah-pee-ah)

Have you ever had hepatitis or cirrhosis?
¿Ha tenido hepatitis o cirrosis?
(Ah teh-nee-doh eh-pah-tee-tees oh see-roh-sees)

Have you ever had joint replacement?
¿Ha tenidole han reemplazado alguna articulación?
(Ah teh-nee-doh-leh ahn rehm-plah-sah-doh ahl-goo-nah ahr-tee-koo-lah-see-ohn)

Have you ever had tuberculosis/lung problems?
¿Ha tenido tuberculosis/problemas con los pulmones?
(Ah teh-nee-doh too-behr-koo-lohs-ees/proh-bleh-mahs kohn lohs pool-moh-nehs)

Have you had a fasting glucose level done?
¿Le han hecho examen de glucosa en ayunas?
(Leh ahn eh-choh ehx-ah-mehn deh gloo-koh-sah ehn ah-yoo-nahs)

Have you had an abortion?
¿Ha tenido abortos?
(Ah teh-nee-doh ah-bohr-tohs)

Have you had any accidents?
¿Ha tenido algún accidente?
(Ah teh-nee-doh ahl-goon ahk-see-dehn-teh)

Have you had any bleeding, swelling or bruising?
¿Ha tenido sangrados, hinchazón o moretones?
(Ah teh-nee-doh sahn-grah-dohs, een-chah-sohn oh moh-reh-toh-nehs)

Have you had any hard blows to your head or chest?
¿Se ha golpeado fuerte la cabeza o el tórax?
(Seh ah gohl-peh-ah-doh foo-ehr-teh lah kah-beh-zah oh ehl toh-rahx)

Have you had anything broken?
¿Ha tenido algo quebrado?
(Ah teh-nee-doh ahl-goh keh-brah-doh)

Have you had blood drawn before?
¿Le han sacado/tomado muestras de
  sangre antes?
*(Leh ahn sah-kah-doh/toh-mah-doh
  moo-ehs-trahs deh sahn-greh ahn-
  tehs)*

Have you had blood transfusion?
¿Ha tenido transfusiones de sangre?
*(Ah teh-nee-doh trahns-foo-see-ohn-
  ehs deh sahn-greh)*

Have you had broken bones?
¿Ha tenido huesos rotos/
  fracturados?
*(Ah teh-nee-doh oo-eh-sohs roh-
  tohs/frahk-too-rah-dohs)*

Have you had cancer?
¿Ha tenido cáncer?
(Ah teh-nee-doh kahn-sehr)

Have you had headaches?
¿Ha tenido dolor de cabeza?
*(Ah teh-nee-doh doh-lohr deh kah-
  beh-sah)*

Have you had neck pain?
¿Ha tenido dolor en el cuello?
*(Ah teh-nee-doh doh-lohr ehn ehl koo-
  eh-yoh)*

Have you had pain in the left arm?
¿Ha sentido dolor en el brazo
  izquierdo?
*(Ah sehn-tee-doh doh-lohr ehn ehl
  brah-soh ees-kee-ehr-doh)*

Have you had reaction to transfusions?
¿Ha tenido reacción a transfusiones?
*(Ah teh-nee-doh reh-ahk-see-ohn ah
  trahns-foo-see-ohn-ehs)*

Have you had rheumatic fever?
¿Ha tenido fiebre reumática?
*(Ah teh-nee-doh fee-eh-breh reh-oo-
  mah-tee-kah)*

Have you had surgeries?
¿Ha tenido operaciones?
*(Ah teh-nee-doh oh-peh-rah-see-ohn-
  ehs)*

Have you had swelling?
¿Ha tenido hinchazón?
(Ah teh-nee-doh een-chah-sohn)

Have you had swelling in your feet?
¿Ha tenido hinchazón en los pies?
*(Ah teh-nee-doh een-chah-sohn ehn
  lohs pee-ehs)*

Have you had swelling in your
  ankles?
¿Ha tenido hinchazón en los
  tobillos?
*(Ah teh-nee-doh een-chah-sohn chn
  lohs toh-bee-yohs)*

Have you had swelling in your
  eyelids?
¿Ha tenido hinchazón en los
  párpados?
*(Ah teh-nee-doh een-chah-sohn ehn
  lohs pahr-pah-dohs)*

Have you had this happen before?
¿Le ha pasado esto antes?
*(Leh ah pah-sah-doh ehs-toh ahn-
  tehs)*

Have you had x-rays?
¿Le han tomado rayos X?
*(Leh ahn toh-mah-doh rah-yohs eh-
  kiss)*

Have you passed out?
¿Se ha desmayado?
(Seh ah dehs-mah-yah-doh)

Have you seen blood in the urine?
¿Ha visto sangre en la orina?
*(Ah bees-toh sahn-greh ehn lah oh-
  ree-nah)*

Having continuous anxiety may cause
  serious problems.
El tener ansiedad continua puede
  llevar a problemas serios.
*(Ehl teh-nehr ahn-see-eh-dahd
  kohn-tee-noo-ah poo-eh-deh yeh-
  bahr ah proh-bleh-mahs seh-ree-
  ohs)*

He also tells her that she must follow directions carefully so that everything turns out alright.
Tambien le dice que debe seguir cuidadosamente las recomendaciones que se le den para que todo salga bien.
(Tahm-bee-ehn leh dee-seh keh deh-beh seh-gheer koo-ee-dah-doh-sah-mehn-teh lahs reh-koh-mehn-dah-see-ohn-ehs keh seh leh dehn pah-rah keh toh-doh sahl-gah bee-ehn)

He assigns a dosage schedule to the order in the computer.
El asigna un horario de dosis a la orden en la computadora.
(Ehl ah-seeg-nah oon oh-rah-ree-oh deh doh-sees ah lah ohr-dehn ehn lah kohm-poo-tah-doh-rah)

He bought me the book.
Me compró el libro.
(Meh kohm-proh ehl lee-broh)

He collected the money from me.
Me cobró el dinero.
(Meh koh-broh ehl dee-neh-roh)

He doesn't speak English, but Spanish.
No habla inglés, sino español.
(Noh ah-blah een-glehs, see-noh ehs-pah-nyohl)

He gave me the money.
Me dió el dinero.
(Meh dee-oh ehl dee-neh-roh)

He had high cholesterol and he had surgery.
Tenía colesterol alto y le hicieron cirugía.
(Teh-nee-ah koh-lehs-teh-rohl ahl-toh ee leh ee-see-eh-rohn see-roo-hee-ah)

He has black hair.
El tiene el pelo negro.
(Ehl tee-ehn-eh ehl peh-loh neh-groh)

He is a barber.
Es barbero.
(Ehs bahr-beh-roh)

He is a hard working barber.
Es un barbero muy trabajador.
(Ehs oon bahr-beh-roh moo-ee trah-bah-hah-dohr)

He is content.
El está contento.
(Ehl ehs-tah kohn-tehn-toh)

He is happy.
El es/está alegre.
(Ehl ehs [ehs-tah] ah-leh-greh)

He is not wearing a green shirt, but a blue one.
No usa camisa verde, sino azul.
(Noh oo-sah kah-mee-sah behr-deh, see-noh ah-sool)

He is sad.
El está triste.
(Ehl ehs-tah trees-teh)

He left without saying anything.
Salió sin decir nada.
(Sah-lee-oh seen deh-seer nah-dah)

He takes the temperature.
Le toma la temperatura.
(Leh toh-mah lah tehm-peh-rah-too-rah.)

He tells her that she will be discharged tomorrow.
Le comunica que mañana será dada de alta.
(Leh koh-moo-nee-kah keh mah-nyah-nah seh-rah dah-dah deh ahl-tah)

He will take you.
El lo llevará.
(Ehl loh yeh-bah-rah)

He will talk to you.
El hablará con usted.
(Ehl ah-blah-rah kohn oos-tehd)

Health insurance?
¿Seguro de salud?
(Seh-goo-roh deh sah-lood)

Hello!
¡Hola!
(Oh-lah)

Hello. I am here to draw your blood.
Hola. Estoy aquí para sacarle una
muestra de sangre.
*(Oh-lah. Ehs-toh-ee ah-kee pah-rah
sah-kahr-leh oo-nah moo-ehs-trah
deh sahn-greh)*

Hello. I am the nurse in charge.
Hola. Yoh soy la enfermera encargada.
*(Oh-lah. Yoh soh-ee lah ehn-fehr-meh-
rah ehn-kahr-gah-dah)*

Hello. I need to take your temperature
and blood pressure.
Hola. Necesito tomarle la
temperatura y la presión de la
sangre.
*(Oh-lah. Neh-seh-see-toh toh-mahr-leh
lah tehm-peh-rah-too-rah ee lah
preh-see-ohn deh lah sahn-greh)*

Hello Mr. Garza, tell me what is wrong.
Hola Sr. Garza, dígame qué le pasa.
*(Oh-lah seh-nyohr Gahr-sah! Dee-gah-
meh, keh leh pah-sah)*

Help him to burp.
Póngalo a repetir/eructar.
*(Pohn-gah-loh ah reh-peh-teer/eh-rook-
tahr)*

Help the patient to identify positive
aspects.
Ayude al paciente a identificar
aspectos positivos.
*(Ah-yoo-deh ahl pah-see-ehn-teh ah
ee-dehn-tee-fee-kahr ahs-pehk-tohs
poh-see-tee-bohs)*

Hemophiliacs and recipients of
contaminated blood.
Hemofílicos y los que reciben
transfusión con sangre
contaminada.
*(Eh-moh-fee-lee-kohs ee los keh reh-
see-behn trahns-foo-see-ohn kohn
sahn-greh kohn-tah-mee-nah-dah)*

Her rings.
Sus anillos.
(Soos ah-nee-yohs)

Here is a glasss of water to rinse with.
Aquí está un vaso de agua para que
se enjuague.
*(Ah-kee ehs-tah oon bah-soh deh ah-
goo-ah pah-rah keh seh ehn-hoo-ah-
geh)*

Here is the bell.
Aquí está la campana.
(Ah-kee ehs-tah lah kahm-pah-nah)

Here is the toilet paper.
Aquí está el papel del
baño/higiénico.
*(Ah-kee ehs-tah ehl pah-pehl dehl
bah-nyoh/ee-hee-eh-nee-koh)*

Here, below the sternum.
Aquí, debajo del esternón.
*(Ah-kee deh-bah-hoh dehl ehs-tehr-
nohn)*

Hi!
¡Hola!
(Oh-lah)

HIV is not transmissible by casual
contact, nor living in the same
house as infected persons.
El VIH no es transmitido en forma
casual, ni por vivir en la misma
casa con personas infectadas.
*(Ehl VIH noh ehs trahns-mee-tee-doh
ehn fohr-mah kah-soo-ahl, nee pohr
bee-beer ehn lah mees-mah kah-sah
kohn pehr-soh-nahs een-fehk-tah-
dahs)*

HIV is not transmissible by coughing,
sneezing, kissing, or swimming with
infected persons.
El VIH no es transmitido en tos,
estornudo, besar, o nadar con
personas infectadas.
*(Ehl VIH noh ehs trahns-mee-tee-doh
ehn tohs, ehs-tohr-noo-doh, beh-
sahr, oh nah-dahr kohn pehr-soh-
nahs een-fehk-tah-dahs)*

HIV is not transmissible by eating food handled by persons with AIDS.
El VIH no es transmitido en comer comida preparada por personas infectadas con SIDA.
(Ehl VIH noh ehs trahns-mee-tee-doh ehn koh-mehr koh-mee-dah preh-pah-rah-dah pohr pehr-soh-nahs een-fehk-tah-dahs kohn see-dah)

Hold it like this.
Manténlo así.
(Mahn-tehn-loh ah-see)

Hold it!
¡Deténlo!
(Deh-tehn-loh)

Hold my finger.
Agarra mi dedo.
(Ah-gah-rah meeh deh-doh)

Hold your breath!
¡No respire!
(Noh rehs-pee-reh)

Hospice offers care from admission through death.
El cuidado del hospicio se da desde el ingreso hasta la muerte.
(Ehl koo-ee-dah-doh dehl ohs-pee-see-oh seh dah dehs-deh ehl een-greh-soh ahs-tah lah moo ehr-teh)

How are you?
¿Cómo está?
(Koh-moh ehs-tah)

How are you, today?
¿Como está hoy?
(Koh-moh ehs-tah oh-ee)

How bad is it?
¿Qué tan mal está?
(Keh tahn mahl ehs-tah)

How did he/she fall?
¿Cómo se cayó?
(Koh-moh seh kah-yoh)

How did this injury happen?
¿Cómo ocurrió está lesión?
(Koh-moh oh-koo-ree-oh ehs-tah leh-see-ohn)

How did you get here?
¿Cómo llegó aquí?
(Koh-moh yeh-goh ah-kee)

How did you move the victim?
¿Cómo movió a la víctima?
(Koh-moh moh-bee-oh ah lah beek-tee-mah)

How did you?
¿Cómo hizo?
(Koh-moh ee-soh)

How do you feel?
¿Cómo te sientes?
(Koh-moh teh see-ehn-tehs)

How do you feel now?
¿Cómo se siente ahora?
(Koh-moh seh see-ehn-teh ah-oh-rah)

How do you get along with your peers?
¿Cómo se lleva usted con sus compañeros?
(Koh-moh seh yeh-bah oos-tehd kohn soos kohm-pah-nyeh-rohs)

How do you like hot dogs?
¿Cómo le gustan los emparedados de salchicha?
(Koh-moh leh goos-tahn lohs ehm-pah-reh-dah-dohs deh sahl-chee-chah)

How do you like the eggs fixed?
¿Cómo le gustan los huevos?
(Koh-moh leh goos-tahn lohs oo-eh-bohs)

How do you like your coffee?
¿Cómo le gusta el café?
(Koh-moh leh goos-tah ehl kah-feh)

How do you spend the day?
¿Cómo pasa el día?
(Koh-moh pah-sah ehl dee-ah)

How far apart are your contractions?
¿Cada cuánto tiempo tiene las contracciones?
(Kah-dah koo-ahn-toh tee-ehm-poh tee-eh-neh lahs kohn-trahk-see-ohn-ehs)

How far?
¿Qué tan lejos?
(Keh tahn leh-hohs)

How is AIDS diagnosed?
¿Cómo se diagnostica el SIDA?
(Koh-moh seh dee-ahg-nohs-tee-kah ehl see-dah)

How is it done?
¿Cómo se hace?
(Koh-moh seh ah-seh)

How long ago?
¿Hace cuánto tiempo?
(Ah-seh koo-ahn-toh tee-ehm-poh)

How long did it last?
¿Cuánto duró?
(Koo-ahn-toh doo-roh)

How long have you been sick?
¿Cuánto tiene de estar enfermo?
(Koo-ahn-toh tee-eh-neh deh ehs-tahr ehn-fehr-moh)

How long have you felt depressed?
¿Desde cuándo se siente deprimido?
(Dehs-deh koo-ahn-doh seh see-ehn-teh deh-pree-mee-doh)

How long?
¿Cuánto tiempo?
(Koo-ahn-toh tee-ehm-poh)

How many boys/girls?
¿Cuántos niños/Cuántas niñas?
(Koo-ahn-tohs nee-nyohs/Koo-ahn-tahs nee-nyahs)

How many cars crashed?
¿Cuántos carros chocaron?
(Koo-ahn-tohs kah-rohs choh-kah-rohn)

How many children do you have?
¿Cuántos niños tiene?
(Koo-ahn-tohs nee-nyohs tee-eh-neh)

How many cigarettes per day?
¿Cuántos cigarrillos por día?
(Koo-ahn-tohs see-gah-ree-yohs pohr dee-ah)

How many cups per day?
Cuántas tazas diarias?
(Koo-ahn-tahs tah-sahs dee-ah-ree-ahs)

How many diapers have you changed since yesterday?
¿Cuántos pañales le ha cambiado desde ayer?
(Koo-ahn-tohs pah-nyah-lehs leh ah kahm-bee-ah-doh dehs-deh ah-yehr)

How many friends do you have?
¿Cuántos amigos tienes?
(Koo-ahn-tohs ah-mee-gohs tee-eh-nehs)

How many glasses of water do you drink?
¿Cuántos vasos de agua toma?
(Koo-ahn-tohs bah-sohs deh ah-goo-ah toh-mah)

How many hours do you sleep?
¿Cuántas horas duermes?
(Koo-ahn-tahs oh-rahs doo-ehr-mehs)

How many hours do you work?
¿Cuántas horas trabaja?
(Koo-ahn-tahs oh-rahs trah-bah-hah)

How many months pregnant?
¿Cuántos meses tiene de embarazo?
(Koo-ahn-tohs meh-sehs tee-eh-neh deh ehm-bah-rah-soh)

How many ounces does he take?
¿Cuántas onzas toma?
(Koo-ahn-tahs ohn-sahs toh-mah)

How many packs a day?
¿Cuántas cajetillas al día?
(Koo-ahn-tahs kah-heh-tee-yahs ahl dee-ah)

How many people were in the car/bus/truck?
¿Cuántas personas estaban en el carro/el autobús/la camioneta?
(Koo-ahn-tahs pehr-soh-nahs ehs-tah-bahn ehn ehl kah-roh/ehl ahoo-toh-boohs/lah kah-mee-oh-neh-tah)

How many persons in your family?
¿Cuántas personas forman su familia?
(Koo-ahn-tahs pehr-soh-nahs fohr-mahn soo fah-mee-lee-ah)

How many pounds have you gained?
¿Cuántas libras a aumentado?
(Koo-ahn-tahs lee-brahs ah ah-oo-mehn-tah-doh)

How many pregnancies have you had?
¿Cuántos embarazos ha tenido?
(Koo-ahn-tohs ehm-bah-rah-sohs ah
  teh-nee-doh)

How many times a day?
¿Cuántas veces al día?
(Koo-ahn-tahs beh-sehs ahl dee-ah)

How many times do you eat per day?
¿Cuántas veces come por dia?
(Koo-ahn-tahs beh-sehs koh-meh pohr
  dee-ah)

How many times does he wake up?
¿Cuántas veces se despierta?
(Koo-ahn-tahs beh-sehs seh dehs-pee-
  ehr-tah)

How many times has he vomited?
¿Cuántas veces ha vomitado?
(Koo-ahn-tahs beh-sehs ah boh-mee-
  tah-doh)

How many years did you go to school?
¿Cuántos años fue a la escuela?
(Koo-ahn-tohs ah-nyohs foo-eh ah lah
  ehs-koo-eh-lah)

How many?
¿Cuántos/Cuántas?
(Koo-ahn-tohs/Koo-ahn-tahs)

How much alcohol do you drink per
  day?
¿Cuánto alcohol toma por día?
(Koo-ahn-toh ahl-kohl toh-mah pohr
  dee-ah)

How much medicine did you take?
¿Cuánta medicina tomó?
(Koo-ahn-tah meh-dee-see-nah toh-
  moh)

How much water do you drink?
¿Cuánta agua toma?
(Koo-ahn-tah ah-goo-ah toh-mah)

How much?
¿Cuánto/Cuánta?
(Koo-ahn-toh/Koo-ahn-tah)

How often do you feed the baby?
¿Qué tan a menudo alimenta al bebé?
(Keh tahn ah meh-noo-doh ah-lee-
  mehn-tah ahl beh-beh)

How often do you have the pain?
¿Qué tan seguido tiene el dolor?
(Keh tahn seh-ghee-doh tee-eh-neh ehl
  doh-lohr)

How often do you urinate?
¿Cuántas veces orina?
(Koo-ahn-tahs beh-sehs oh-ree-nah)

How old are you/they?
¿Cuántos años tiene/tienen?
(Koo-ahn-tohs ah-nyohs /tee-eh-
  neh/tee-eh-nehn)

How serious is AIDS?
¿Qué tan serio es el SIDA?
(Keh tahn seh-ree-oh ehs ehl
  see-dah)

How severe is the pain?
¿Qué tan severo es el dolor?
(Keh tahn seh-beh-roh ehs ehl doh-lohr)

How?
¿Cómo?
(Koh-moh)

I also need a urine sample.
También necesito una muestra de
  orina.
(Tahm-bee-ehn neh-seh-see-toh oo-nah
  moo-ehs-trah deh oh-ree-nah)

I am 44 years old.
Tengo cuarenta y cuatro años.
(Tehn-goh koo-ah-rehn-tah ee koo-ah-
  troh ah-nyohs)

I am afraid to get lost.
Tengo miedo de perderme.
(Tehn-goh mee-eh-doh deh pehr-dehr-
  meh)

I am back.
Ya regresé.
(Yah reh-greh-seh)

I am continuously. . .
Continuamente estoy. . .
(Kohn-tee-noo-ah-mehn-teh ehs-tohy)

I am Dr. Blanco.
Yo soy el doctor Blanco.
(Yoh soh-ee ehl dohk-tohr Blahn-koh)

I am fine, doctor, thank you! I feel like new.
¡Muy bien, doctor, gracias! Me siento como nuevo.
(Moo-ee bee-ehn, dohk-tohr, grah-see-ahs. Meh see-ehn-toh koh-moh noo-eh-boh)

I am going to ask many/some questions!
¡Voy a hacerle muchas/unas preguntas!
(Boh-ee ah ah-sehr-leh moo-chahs/oo-nahs preh-goon-tahs)

I am going to auscultate.
Voy a auscultar/escuchar.
(Boh-ee ah ah-oos-kool-tahr/ehs-koo-chahr)

I am going to call the radiologist.
Voy a llamar al radiólogo.
(Boh-ee ah yah-mahr ahl rah-dee-oh-loh-goh)

I am going to check how strong your abdominal muscle is.
Voy a ver la fuerza del músculo abdominal.
(Boh-ee ah behr lah foo-ehr-sah dehl moos-koo-loh ahb-doh-mce-nahl)

I am going to check the arm.
Voy a revisar tu brazo.
(Boh-ee ah reh-bee-sahr too brah-soh)

I am going to check the oxygen tank.
Voy a checar el tanque de oxígeno.
(Boh-ee ah cheh-kahr ehl tahn-keh deh ohx-ee-heh-noh)

I am going to check your ears.
Voy a revisar tus orejas.
(Boh-ee ah reh-bee-sahr tuos oh-reh-hahs)

I am going to check your eyes.
Voy a revisar tus ojos.
(Boh-ee ah reh-bee-sahr toos oh-hohs)

I am going to check your gums.
Voy a revisar tus encías.
(Boh-ee ah reh-bee-sahr toos ehn-see-ahs)

I am going to check your hand.
Voy a revisar tu mano.
(Boh-ee ah reh-bee-sahr too mah-noh)

I am going to check your head.
Voy a revisar tu cabeza.
(Boh-ee ah reh-bee-sahr too kah-beh-sah)

I am going to check your liver.
Voy a revisar tu hígado.
(Boh-ee ah reh-bee-sahr too ee-gah-doh)

I am going to check your mouth.
Voy a revisar tu boca.
(Boh-ee ah reh-bee-sahr tooh boh-kah)

I am going to check your nose.
Voy a revisar la nariz.
(Boh-ee ah reh-bee-sahr lah nah-rees)

I am going to check your teeth.
Voy a revisar tus dientes.
(Boh-ee ah reh-bee-sahr toos dee-ehn-tehs)

I am going to check your throat.
Voy a revisar la garganta.
(Boh-ee ah reh-bee-sahr lah gahr-gahn-tah)

I am going to clean your teeth.
Voy a limpiarle los dientes.
(Boh-ee ah leem-pee-ahr-leh lohs dee-ehn-tehs)

I am going to collect a stool sample.
Voy a recoger una muestra de excremento.
(Boh-ee ah reh-koh-hehr oo-nah moo-ehs-trah deh ehx-kreh-mehn-toh)

I am going to cover you with a sheet.
Voy a cubrirlo con una sábana.
(Boh-ee ah koo-breer-loh kohn oo-nah sah-bah-nah)

I am going to cover you.
Lo voy a cubrir.
(Loh boh-ee ah koo-breer)

I am going to examine the genitalia.
Voy a examinar los genitales.
(Boh-ee ah ehx-ah-mee-nahr lohs heh-nee-tah-lehs)

I am going to examine the leg.
Voy a examinar tu pierna.
(Boh-ee ah ehx-ah-mee-nahr too pee-ehr-nah)

I am going to examine the rectum.
Voy a examinar el recto.
(Boh-ee ah ehx-ah-mee-nahr ehl rehk-toh)

I am going to examine you.
Voy a examinarlo.
(Boh-ee ah ehx-ah-mee-nahr-loh[lah])

I am going to examine your back.
Voy a examinar tu espalda.
(Boh-ee ah ehx-ah-mee-nahr too ehs-pahl-dah)

I am going to examine your foot.
Voy a examinar tu pie.
(Boh-ee ah ehx-ah-mee-nahr too pee-eh)

I am going to examine your nailbeds.
Voy a examinar la base de tus uñas.
(Boh-ee ah ehx-ah-mee-nahr lah bah-seh deh toos oo-nyahs)

I am going to explain the collection of urine.
Le voy a explicar la colección de orina.
(Leh boh-ee ah ehx-plee-kahr lah koh-lehk-see-ohn deh oh-ree-nah)

I am going to get a wheelchair.
Voy a traer una silla de ruedas.
(Boh-ee ah trah-ehr oo-nah see-yah deh roo-eh-dahs)

I am going to give you a list.
Voy a darle una lista.
(Boh-ee ah dahr-leh oo-nah lees-tah)

I am going to give you a tour of the floor.
Voy a darle un recorrido por el piso.
(Boh-ee ah dahr-leh oon reh-koh-ree-doh pohr ehl pee-soh)

I am going to help you.
Voy a ayudarlo.
(Boh-ee ah ah-yoo-dahr-loh)

I am going to help you lie on the stretcher.
Voy a ayudarlo a acostarse en la camilla.
(Boh-ee ah ah-yoo-dahr-loh ah ah-kohs-tahr-seh ehn lah kah-mee-yah)

I am going to hit gently.
Voy a darle golpecitos.
(Boh-ee ah dahr-leh gohl-peh-see-tohs)

I am going to insert your dentures.
Voy a ponerle la dentadura.
(Boh-ee ah poh-nehr-leh lah dehn-tah-doo-rah)

I am going to let you rest.
Voy a dejarlo descansar.
(Boh-ee ah deh-hahr-loh dehs-kahn-sahr)

I am going to lift your sleeve.
Voy a levantar la manga.
(Boh-ee ah leh-bahn-tahr lah mahn-gah)

I am going to listen to the baby's heart beat.
Voy a escuchar el latido del corazón del bebé.
(Boh-ee ah ehs-koo-chahr ehl lah-tee-doh dehl koh-rah-sohn dehl beh-beh)

I am going to listen to the lungs.
Voy a oír los pulmones.
(Boh-ee ah oh-eer lohs pool-moh-nehs)

I am going to listen to your heart.
Voy a escuchar el corazón.
(Boh-ee ah ehs-koo-chahr ehl koh-rah-sohn)

I am going to listen to your heartbeat.
Voy a oír tu pulso apical/los latidos del corazón.
(Boh-ee ah oh-eer too pool-soh ah-pee-kahl/lohs lah-tee-dohs dehl koh-rah-sohn)

I am going to observe the jugular vein.
Voy a observar tu vena yugular.
(Boh-ee ah ohb-sehr-bahr too beh-nah yoo-goo-lahr)

I am going to palpate deeply.
Voy a palpar hondo.
(Boh-ee ah pahl-pahr ohn-doh)

I am going to palpate it.
Voy a palparla.
(Boh-ee ah pahl-pahr-lah)

I am going to palpate lightly.
Voy a palpar/tocar ligero.
(Boh-ee ah pahl-pahr/toh-kahr lee-heh-roh)

I am going to palpate the axillary nodes.
Voy a palpar los nodos de la axila.
(Boh-ee ah pahl-pahr lohs noh-dohs deh lah ahx-ee-lah)

I am going to palpate the breast.
Voy a palpar el seno.
(Boh-ee ah pahl-pahr ehl seh-noh)

I am going to palpate the groin.
Voy a palpar las ingles.
(Boh-ee ah pahl-pahr lahs een-glehs)

I am going to palpate the shoulder.
Voy a palpar tu hombro.
(Boh-ee ah pahl-pahr too ohm-broh)

I am going to palpate with both hands.
Voy a palpar/tocar con las dos manos.
(Boh-ee ah pahl-pahr/toh-kahr kohn lahs dohs mah-nohs)

I am going to palpate your carotid pulse.
Voy a palpar tu pulso en la carótida/en el cuello.
(Boh-ee ah pahl-pahr too pool-soh ehn lah kah-roh-tee-dah/ehn ehl koo-eh-yoh)

I am going to palpate your chest.
Voy a palpar el pecho.
(Boh-ee ah pahl-pahr ehl peh-choh)

I am going to palpate your elbow.
Voy a palpar tu codo.
(Boh-ee ah pahl-pahr too koh-doh)

I am going to palpate your feet and ankles.
Voy a palpar tus pies y tobillos.
(Boh-ee ah pahl-pahr toos pee-ehs ee toh-bee-yohs)

I am going to palpate your knees.
Voy a palpar tus rodillas.
(Boh-ee ah pahl-pahr toos roh-dee-yahs)

I am going to palpate your nodes.
Voy a palpar tus nodos.
(Boh-ee ah pahl-pahr toos noh-dohs)

I am going to press on your big toe.
Voy a apretar tu dedo grueso.
(Boh-ee ah ah-preh-tahr too deh-doh groo-eh-soh)

I am going to put on a bandage/Bandaid.
Voy a ponerle una cinta adhesiva/bandaid.
(Boh-ee ah poh-nehr-leh oo-nah seen-tah ah-deh-see-bah/bahn-dah-eed)

I am going to put a splint on the leg.
Voy a ponerle una tablilla en la pierna.
(Boh-ee ah poh-nehr-leh oo-nah tah-blee-yah ehn lah pee-ehr-nah)

I am going to take x-rays of the abdomen first.
Voy a tomar rayos X del abdomen primero.
(Boh-ee ah toh-mahr rah-yohs eh-kiss dehl ahb-doh-mehn pree-meh-roh)

I am going to take x-rays.
Le tomaré radiografías.
(Leh toh-mah-reh rah-dee-oh-grah-fee-ahs)

I am going to take the radial pulse.
Voy a tomar tu pulso radial.
(Boh-ee ah toh-mahr too pool-soh rah-dee-ahl)

I am going to take your blood pressure and the pulse.
Voy a tomar la presión y el pulso.
(Boh-ee ah toh-mahr lah preh-see-ohn ee ehl pool-soh)

I am going to tap.
Voy a percutir/golpear.
(Boh-ee ah pehr-koo-teer/gohl-peh-ahr)

I am going to use local anesthetic.
Voy a usar anestesia local.
(Boh-ee ah oo-sahr ah-nehs-teh-see-ah loh-kahl)

I am here to care for your husband.
Estoy aquí para cuidar a su esposo.
(Ehs-toh-ee ah-kee pah-rah koo-ee-dahr ah soo ehs-poh-soh)

I am here to examine the baby.
Estoy aquí para examinar al bebé.
(Ehs-toh-ee ah-kee pah-rah ehx-ah-mee-nahr ahl beh-beh)

I am here to help you with exercises.
Estoy aquí para ayudarlo con ejercicios.
(Ehs-toh-ee ah-kee pah-rah ah-yoo-dahr-loh kohn eh-hehr-see-see-ohs)

I am hurting a lot.
Tengo mucho dolor.
(Tehn-goh moo-choh doh-lohr)

I am Mexican.
Soy Mexicana.
(Soh-ee Meh-hee-kah-nah)

I am not well.
No estoy bien.
(Noh ehs-toh-ee bee-ehn)

I am pre-diabetic. I control it with diet.
Soy prediabética. Me controlo con dieta.
(Soh-ee preh-dee-ah-beh-tee-kah. Meh kohn-troh-loh kohn dee-eh-tah)

I am putting a casette under your waist.
Estoy poniendo una casetera abajo de la cintura.
(Ehs-toh-ee poh-nee-ehn-doh oo-nah kah-seh-teh-rah ah-bah-hoh deh lah seen-too-rah)

I am putting on a temporary filling.
Le aplicaré empaste temporal.
(Leh ah-plee-kah-reh ehm-pahs-teh tehm-poh-rahl)

I am sorry, no toothpicks.
Lo siento, no hay palillos.
(Loh see-ehn-toh, noh ah-ee pah-lee-yohs)

I am the dentist.
Yo soy el/la dentista.
(Yoh soh-ee ehl/lah dehn-tees-tah)

I am the doctor (female).
Yo soy la doctora.
(Yoh soh-ee lah dohk-tohr-ah)

I am the doctor (male).
Yo soy el doctor.
(Yoh soh-ee ehl dohk-tohr)

I am the medical student.
Yo soy el/la estudiante de medicina.
(Yoh soh-ee ehl/lah ehs-too-dee-ahn-teh deh meh-dee-see-nah)

I am the nurse.
Yo soy el/la enfermero(a).
(Yoh soh-ee ehl/lah ehn-fehr-meh-roh[rah])

I am the social worker.
Yo soy el/la trabajador(a) social.
(Yoh soh-ee ehl/lah trah-bah-hah-dohr[-dohra] soh-see-ahl)

I am the technician.
Yo soy el técnico/la técnica.
(Yoh soh-ee ehl tehk-nee-koh/lah tehk-nee-kah)

I am the therapist.
Yo soy el/la terapista.
(Yoh soh-ee ehl/lah teh-rah-pees-tah)

I am through.
Ya terminé.
(Yah tehr-mee-neh)

I am very healthy!
¡Estoy muy sano!
(Ehs-toh-ee moo-ee sah-noh)

I can do that.
Puedo hacerlo.
(Poo-eh-doh ah-sehr-loh)

I can help you to sit down.
Le puedo ayudar a sentarse.
(Leh poo-eh-doh ah-yoo-dahr ah sehn-tahr-seh)

I can stop.
Puedo pararme.
(Poo-eh-doh pah-rahr-meh)

I cannot read English, can you help me?
¿No puedo leer inglés, puede ayudarme?
(Noh poo-eh-doh leh-ehr een-glehs, poo-eh-deh ah-yoo-dahr-meh)

I certify that I have been informed of
the treatment and have been told of
the benefits and risks.
Yo certifico que me han informado
acerca del tratamiento y me han
dicho sus beneficios y riesgos.
*(Yoh sehr-tee-fee-koh keh meh ahn
een-fohr-mah-doh dehl trah-tah-
mee-ehn-toh ee meh ahn dee-choh soos
beh-neh-fee-see-ohs ee ree-ehs-gohs)*

I charged.
Yo cobré.
(Yoh koh-breh)

I checked your x-rays.
Revisé sus radiografías.
*(Reh-bee-seh soos rah-dee-oh-grah-fee-
ahs)*

I consent to the treatment in addition
to or different from those now being
planned.
Doy permiso para el tratamiento en
adición o diferente del tratamiento
planeado.
*(Doh-ee pehr-mee-soh pah-rah ehl trah-
tah-mee-ehn-toh ehn ah-dee-see-ohn
oh dee-feh-rehn-teh dehl trah-tah-
mee-ehn-toh plah-neh-ah-doh)*

I don't want.
No quiero.
(Noh kee-eh-roh)

I don't have a pen either.
Tampoco tengo una pluma.
*(Tahm-poh-koh tehn-goh oo-nah ploo-
mah)*

I don't know.
No sé.
(Noh seh)

I don't like to study, but (rather) to go
to the theater.
No me gusta estudiar, sino ir al
teatro.
*(Noh meh goos-tah ehs-too-dee-ahr,
see-noh eer ahl teh-ah-troh)*

I don't think so.
No lo creo.
(Noh loh kreh-oh)

I don't like it.
No me gusta.
(Noh meh goos-tah)

I feel dizzy.
Me siento mareado.
(Meh see-ehn-toh mah-reh-ah-doh)

I feel overwhelmed, anxious.
Me siento abatido, ansioso.
*(Meh see-ehn-toh ah-bah-tee-doh ahn-
see-oh-soh)*

I go downtown (on) Tuesdays.
Los martes voy al centro.
(Lohs mahr-tehs boh-ee ahl sehn-troh)

I go to sleep at eleven.
Me duermo a las once.
(Meh doo-ehr-moh ah lahs ohn-seh)

I have a gown.
Tengo una bata.
(Tehn-goh oo-nah bah-tah)

I have a piece of paper.
Tengo un pedazo de papel.
*(Tehn-goh oon peh-dah-soh deh pah-
pehl)*

I have been sick all morning.
Me he sentido mal toda la mañana.
*(Meh eh sehn-tee-doh mahl toh-dah
lah mah-nyah-nah)*

I have diarrhea and stomach pains.
Tengo diarrea y dolores de estómago.
*(Tehn-goh dee-ah-reh-ah ee doh-loh-
rehs deh ehs-toh-mah-goh)*

I have finished the exam.
Terminé de revisarte.
(Tehr-mee-neh deh reh-bee-sahr-teh)

I have first-hand information.
Tengo información de primera.
*(Tehn-goh een-fohr-mah-see-ohn deh
pree-meh-rah)*

I have looked at the information we
discussed yesterday.
He revisado la información que
discutimos ayer.
*(Heh reh-bee-sah-doh lah een-fohr-
mah-see-ohn keh dees-koo-tee-mohs
ah-yehr)*

I have nausea and fever.
Tengo náusea y fiebre.
(Tehn-goh nah-oo-seh-ah ee fee-eh-breh)

I have nausea, vomiting, fever, and
general malaise.
Tengo náuseas, vómito, fiebre y
malestar general.
*(Tehn-goh nah-oo-seh-ahs, boh-mee-
toh, fee-eh-breh ee mahl-ehs-tahr
heh-neh-rahl)*

I have neither paper nor pencil.
No tengo ni papel ni lápiz.
(Noh tehn-goh nee pah-pehl nee lah-pees)

I have noticed some difficulty
breathing for the last two days.
Me he dado cuenta de alguna
dificultad para respirar en los
últimos dos días.
*(Meh eh dah-doh koo-ehn-tah deh
ahl-goo-nah dee-fee-koohl-tahd pah-
rah rehs-pee-rahr ehn lohs ool-tee-
mohs dohs dee-ahs)*

I have pain.
Tengo dolor.
(Tehn-goh doh-lohr)

I have some paper.
Tengo papel.
(Tehn-goh pah-pehl)

I have the bedpan.
Tengo el bacín/pato.
(Tehn-goh ehl bah-seen/pah-toh)

I have to assess first.
Necesito evaluar primero.
*(Neh-seh-see-toh eh-bah-loo-ahr pree-
meh-roh)*

I have to call your parents.
Tengo que llamar a sus padres.
*(Tehn-goh keh yah-mahr ah soos pah-
drehs)*

I have to enter the information in the
computer.
Tengo que poner la información en
la computadora.
*(Tehn-goh keh poh-nehr lah een-fohr-
mah-see-ohn ehn lah kohm-poo-tah-
doh-rah)*

I have to take out your tooth.
Tengo que extraer/sacar el diente.
*(Tehn-goh keh ehx-trah-ehr/sah-kahr
ehl dee-ehn-teh)*

I hope you do well.
Que siga bien.
(Keh see-gah bee-ehn)

I like green (that which is green).
Me gusta lo verde.
(Meh goos-tah loh behr-deh)

I like red (that which is red).
Me gusta lo rojo.
(Meh goos-tah loh roh-hoh)

I like summer.
Me gusta el verano.
(Meh goos-tah ehl beh-rah-noh)

I need better directions.
Necesito mejores direcciones.
*(Neh-seh-see-toh meh-hoh-rehs dee-
rehk-see-ohn-ehs)*

I need for you to sign this permission
slip so that the procedure might be
done.
Necesito que firme usted el permiso,
para realizar este estudio.
*(Neh-seh-see-toh keh feer-meh oos-
tehd ehl pehr-mee-soh, pah-rah
reh-ah-lee-sahr ehs-teh ehs-too-dee-
oh)*

I need to ask you some questions.
Necesito hacerle unas preguntas.
*(Neh-seh-see-toh ah-sehr-leh oo-nahs
preh-goon-tahs)*

I need to cut the pant.
Necesito cortar el pantalón.
*(Neh-seh-see-toh kohr-tahr ehl pahn-
tah-lohn)*

I need to go to the surgery clinic.
Necesito ir a la clínica de cirugía.
*(Neh-seh-see-toh eer ah lah klee-nee-
kah deh see-roo-hee-ah)*

I need to see Doctor White.
Necesito ver al Doctor White.
*(Neh-seh-see-toh behr ahl dohk-tohr
White)*

I need to see if you are hurt.
Necesito ver si está lastimado.
*(Neh-seh-see-toh behr see ehs-tah
lahs-tee-mah-doh)*

I need to see the injured.
Necesito ver al accidentado.
*(Neh-seh-see-toh behr ahl ahk-see-
dehn-tah-doh)*

I need to use a tourniquet.
Necesito usar un torniquete/una
ligadura.
*(Neh-seh-see-toh oo-sahr oon tohr-nee-
keh-teh/oon-ah lee-gah-doo-rah)*

I need two tubes of blood.
Necesito dos tubos de sangre.
*(Neh-seh-see-toh dohs too-bohs deh
sahn-greh)*

I never have headaches!
¡Nunca tengo dolor de cabeza!
*(Noon-kah tehn-goh doh-lohr deh kah-
beh-sah)*

I pulled your tooth.
Le saqué el diente.
(Leh sah-keh ehl dee-ehn-teh)

I see from your history that weight has
always been a problem.
Veo en su historia que su peso
siempre ha sido un problema.
*(Beh-oh ehn soo ees-toh-ree-ah keh soo
peh-soh see-ehm-preh ah see-doh
oon proh-bleh-mah)*

I see how good she is.
Ya veo lo buena que es.
(Yah beh-oh loh boo-eh-nah keh ehs)

I see no one (here).
No veo a nadie (aquí).
(Noh beh-oh ah nah-dee-eh [ah-kee])

I see your sister and grandfather had
diabetes.
Veo que su hermana y abuelo tenían
diabetes.
*(Beh-oh keh soo ehr-mah-nah ee ah-
boo-eh-loh teh-nee-ahn dee-ah-beh-
tehs)*

I see.
Ya veo.
(Yah beh-oh)

I think it is broken.
Creo que está rota.
(Kreh-oh keh ehs-tah roh-tah)

I think the same as you.
Pienso lo mismo que usted.
*(Pee-ehn-soh loh mees-moh keh oos-
tehd)*

I want something to drink (eat)!
¡Yo quiero algo de tomar/beber
(comer)!
*(Yoh kee-eh-roh ahl-goh deh
toh-mahr/beh-behr[koh-mehr])*

I want something to read!
¡Yo quiero algo de leer!
(Yoh kee-eh-roh ahl-goh deh leh-ehr)

I want to be a good nurse.
Quiero ser una buena enfermera.
*(Kee-eh-roh sehr oo-nah boo-eh-nah
ehn-fehr-meh-rah)*

I want to be a nurse.
Quiero ser una enfermera.
*(Kee-eh-roh sehr oo-nah ehn-fehr-meh-
rah)*

I want to brush your teeth.
Quiero limpiarle los dientes.
*(Kee-eh-roh leem-pee-ahr-leh lohs dee-
ehn-tehs)*

I want to do some testing.
Quiero hacer una prueba.
*(Kee-eh-roh ah-sehr oon-ah proo-eh-
bah)*

I want to examine the older child.
Quiero examinar al niño mayor.
*(Kee-eh-roh ehx-ah-mee-nahr ahl nee-
nyoh mah-yohr)*

I want to hear the abdomen.
Quiero escuchar el abdomen.
*(Kee-eh-roh ehs-koo-chahr ehl ahb-
doh-mehn)*

I want to hear your heart.
Quiero escuchar el corazón.
(Kee-eh-roh ehs-koo-chahr ehl koh-rah-sohn)

I want to hear your lungs.
Quiero escuchar los pulmones.
(Kee-eh-roh ehs-koo-chahr lohs pool-moh-nehs)

I want to help you stand up.
Quiero ayudarlo a sentarse.
(Kee-eh-roh ah-yoo-dahr-loh ah sehn-tahr-seh)

I want to review our services.
Quiero repasar nuestros servicios.
(Kee-eh-roh reh-pah-sahr noo-ehs-trohs sehr-bee-see-ohs.

I want to see if the x-rays are good.
Quiero ver si los rayos X salieron bien.
(Kee-eh-roh behr see lohs rah-yohs eh-kiss sah-lee-eh-rohn bee-ehn)

I want to take a sample of blood from your finger.
Quiero tomar una muestra de sangre del dedo.
(Kee-eh-roh toh-mahr oo-nah moo-ehs-trah deh sahn-greh del deh-doh)

I want to talk about bacterial plaque.
Quiero platicar acerca de la placa bacteriana.
(Kee-eh-roh plah-tee-kahr ah-sehr-kah deh lah plah-kah bahk-teh-ree-ah-nah)

I want to talk to you.
Quiero hablar con usted.
(Kee-eh-roh ah-blahr kohn oos-tehd)

I want to test the sugar level.
Quiero checar el nivel de azúcar.
(Kee-eh-roh cheh-kahr ehl nee-behl deh ah-soo-kahr)

I want you to chew on them for four minutes.
Quiero que las muerda por cuatro minutos.
(Kee-eh-roh keh lahs moo-ehr-dah pohr koo-ah-troh mee-noo-tohs)

I want you to do each exercise three times a day.
Quiero que haga cada ejercicio tres veces al día.
(Kee-eh-roh keh ah-gah kah-dah eh-hehr-see-see-oh trehs beh-sehs ahl dee-ah)

I want you to use a cane.
Quiero que use un bastón.
(Kee-eh-roh keh oo-seh oon bahs-tohn)

I want you to write your name and today's date.
Quiero que escriba su nombre y la fecha de hoy.
(Kee-eh-roh keh ehs-kree-bah soo nohm-breh ee lah feh-chah deh oh-ee)

I was doing nothing.
No estaba haciendo nada.
(Noh ehs-tah-bah ah-see-ehn-doh nah-dah)

I was just sitting, watching television when the pain started.
Sólo estaba sentado, viendo televisión cuando comenzó el dolor.
(Soh-loh ehs-tah-bah sehn-tah-doh, bee-ehn-doh teh-leh-bee-see-ohn koo-ahn-doh koh-mehn-soh ehl doh-lohr)

I was told to come here.
Me dijeron que viniera aquí.
(Meh dee-heh-rohn keh bee-nee-eh-rah ah-kee)

I will ask you to void.
Le diré que orine.
(Leh dee-reh keh oh-ree-neh)

I will give you a bath.
Voy a bañarlo.
(Boh-ee ah bah-nyahr-loh)

I will place the saliva ejector in between the trays so that you will not swallow any of the fluoride.
Pondré el extractor de saliva en medio de las bandejas, para que no se trague el fluoruro.
(Pohn-dreh ehl ehx-trahk-tohr deh sah-lee-bah ehn meh-dee-oh deh lahs bahn-deh-hahs, pah-rah keh noh seh trah-geh ehl floh-roo-roh)

I will place the trays over the teeth.
Pondré las bandejas sobre los
dientes.
*(Pohn-dreh lahs bahn-deh-hahs soh-
breh lohs dee-ehn-tehs)*

I will remind you during the day.
Le recordaré durante el día.
*(Leh reh-kohr-dah-reh doo-rahn-teh
ehl dee-ah)*

I will return.
Regresaré/volveré.
(Reh-greh-sah-reh/bohl-beh-reh)

I will return in ten minutes.
Volveré en diez minutos.
*(Bohl-beh-reh chn dee-ehs mee-noo-
tohs)*

I will return in two days.
Regresaré en dos días.
(Reh-greh-sah-reh ehn dohs dee-ahs)

I will return shortly.
Regresaré en seguida.
(Reh-greh-sah-reh ehn seh-gee-dah)

I will return tomorrow.
Regresaré mañana.
(Reh-greh-sah-reh mah-nyah-nah)

I will return to ask you more
questions.
Regresaré para hacerle más
preguntas.
*(Reh-greh-sah-reh pah-rah ah-sehr-leh
mahs preh-goon-tahs)*

I will see the strength of the
abdominal muscle.
Veré la fuerza del músculo
abdominal.
*(Beh-reh lah foo-ehr-sah dehl moos-
koo-loh ahb-doh-mee-nahl)*

I will see you (f).
La veré.
(Lah beh-reh)

I will see you tomorrow.
La veré mañana.
(Lah beh-reh mah-nyah-nah)

I will see you tomorrow at nine (m).
Lo veré mañana a las nueve.
*(Loh beh-reh mah-nyah-nah ah lahs
noo-eh-beh)*

I will show you your room.
Le mostraré su cuarto.
(Leh mohs-trah-reh soo koo-ahr-toh)

I will start by taking vital signs.
Empezaré por tomar los signos
vitales.
*(Ehm-peh-sah-reh pohr toh-mahr lohs
seeg-nohs bee-tah-lehs)*

I will take your blood pressure.
Tomaré tu presión de sangre.
*(Toh-mah-reh too preh-see-ohn deh
sahn-greh)*

I will talk to you every day.
Hablaré con usted todos los días.
*(Ah-blah-reh kohn oos-tehd toh-dohs
lohs dee-ahs)*

I will talk to your mother again.
Hablaré con tu mamá otra vez.
*(Ah-blah-reh kohn too mah-mah oh-
trah behs)*

I will use local anesthetic.
Le pondré/aplicaré anestesia local.
*(Leh pohn-dreh/ah-plee-kah-reh ah-
nehs-teh-see-ah loh-kahl)*

I will use resins.
Usaré resinas.
(Oo-sah-reh reh-see-nahs)

I will wake you up in the morning.
La despertaré en la mañana.
*(Lah dehs-pehr-tah-reh ehn lah mah-
nyah-nah)*

I wish you would leave me alone.
Deseo que ustedes me dejen solo.
*(Deh-seh-oh keh oos-teh-dehs meh
deh-hehn soh-loh)*

I would like to talk to you!
¡Me gustaría hablar contigo!
*(Meh goos-tah-ree-ah ah-blahr kohn-
tee-goh)*

356 ✦ Índice de Frases y Oraciones

Identify appropriate nursing interventions during the preoperative and postoperative phases of care.

Identifique las intervenciones y cuidados del paciente en el proceso preoperatorio y postoperatorio.

(Ee-dehn-tee-fee-keh lahs een-tehr-behn-see-oh-nehs ee koo-eeh-dah-dohs dehl pah-see-ehn-teh ehn ehl proh-seh-soh preh-oh-peh-rah-toh-ree-oh ee pohst-oh-peh-rah-toh-ree-oh)

Identify clinical indications for amputations.

Identifique las indicaciones clínicas para amputaciones.

(Ee-dehn-tee-fee-keh lahs een-dee-kah-see-oh-nehs klee-nee-kahs pah-rah ahm-poo-tah-see-oh-nehs)

If it hurts, tell me.

Si duele, avísame.

(See doo-eh-leh, ah-bee-sah-meh)

If it is a lot, or there is fever, go to the hospital right away.

Si es abundante, o aparece fiebre, acuda inmediatamente al hospital.

(See ehs ah-boon-dahn-teh, oh ah-pah-reh-seh fee-eh-breh, ah-koo-dah een-meh-dee-ah-tah-mehn-teh ahl ohs-pee-tahl)

If it is far, could I drive?

¿Si está lejos, podría manejar?

(See ehs-tah leh-hohs, poh-dree-ah mah-neh-hahr)

If it is something you cannot control ignore it!

¡Si es algo que no puede controlar ignórelo!

(See ehs ahl-goh keh noh poo-eh-deh kohn-troh-lahr eeg-noh-reh loh)

If nurses find expired items on the unit, they return them to the pharmacy for replacement.

Si las enfermeras encuentran artículos con fecha vencida, los regresan a la farmacia donde son reemplazados.

(See lahs ehn-fehr-meh-rahs ehn-koo-ehn-trahn ahr-tee-koo-lohs kohn feh-chah behn-see-dah, lohs reh-greh-sahn ah lah fahr-mah-see-ah dohn-deh sohn reh-ehm-plah-sah-dohs)

If you are unable to sign the consent, a relative can sign it.

Si no puede firmar el consentimiento un pariente lo puede firmar.

(See noh poo-eh-deh feer-mahr ehl kohn-sehn-tee-mee-ehn-toh, oon pah-ree-ehn-teh loh poo-eh-deh feer-mahr)

If you do not have ice in the bucket, please call me.

Si no tiene hielo en la tina, llámeme.

(See noh tee-eh-neh ee-eh-loh ehn lah tee-nah, yah-meh-meh)

If you do not understand, please let me know.

Si no entiende, dígame por favor.

(See noh ehn-tee-ehn-deh, dee-gah-meh pohr fah-bohr)

If you follow these recommendations, everything will be all right.

Si usted sigue estos consejos, todo saldrá con éxito.

(See oos-tehd see-geh ehs-tohs kohn-seh-hohs, toh-doh sahl-drah kohn ehx-ee-toh)

If you have additional questions, call me and I will return and answer them all.

Si tiene preguntas adicionales, llameme y vendré para contestarlas.

(See tee-eh-neh preh-goon-tahs ah-dee-see-oh-nah-lehs, yah-meh-meh ee behn-dreh pah-rah kohn-tehs-tahr-lahs)

If you have been here, I need your card.
Si ha estado aquí, necesito su tarjeta.
(See ah ehs-tah-doh ah-kee, neh-seh-see-toh soo tahr-heh-tah)

If you haven't, please fill out these papers.
Si no, por favor llene estos papeles.
(See noh, pohr fah-bohr yeh-neh ehs-tohs pah-peh-lehs)

If you have questions, please let me know.
Si tiene preguntas, por favor avíseme.
(See tee-eh-neh preh-goon-tahs, pohr fah-bohr ah-bee-seh-meh)

If you need more sheets, call the assistant.
Si necesita más sábanas, llame a la asistente.
(See neh-seh-see-tah mahs sah-bah-nahs, yah-meh ah lah ah-sees-tehn-teh)

If you notice fever or any problems in the incision, go to my office immediately.
Si nota fiebre o problemas en la herida, vaya inmediatamente a mi oficina.
(See noh-tah fee-eh-breh oh proh-bleh-mahs ehn lah eh-ree-dah, bah-yah een-meh-dee-ah-tah-mehn-teh ah mee oh-fee-see-nah)

If you react to the medicine call your physician.
Si reacciona mal al medicamento llame a su médico.
(See reh-ahk-see-ohn-ah mahl ahl meh-dee-kah-mehn-toh yah-meh ah soo meh-dee-koh)

If you see anything wrong, take him to the doctor.
Si nota algo malo, llévelo a su doctor.
(See noh-tah ahl-goh mah-loh, yeh-beh-loh ah soo dohk-torh)

If you want to watch TV, you have to pay a fee.
Si quiere ver el televisor, tiene que pagar una cuota.
(See kee-eh-reh behr ehl teh-leh-bee-sohr, tee-eh-neh keh pah-gahr oo-nah koo-oh-tah)

If your behavior changes you must go to a specialist.
Si continúa con cambios en su persona debe acudir con un especialista.
(See kohn-tee-noo-ah kohn kahm-bee-ohs ehn soo pehr-soh-nah deh-beh ah-koo-deer kohn oon ehs-peh-see-ah-lees-tah)

If your partner is in a high risk group, cease sexual relations.
Si su compañera está en el grupo de alto riesgo, suspenda las relaciones sexuales.
(See soo kohm-pah-nyeh-rah ehs-tah ehn ehl groo-poh deh ahl-toh ree-ehs-goh, soos-pehn-dah lahs reh-lah-see-ohn-ehs sehx-oo-ahl-ehs)

I'll call for a wheelchair.
Llamaré por una silla de ruedas.
(Yah-mah-reh pohr oo-nah see-yah deh roo-eh-dahs)

I'm 53.
Tengo cincuenta y tres años.
(Tehn-goh seen-koo-ehn-tah ee trehs ah-nyos)

I'm a paramedic.
Soy paramédico.
(Soh-ee pahr-ah-meh-dee-koh)

I'm going to clean your teeth.
Voy a limpiarle los dientes.
(Boh-ee ah leem-pee-ahr-leh lohs dee-ehn-tehs)

I'm going to polish your teeth.
Voy a pulir sus dientes.
(Boh-ee ah poo-leer soos dee-ehn-tehs)

I'm going to take x-rays.
Le tomaré radiografías.
(Leh toh-mah-reh rah-dee-oh-grah-fee-ahs)

I'm going to test your muscle strength.
Voy a medir la fuerza del músculo.
(Boh-ee ah meh-deer lah foo-ehr-sah dehl moos-koo-loh)

In case of a medication error, the doctor is notified.
En caso de error en el medicamento, se notifica al doctor.
(Ehn kah-soh deh eh-rohr ehn ehl meh-dee-kah-mehn-toh, seh noh-tee-fee-kah ahl dohk-tohr)

In case of fire, take the stairs.
En caso de fuego, tome las escaleras.
(Ehn kah-soh deh foo-eh-goh, toh-meh lahs ehs-kah-leh-rahs)

In that case, tell me your whole name.
En ese caso, dígame su nombre completo.
(Ehn eh-seh kah-soh, dee-gah-meh soo nohm-breh kohm-pleh-toh)

In your case, eat nothing after eight tonight.
En su caso, no coma nada después de las ocho de la noche.
(Ehn soo kah-soh, noh koh-mah nah-dah dehs-poo-ehs deh lahs oh-choh deh lah noh-cheh)

Indications and incidence.
Indicaciones e incidencias.
(Een-dee-kah-see-oh-nehs eh een-see-dehn-see-ahs)

Indigestion or difficulty swallowing.
Indigestión o dificultad al tragar.
(Een-dee-hehs-tee-ohn oh dee-fee-kool-tahd ahl trah-gahr)

Infected persons can transmit the virus.
Las personas infectadas pueden transmitir el virus.
(Lahs pehr-soh-nahs een-fehk-tah-dahs poo-eh-dehn trahns-mee-teer ehl bee-roos)

Insert the floss gently between the teeth.
Meta el hilo suavemente en medio de los dientes.
(Meh-tah ehl ee-loh soo-ah-beh-mehn-teh ehn meh-dee-oh deh lohs dee-ehn-tehs)

Is he at work?
¿Está trabajando?
(Ehs-tah trah-bah-hahn-doh)

Is he breast feeding?
¿Está tomando pecho?
(Ehs-tah toh-mahn-doh peh-choh)

Is he coughing?
¿Está tosiendo?
(Ehs-tah toh-see-ehn-doh)

Is he eating well?
¿Está comiendo bien?
(Ehs-tah koh-mee-ehn-doh bee-ehn)

Is he hyperactive?
¿Es inquieto/latoso?
(Ehs een-kee-eh-toh/lah-toh-soh)

Is he sleeping well?
¿Está durmiendo bien?
(Ehs-tah door-mee-ehn-doh bee-ehn)

Is he taking formula?
¿Está tomando formula?
(Ehs-tah toh-mahn-doh fohr-moo-lah)

Is he urinating well?
¿Orina bien?
(Oh-ree-nah bee-ehn)

Is he with you?
¿El viene con usted?
(Ehl bee-ehn-eh kohn oos-tehd)

Is it a dry cough?
¿Es tos seca?
(Ehs tohs seh-kah)

Is it a house?
¿Es una casa?
(Ehs oo-nah kah-sah)

Is it a lot?
¿Es mucho?
(Ehs moo-choh)

Is it far?
¿Está lejos?
(Ehs-tah leh-hohs)

Is it here in town?
¿Está en esta ciudad?
(Ehs-tah ehn ehs-tah see-oo-dahd)

Is it the same color?
¿Es del mismo color?
(Ehs dehl mees-moh koh-lohr)

Is parking available?
¿Hay estacionamiento?
(Ah-ee ehs-tah-see-ohn-ah-mee-ehn-toh)

Is someone with you?
¿Hay alguien con usted?
(Ah-ee ahl-ghee-ehn kohn oos-tehd)

Is that a lot?
¿Es mucho?
(Ehs moo-choh)

Is that an apartment?
¿Es apartamento?
(Ehs ah-pahr-tah-mehn-toh)

Is that enough?
¿Es mucho/suficiente?
(Ehs moo-choh/soo-fee-see-ehn-teh)

Is that right?
¿Es cierto?
(Ehs see-ehr-toh)

Is that too much?
¿Es mucho/demasiado?
(Ehs moo-choh/deh-mah-see-ah-doh)

Is the pain in one place?
¿El dolor es fijo?
(Ehl doh-lohr ehs fee-hoh)

Is the pain localized in the same place?
¿El dolor está fijo en el mismo lugar?
(Ehl doh-lohr ehs-tah fee-hoh ehn ehl mees-moh loo-gahr)

Is the pain sharp?
¿El dolor es agudo?
(Ehl doh-lohr ehs ah-goo-doh)

Is the pain there all the time, or does it come and go?
¿Está el dolor allí todo el tiempo, o va y viene?
(Ehs-tah ehl doh-lohr ah-yee toh-doh ehl tee-ehm-poh, oh bah ee bee-ehn-eh)

What is the danger from donated blood?
¿Qué peligro hay por sangre donada?
(Keh peh-lee-groh ah-ee pohr sahn-greh doh-nah-dah)

Is there a laboratory test for AIDS?
¿Hay pruebas de laboratorio para detectar el SIDA?
(Ah-ee proo-eh-buhs deh lah-boh-rah-toh-ree-oh pah-rah deh-tehk-tahr ehl see-dah)

Is there a policeman?
¿Hay un policía?
(Ah-ee oon poh-lee-see-ah)

Is there any pain?
¿Tiene algún dolor?
(Tee-eh-neh ahl-goon doh-lohr)

Is there any thing that worries you?
¿Hay algo que te/le preocupa?
(Ah-ee ahl-goh keh teh/leh preh-oh-koo-pah)

Is there anything else bothering you?
¿Hay otra cosa que le moleste?
(Ah-ee oh-trah koh-sah keh leh moh-lehs-teh)

Is there numbness/a tingling
sensation/burning in your
leg/arm/foot/hand?
¿Está entumecido/adormecido/tiene
ardor en su
pierna/brazo/pie/mano?
(Ehs-tah ehn-too-meh-see-doh/ah-
dohr-meh-see-doh/tee-eh-neh ahr-
dohr ehn soo pee-ehr-nah/brah-
soh/pee-eh/mah-noh)

Is this____Hospital?
¿Es este el Hospital____?
(Ehs ehs-teh ehl ohs-pee-tahl____)

Is this your first suicide attempt?
¿Es este su primer intento de
suicidio?
(Ehs ehs-teh soo pree-mehr een-tehn-
toh deh soo-ee-see-dee-oh)

Is this your first time in the hospital?
¿Es su primera vez en el hospital?
(Ehs soo pree-meh-rah behs ehn ehl
ohs-pee-tahl)

Is your appetite bad?
¿Tiene mal apetito?
(Tee-eh-neh mahl ah-peh-tee-toh)

Is your family in the city?
¿Está su familia en la ciudad?
(Ehs-tah soo fah-mee-lee-ah ehn lah
see-oo-dahd)

Is your family in town?
¿Está su familia en la ciudad?
(Ehs-tah soo fah-mee-lee-ah ehn lah
see-oo-dahd)

Is your water bag broken?
¿Se reventó su bolsa de agua?
(Seh reh-behn-toh soo bohl-sah deh
ah-goo-ah)

It also causes pyorrhea and tooth loss.
Causa también pérdida de dientes y
piorrea.
(Kah-oo-sah tahm-bee-ehn pehr-dee-
dah deh dee-ehn-tehs ee pee-oh-reh-
ah)

It belongs to the doctor.
Es del doctor.
(Ehs dehl dohk-tohr)

It belongs to the teacher.
Es de la maestra.
(Ehs deh lah mah-ehs-trah)

It can cause drowsiness.
Le puede causar somnolencia.
(Leh poo-eh-deh kah-oo-sahr sohm-
noh-lehn-see-ah)

It causes dental caries.
Causa caries dental.
(Kah-oo-sah kah-ree-ehs dehn-tahl)

It feels like a board.
Se siente como una tabla.
(Seh see-ehn-teh koh-moh oo-nah tah-
blah)

It has been.
Ha sido.
(Ah see-doh)

It has the film inside.
Tiene la película adentro.
(Tee-eh-neh lah peh-lee-koo-lah ah-
dehn-troh)

It hurts when I let go?
¿Duele cuando dejo ir?
(Doo-eh-leh koo-ahn-doh deh-hoh
eehr)

It hurts when I press?
¿Duele cuando aplano?
(Doo-eh-leh koo-ahn-doh ah-plah-noh)

It is 100 degrees.
Es de cien grados.
(Ehs deh see-ehn grah-dohs)

It is a procedure used to see how open
the veins are throughout the leg.
Es un procedimiento para valorar las
venas de su pierna.
(Ehs oon proh-seh-dee-mee-ehn-toh
pah-rah bah-loh-rahr lahs beh-nahs
deh soo pee-ehr-nah)

It is a six-story building.
Es un edificio de seis pisos.
(Ehs oon eh-dee-fee-see-oh deh seh-ees pee-sohs)

It is also an imbalance between the availability and the requirements of insulin.
Es también un desequilibrio entre la disponibilidad y los requerimientos de insulina.
(Ehs tahm-bee-ehn oon deh-seh-kee-lee-bree-oh ehn-treh la dees-poh-nee-bee-lee-dahd ee lohs reh-keh-ree-mee-ehn-tohs deh een-soo-lee-nah)

It is not as bad when I stay still, but it hurts a lot if I try to move the leg.
No está tan mal cuando estoy quieto, pero me duele mucho si trato de mover la pierna.
(Noh ehs-tah tahn mahl koo-ahn-doh ehs-toh-ee kee-eh-toh, peh-roh meh doo-eh-leh moo-choh see trah-toh deh moh-behr lah pee-ehr-nah)

It is one o'clock.
Es la una.
(Ehs lah oo-nah)

It is open seven AM to twelve midnight.
Está abierta de siete de la mañana a doce de la noche/a medianoche.
(Ehs-tah ah-bee-ehr-tah deh see-eh-teh deh lah mah-nyah-nah ah doh-seh deh lah noh-cheh/Ah meh-dee-ah-noh-cheh)

It is open from seven AM to one AM.
Está abierta de las siete de la mañana a la una de la mañana.
(Ehs-tah ah-bee-ehr-tah deh lahs see-eh-teh deh lah mah-nyah-nah ah lah oo-nah deh lah mah-nyah-nah)

It is open Saturday, Sunday, and holidays.
Está abierta los sábados, domingos, y dias festivos.
(Ehs-tah ah-bee-ehr-tah lohs sah-bah-dohs, doh-meen-gohs ee dee-ahs fehs-tee-bohs)

It is the next day.
Es el día siguiente.
(Ehs ehl dee-ah see-ghee-ehn-teh)

It is time to go.
Es tiempo de ir.
(Ehs tee-ehm-poh deh eer)

It keeps the food warm.
Guarda la comida tibia.
(Goo-ahr-dah lah koh-mee-dah tee-bee-ah).

It looked as if a professional had made it.
Parece como si un profesional lo hubiera hecho.
(Pah-reh-seh koh-moh see oon proh-feh-see-oh-nahl loh oo-bee-eh-rah heh-choh)

It sounds good.
Se oye bien.
(Seh oh-yeh bee-ehn)

It takes ten minutes.
Se toma diez minutos.
(Seh toh-mah dee-ehs mee-noo-tohs)

It will also help if you have any teeth that are sensitive.
Ayudará también si los dientes están sensibles.
(Ah-yoo-dah-rah tahm-bee-ehn see-lohs dee-ehn-tehs ehs-tahn sehn-see-blehs)

It will take a minute.
Tomará un minuto.
(Toh-mah-rah oon mee-noo-toh)

It will take ten minutes.
Se tomará diez minutos.
(Seh toh-mah-rah dee-ehs mee-noo-tohs)

It's not helping me.
No me está ayudando.
(Noh meh ehs-tah ah-yoo-dahn-doh)

It's in the middle of the wall.
Está a la mitad de la pared.
(Ehs-tah ah lah mee-tahd deh lah pah-rehd)

It's not very far.
No está muy lejos.
(Noh ehs-tah moo-ee leh-hohs)

It's nothing/You are welcome.
De nada.
(Deh nah-dah)

I'm not going today.
Hoy no voy a ir.
(Oh-ee noh boh-ee ah eer)

Jump with one foot.
Brinca con un pie.
(Breen-kah kohn oon pee-eh)

Keep a general hygiene: bath, nail cutting, sleep.
Medidas de higiene general: baño, recorte de uñas, dormir.
(Meh-dee-dahs deh ee-hee-eh-neh heh-neh-rahl: bah-nyo, reh-kohr-teh deh oo-nyahs, dohr-meer)

Keep moving.
Siga moviéndose.
(See-gah moh-bee-ehn-doh-seh)

Keep quiet.
Estése quieto/No se mueva.
(Ehs-teh-seh kee-eh-toh)/Noh seh moo-eh-bah)

Keep the area clean.
Mantenga el área limpia.
(Mahn-tehn-gah ehl ah-reh-ah leem-pee-ah)

Keep the baby awake.
Mantenga al bebé despierto.
(Mahn-tehn-gah ahl beh-beh dehs-pee-ehr-toh)

Keep the leg straight.
Mantenga la pierna derecha.
(Mahn-tehn-gah lah pee-ehr-nah deh-reh-chah)

Keep the oxygen equipment at least ten feet away from stoves, furnaces and water heaters.
Guarde el equipo de oxígeno al menos diez pies de estufas, calentadores o calentador de agua.
(Goo-ahr-deh ehl eh-kee-poh deh ohx-ee-heh-noh ahl meh-nohs dee-ehs pee-ehs deh ehs-too-fahs, kah-lehn-tah-doh-rehs o kah-lehn-tah-dohr deh-ah-goo-ah)

Keep the siderails up at night.
Mantenga los barandales levantados durante la noche.
(Mahn-tehn-gah lohs bah-rahn-dah-lehs leh-bahn-tah-dohs doo-rahn-teh lah noh-cheh)

Keep your feet together.
Mantenga los pies juntos.
(Mahn-tehn-gah lohs pee-ehs hoon-tohs)

Keep your leg elevated.
Mantenga la pierna elevada.
(Mahn-tehn-gah lah pee-ehr-nah eh-leh-bah-dah)

Kitchen personnel bring the food trays.
Los empleados de la cocina traen las bandejas con comida.
(Lohs ehm-pleh-ah-dohs deh lah koh-see-nah trah-ehn lahs bahn-deh-hahs kohn koh-mee-dah)

Kneel down!
¡Póngase de rodillas!
(Pohn-gah-seh deh roh-dee-yahs)

Know sexual background/habits of partners.
Conozca los hábitos sexuales de su pareja.
(Koh-nohs-kah lohs ah-bee-tohs sex-oo-ah-lehs deh soo pah-reh-hah)

Later on, they will take x-rays.
Más tarde, le van a tomar rayos X.
(Mahs tahr-deh leh bahn ah toh-mahr rah-yohs eh-kiss)

Lay down so I can examine you.
Acuéstese para explorarlo.
(Ah-koo-ehs-teh-seh pah-rah ehx-ploh-rahr-loh)

Leave behind.
Abandonar.
(Ah-bahn-doh-nahr)

Leave the area uncovered.
Deje el área descubierta.
(Deh-heh ehl ah-reh-ah dehs-koo-bee-ehr-tah)

Left. . .
Izquierdo. . .
(Ees-kee-ehr-doh)

Lescol for the cholesterol and naproxin for my aches.
Lescol para el colesterol y naproxeno para mis dolores.
(Lehs-kohl pah-rah ehl koh-lehs-teh-rohl ee nah-prohx-eh-noh pah-rah mees doh-loh-rehs)

Let it go.
Déjalo ir.
(Deh-hah-loh eer)

Let it out slowly.
Déjalo ir despacio.
(Deh-hah-loh eer dehs-pah-see-oh)

Let it out.
Exhala.
(Ehx-ah-lah)

Let me go through.
Déjeme pasar.
(Deh-heh-meh pah-sahr)

Let me know how you feel.
Dígame como se siente.
(Dee-gah-meh koh-moh seh see-ehn-teh)

Let me see.
Déjeme ver.
(Deh-heh-meh behr)

Let me show you the correct way to floss.
Déjeme enseñarle la manera correcta de usar el hilo.
(Deh-heh-meh ehn-seh-nyahr-leh lah mah-neh-rah koh-rehk-tah deh oo-sahr ehl ee-loh)

Let me show you with your toothbrush a way that will help you remove the plaque.
Déjeme enseñarle con su cepillo una manera que le ayudará a quitar la placa.
(Deh-heh-meh ehn-seh-nyahr-leh kohn soo seh-pee-yoh oo-nah mah-neh-rah keh leh ah-yoo-dahr-ah ah kee-tahr lah plah-kah)

Let's go over the consent form.
Vamos a ver la forma de consentimiento.
(Bah-mohs ah behr lah fohr-mah deh kohn-sehn-tee-mee-ehn-toh)

Let's see how far you can walk.
Vamos a ver que tan lejos puede caminar.
(Bah-mohs a behr keh tahn leh-hohs poo-eh-deh kah-mee-nahr)

Let's walk.
Vamos a caminar.
(Bah-mohs ah kah-mee-nahr)

Lie down (please)!
¡Acuéstese (por favor)!
(Ah-koo-ehs-teh-seh [pohr fah-bohr])

Lift the foot.
Levante el pie.
(Leh-bahn-teh ehl pee-eh)

Lift your arm(s).
Levanta tu/los brazo(s).
(Leh-bahn-tah too/lohs brah-soh[s])

Lift your foot.
Levanta tu pie.
(Leh-bahn-tah too pee-eh)

Lift your hand.
Levanta tu mano.
(Leh-bahn-tah too mah-noh)

Lift your head.
Levanta la cabeza.
(Leh-bahn-tah lah kah-beh-sah)

Lift your leg.
Levanta la pierna.
(Leh-bahn-tah lah pee-ehr-nah)

Lift your right arm.
Levante el brazo derecho.
(Leh-bahn-teh ehl brah-soh deh-reh-choh)

Lift your right foot.
Levante el pie derecho.
(Leh-bahn-teh ehl pee-eh deh-reh-choh)

Lips should not be dry.
Los labios no deben estar secos.
(Lohs lah-bee-ohs noh deh-behn ehs-tahr seh-kohs)

Listen!
¡Escuche/Oiga!
(Ehs-koo-cheh/Oh-ee-gah)

Look down.
Mira hacia abajo.
(Mee-rah ah-see-ah ah-bah-hoh)

Look straight ahead.
Mira hacia adelante.
(Mee-rah ah-see-ah ah-deh-lahn-teh)

Look straight at the light.
Mira directo a la luz.
(Mee-rah dee-rehk-toh ah lah loos)

Look up.
Mira hacia arriba.
(Mee-rah ah-see-ah ah-ree-bah)

Look up/down.
Mira arriba/abajo.
(Mee-rah ah-ree-bah/ah-bah-hoh)

Lot number?
¿Número de lote?
(Noo-meh-roh deh loh-teh)

Lower extremities?
¿Extremidades inferiores?
(Ehx-treh-mee-dah-dehs een-feh-ree-oh-rehs)

Lower the foot.
Baja el pie.
(Bah-hah ehl pee-eh)

Lower your head.
Baja la cabeza.
(Bah-hah lah kah-beh-sah)

Lower your legs.
Baje las piernas.
(Bah-heh lahs pee-ehr-nahs)

Lower!
¡Baje!
(Bah-heh)

Lump in breast or elsewhere.
Bolita en el pecho o en otra parte.
(Boh-lee-tah ehn ehl peh-choh oh ehn oh-trah pahr-teh)

Maintain it like this.
Mantenlo así.
(Mahn-tehn-loh ah-see)

Make a fist!
¡Cierre la mano/Haga un puño!
(See-eh-reh lah mah-noh/Ah-gah oon poo-nyoh)

Make some room!
¡Haga lugar!
(Ah-gah loo-gahr)

Make sure that you point the
  toothbrush toward the gumline.
Asegure que el cepillo apunte contra
  la encía.
(Ah-seh-goo-reh keh ehl seh-pee-yoh ah-poon-teh kohn-trah lah ehn-see-ah)

Make the baby burp.
Haga que el bebé eructe/repita.
(Ah-gah keh ehl beh-beh eh-rook-teh/reh-pee-tah)

Make your home pleasant and
  cheerful.
Haga su hogar placentero y alegre.
(Ah-gah soo oh-gahr plah-sehn-teh-roh ee ah-leh-greh)

Mary has a broken foot.
María tiene el pie quebrado.
(Mah-ree-ah tee-eh-neh ehl pee-eh keh-brah-doh)

May I help you?
¿Puedo ayudarlo?
(Poo-eh-doh ah-yoo-dahr-loh)

May I join you?
¿Lo/La puedo acompañar?
(Loh/Lah poo-eh-doh ah-kohm-pah-nyahr)

Medicaid?
¿Medicaid?
(Meh-dee-keh-eed)

Mental status examination.
Examen del estado mental.
(Ehx-ah-mehn dehl ehs-tah-doh mehn-tahl)

Moist cough?
¿Tos húmeda?
(Tohs oo-meh-dah)

Monthly, the pharmacy staff inspects the medication area.
Cada mes, los empleados de la farmacia inspeccionan el área de medicamentos.
(Kah-dah mehs lohs ehm-pleh-ah-dohs deh lah fahr-mah-see-ah eens-pehk-see-ohn-ahn ehl ah-reh-ah deh meh-dee-kah-mehn-tohs)

Most have no symptoms.
La mayoría no tiene síntomas.
(Lah mah-yoh-ree-ah noh tee-eh-neh seen-toh-mahs)

Move carefully!
¡Muévase con cuidado!
(Moo-eh-bah-seh kohn koo-ee-dah-doh)

Move it side to side.
Muévela de lado a lado.
(Moo-eh-beh-lah deh lah-doh ah lah-doh)

Move your eyes.
Mueva sus ojos.
(Moo-eh-bah soos oh-hohs)

Move your head to say yes or no.
Mueva la cabeza para decir sí o no.
(Moo-eh-bah lah kah-beh-sah pah-rah deh-seer see oh noh)

Move your leg backward.
Mueve tu pierna para atrás.
(Moo-eh-beh too pee-ehr-nah pah-rah ah-trahs)

Move your leg forward.
Mueve tu pierna para adelante.
(Moo-eh-beh too pee-ehr-nah pah-rah ah-deh-lahn-teh)

Move your leg.
Mueve tu pierna.
(Moo-ch-beh too pee-ehr-nah)

Move!
¡Mueva!
(Moo-eh-bah)

Mr. Garza, you probably have appendicitis.
Señor Garza, probablemente tenga apendicitis.
(Seh-nyohr Gahr-sah, proh-bah-bleh-mehn-teh tehn-gah ah-pehn-dee-see-tees)

Mr. Gomez left yesterday.
El señor Gómez salió ayer.
(Ehl seh-nyohr Goh-mehs sah-lee-oh ah-yehr)

Mr. Martinez arrives at the department.
El senor Martinez llega al departamento.
(Ehl seh-nyohr Mahr-tee-nehs yeh-gah ahl deh-pahr-tah-mehn-toh)

Mr. Ríos, How are you?
Señor Ríos, cómo está?
(Seh-nyohr Ree-ohs, koh-moh ehs-tah)

Mrs. García, tomorrow you will be discharged from the hospital.
Señora García, mañana sale usted del hospital.
(Seh-nyoh-rah Gahr-see-ah, mah-nyah-nah sah-leh oos-tehd dehl ohs-pee-tahl)

Mrs. Garza, the doctor ordered blood samples.
Señora Garza, el doctor ordenó muestras de sangre.
(Seh-nyoh-rah Gahr-sah, ehl dohk-tohr ohr-deh-noh moo-ehs-trahs deh sahn-greh)

Mrs. Garza, I want you to get up and go to the bathroom to urinate.
Señora Garza, Quiero que se levante y vaya al baño a orinar.
(Seh-nyoh-rah Gahr-sah, Kee-eh-roh keh seh leh-bahn-teh ee bah-yah ahl bah-nyoh ah oh-ree-nahr)

Mrs. Ortiz, take this pill every eight hours for ten days.
Señora Ortiz, tome esta pastilla cada ocho horas por diez días.
(Seh-nyoh-rah Ohr-tees, toh-meh ehs-tah pahs-tee-yah kah-dah oh-choh oh-rahs pohr dee-ehs dee-ahs)

Mrs. Ortiz, you need to go to the hospital.
Señora Ortiz, necesita ir al hospital.
(Seh-nyoh-rah Ohr-tees, neh-seh-see-tah eer ahl ohs-pee-tahl)

Mrs. Vargas, I need to help you change clothes.
Señora Vargas, necesito ayudarle a cambiar la ropa.
(Seh-nyoh-rah Bahr-gahs, neh-seh-see-toh ah-yoo-dahr-leh ah kahm-bee-ahr lah roh-pah)

My agency asked me to visit you.
Mi agencia me pidió que la visitara.
(Mee ah-hehn-see-ah meh pee-dee-oh keh lah bee-see-tah-rah)

My daughter will be here.
Mi hija estará aquí.
(Mee ee-hah ehs-tah-rah ah-kee)

My friend speaks French.
Mi amigo habla francés.
(Mee ah-mee-goh ah-blah frahn-sehs)

The whole book is in German.
Todo el libro está en alemán.
(Toh-doh ehl lee-broh ehs-tah ehn ah-leh-mahn)

My grandfather died from complications of an amputation because of DM.
Mi abuelo murió por complicaciones de una amputación debida a DM.
(Mee ah-boo-eh-loh moo-ree-oh pohr kohm-plee-kah-see-oh-nehs deh oo-nah ahm-poo-tah-see-ohn deh-bee-dah ah Deh Emeh)

My left leg hurts.
Me duele la pierna izquierda.
(Meh doo-eh-leh lah pee-ehr-nah ees-kee-ehr-dah)

My name is. . .
Mi nombre es. . ./Me llamo. . .
(Mee nohm-breh ehs/Mee yah-moh)

My name is John.
Me llamo Juan.
(Meh yah-moh Joo-ahn)

My nose is prettier than yours.
Mi nariz es más bonita que la tuya.
(Mee nah-rees ehs mahs boh-nee-tah keh lah too-yah)

My sister is now being treated.
Mi hermana está en tratamiento.
(Mee ehr-mah-nah ehs-tah ehn trah-tah-mee-ehn-toh)

My wife just had a baby.
Mi esposa tuvo un bebé.
(Mee ehs-poh-sah too-boh oon beh-beh)

Nagging cough or horseness.
Tos persistente o afónico.
(Tohs pehr-sees-tehn-teh oh ah-foh-nee-koh)

Name of the drug.
Nombre de la droga/del medicamento.
(Nohm-breh deh lah droh-gah/dehl meh-dee-kah-mehn-toh)

Never mind.
No importa.
(Noh eem-pohr-tah)

Never?
¿Nunca?
(Noon-kah)

No, I just don't want to go.
No, sólo que no quiero ir.
(Noh, soh-loh keh noh kee-eh-roh eer)

No problem!
¡No hay problema!
(Noh ah-ee proh-bleh-mah)

No smoking.
No se permite fumar.
(Noh seh pehr-mee-teh foo-mahr)

No, but there is a test for antibodies.
No, pero hay prueba de anticuerpos.
(Noh, peh-roh ah-ee prooh-eh-bah deh
  ahn-tee-koo-ehr-pohs)

No, I do not speak English.
No, no hablo inglés.
(Noh, noh ah-bloh cen-glehs)

No, I do not speak Spanish.
No, no hablo español.
(Noh, noh ah-bloh ehs-pah-nyohl)

No, I don't think so.
No, no lo creo.
(Noh, noh loh kreh-oh)

No, I don't understand.
No, no comprendo/no entiendo.
(Noh, noh kohm-prehn-doh/noh ehn-
  tee-ehn-doh)

No, I have not noticed any.
No, no me he dado cuenta de
  ninguna cosa.
(Noh, noh meh eh dah-doh koo-ehn-
  tah deh neen-goo-nah koh-sah)

No, it moved to the right side.
No, se recorrió al lado derecho.
(Noh, seh reh-koh-ree-oh ahl lah-doh
  deh-reh-choh)

No, never.
No, nunca.
(Noh, noon-kah)

No, not that I know of.
No, que yo sepa.
(Noh, keh yoh seh-pah)

No. We control the amount of
  radiation you receive.
No. Controlamos la cantidad de
  radiación que recibe.
(Noh. Kohn-troh-lah-mohs lah kahn-
  tee-dahd deh rah-dee-ah-see-ohn
  keh reh-see-beh)

No/yes.
No/sí.
(Noh/see)

None!
¡Ninguno!
(Neen-goo-noh)

Normal rectal temperature should be
  100.4 degrees Fahrenheit.
La temperatura normal en el recto es
  de cien punto quatro grados
  Fahrenheit.
(Lah tehm-peh-rah-too-rah nohr-mahl
  ehn ehl rehk-toh ehs deh see-ehn
  poon-toh koo-ah-troh grah-dohs
  Fah-rehn-heh-eet)

Not at all.
De ningún modo.
(Deh neen-goon moh-doh)

Not right now, but I will discuss it
  with my family.
No por ahora, pero lo discutiré con
  mi familia.
(Noh pohr ah-oh-rah, peh-roh loh
  dees-koo-tee-reh kohn mee fah-mee-
  lee-ah)

Nothing seems to make it better or
  worse.
Nada parece hacerlo peor o mejor.
(Nah-dah pah-reh-seh ah-sehr-loh
  peh-ohr oh meh-hohr)

Now, follow my commands.
Ahora, siga mis órdenes.
(Ah-oh-rah see-gah mees ohr-deh-
  nehs)

Now I am going to give you some
  fluoride.
Ahora voy a darle fluoruro.
(Ah-oh-rah boh-ee ah dahr-leh floh-
  roo-roh)

Now I need to x-ray the chest.
Ahora necesito tomar radiografía del
  pecho.
(Ah-oh-rah neh-seh-see-toh toh-mahr
  rah-dee-oh-grah-fee-ah dehl peh-
  choh)

Now raise the left arm.
Ahora levante el brazo izquierdo.
(Ah-oh-rah leh-bahn-teh ehl brah-soh
  ees-kee-ehr-doh)

Now you can change clothes.
Ahora se puede cambiar de ropa.
(Ah-oh-rah seh poo-eh-deh kahm-bee-
  ahr deh roh-pah)

Now, bend over.
Ahora, agáchate.
(Ah-oh-rah, ah-gah-chah-teh)

Now, I am going to examine your abdomen.
Ahora, voy a revisar tu abdomen/vientre.
(Ah-oh-rah boh-ee ah reh-bee-sahr too ahb-doh-mehn/bee-ehn-treh)

Now, I am going to examine your chest.
Ahora, voy a revisar tu pecho.
(Ah-oh-rah boh-ee ah reh-bee-sahr too peh-choh)

Now, I am going to examine your skin.
Ahora, voy a revisar tu piel.
(Ah-oh-rah boh-ee ah reh-bee-sahr too pee-ehl)

Now, raise the left arm.
Ahora, levante el brazo izquierdo.
(Ah-oh-rah, leh-bahn-teh ehl brah-soh ees-kee-ehr-doh)

Now, stand up and walk.
Ahora, levántese y camine.
(Ah-oh-rah, leh-bahn-teh-seh ee kah-mee-neh)

Now, stand up!
Ahora, ¡levántate!
(Ah-oh-rah, leh-bahn-tah-teh)

Now, take a deep breath.
Ahora, respira hondo/profundo.
(Ah-oh-rah, rehs-pee-rah ohn-doh/proh-foon-doh)

Now, turn to the screen.
Ahora, voltee hacia la placa.
(Ah-oh-rah, bohl-teh-eh ah-see-ah lah plah-kah)

Number of patients.
Número de pacientes.
(Noo-meh-roh deh pah-see-ehn-tehs)

Nurses control narcotic records on the unit.
Las enfermeras controlan archivos de narcóticos en el piso.
(Lahs ehn-fehr-meh-rahs kohn-troh-lahn ahr-chee-bohs deh nahr-koh-tee-kohs ehn ehl pee-soh)

Nursing care of the patient.
Cuidados del paciente.
(Koo-ee-dah-dohs dehl pah-see-ehn-teh)

Nursing staff take STAT orders to the pharmacy.
Las enfermeras llevan órdenes urgentes a la farmacia.
(Lahs ehm-fehr-meh-rahs yeh-bahn ohr-deh-nehs oor-hehn-tehs ah lah fahr-mah-see-ah)

Observe blood pressure, pulse, and the level of urine.
Observe la presión de la sangre, el pulso y el nivel de la orina.
(Ohb-sehr-beh lah preh-see-ohn deh lah sahn-greh, ehl pool-soh ee ehl nee-behl deh lah oh-ree-nah)

Observe the patient's mental status.
Observe el estado mental del paciente.
(Ohb-sehr-beh ehl ehs-tah-doh mehn-tahl dehl pah-see-ehn-teh)

Occasionally.
Ocasionalmente.
(Oh-kah-see-ohn-ahl-mehn-teh)

Of course.
Desde luego.
(Dehs-deh loo-eh-goh)

Often, two times per week.
Seguido, dos veces por semana.
(Seh-gee-doh, dohs beh-sehs pohr seh-mah-nah)

On the one hand.
Por un lado.
(Pohr oon lah-doh)

Once in a while.
De vez en cuando.
(Deh behs ehn koo-ahn-doh)

One and a half.
Una y media.
(Oo-nah ee meh-dee-ah)

One more time.
Una vez más.
(Oo-nah behs mahs)

Only at parties.
Sólo en las fiestas.
(Soh-loh ehn lahs fee-ehs-tahs)

Only five minutes.
Sólo cinco minutos.
(Soh-loh seen-koh mee-noo-tohs)

Open again.
Abrela otra vez.
(Ah-breh-lah oh-trah behs)

Open the fingers wide.
Separa bien los dedos.
(Seh-pah-rah bee-ehn lohs deh-dohs)

Open your eyes!
¡Abra los ojos!
(Ah-brah lohs oh-hohs)

Open your hand!
¡Abra la mano!
(Ah-brah lah mah-noh)

Open your mouth, please.
Abra la boca, por favor.
(Ah-brah lah boh-kah, pohr fah-bohr)

Open!
¡Abra!
(Ah-brah)

Other recommendations.
Otras recomendaciones.
(Oh-trahs reh-koh-mehn-dah-see-oh-nehs)

Outpatient prescriptions are also dispensed.
Las recetas para pacientes de consulta externa se surten también.
(Lahs reh-seh-tahs pah-rah pah-see-ehn-tehs deh kohn-sool-tah ehx-tehr-nah seh soor-tehn tahm-bee-ehn)

Outpatient prescriptions are filled by the pharmacy.
Las recetas para pacientes de consulta externa se distribuyen por la farmacia.
(Lahs reh-seh-tahs pah-rah pah-see-ehn-tehs deh kohn-sool-tah ehx-tehr-nah seh dees-tree-boo-yehn pohr lah fahr-mah-see-ah)

Over the stool.
Sobre el taburete.
(Soh-breh ehl tah-boo-reh-teh)

Pain at the waist?
¿Dolor en la cintura?
(Doh-lohr ehn lah seen-too-rah)

Pain?
¿Dolor?
(Doh-lohr)

Palpitations?
¿Palpitaciones?
(Pahl-pee-tah-see-ohn-ehs)

Pardon me!
¡Perdóneme!
(Pehr-doh-neh-meh)

Pat his back gently.
Dé palmaditas en la espalda.
(Deh pahl-mah-dee-tahs ehn lah ehs-pahl-dah)

Pay attention to the following signs so you can detect cancer early.
Preste atención a las siguientes señas para que detecte el cáncer oportunamente.
(Prehs-teh ah-tehn-see-ohn ah lahs see-gee-ehn-tehs seh-nyahs pah-rah keh deh-tehk-teh ehl kahn-sehr oh-pohr-too-nah-mehn-teh)

Peanut butter sandwich.
Lonche de crema de cacahuate.
(Lohn-cheh deh kreh-mah deh kah-kah-oo-ah-teh)

Perform monthly self breast exam.
Haga un autoexamen del pecho cada mes.
(Ah-gah-seh oon ah-oo-toh ehx-ah-mehn dehl peh-choh kah-dah mehs)

Phone for local calls.
Teléfono para llamadas locales.
(Teh-leh-foh-noh pah-rah yah-mah-dahs loh-kah-lehs)

Place a light in the hallway.
Ponga una luz en el pasillo.
(Pohn-gah oo-nah loos ehn ehl pah-see-yoh)

Place the sling in the right arm.
Ponga el cabestrillo en el brazo derecho.
(Pohn-gah ehl kah-behs-tree-yoh ehn ehl brah-soh deh-reh-choh)

Place the urine in the brown plastic bottle.
Ponga la orina en la botella de plástico café.
(Pohn-gah lah oh-ree-nah ehn lah boh-teh-yah deh plahs-tee-koh kah-feh)

Place your arm around my waist.
Ponga su brazo alrededor de mi cintura.
(Pohn-gah soo brah-soh ahl-reh-deh-dohr deh mee seen-too-rah)

Place your arms behind the back.
Ponga los brazos atrás.
(Pohn-gah lohs brah-sohs ah-trahs)

Place your feet here.
Ponga los pies aquí.
(Pohn-gah lohs pee-ehs ah-kee)

Place your foot on the opposite knee.
Pon tu pie sobre la rodilla opuesta.
(Pohn too pee-eh soh-breh lah roh-dee-yah oh-poo-ehs-tah)

Place your hands behind your head.
Pon tus manos atrás de tu cabeza.
(Pohn toos mah-nohs ah-trahs deh too kah-beh-sah)

Plan an adequate diet.
Planear alimentos adecuados.
(Plah-neh-ahr ah-lee-mehn-tohs ah-deh-koo-ah-dohs)

Plaque can be prevented by brushing and flossing.
La placa se evita usando hilo dental y cepillo.
(Lah plah-kah seh eh-bee-tah oo-sahn-doh ee-loh dehn-tahl ee seh-pee-yoh)

Plaque gets in between the teeth where the brush cannot reach.
La placa entra en medio de los dientes donde no alcanza el cepillo.
(Lah plah-kah ehn-trah ehn meh-dee-oh deh lohs dee-ehn-tehs dohn-deh noh ahl-kahn-zah ehl seh-pee-yoh)

Plaque is a sticky, colorless layer of bacteria.
La placa es una capa pegajosa sin color y con bacterias.
(Lah plah-kah ehs oo-nah kah-pah peh-gah-hoh-sah seehn koh-lohr ee kohn bahk-teh-ree-ahs)

Please breathe normally.
Por favor, respire normal.
(Pohr fah-bohr, rehs-pee-reh nohr-mahl)

Please cross your leg.
Por favor, cruce la pierna.
(Pohr fah-bohr, kroo-seh lah pee-ehr-nah)

Please do the following:
Por favor, haga lo siguiente:
(Pohr fah-bohr, ah-gah loh see-gee-ehn-teh)

Please don't move.
Por favor, no se mueva.
(Pohr fah-bohr noh seh moo-eh-bah)

Please keep your appointment.
Por favor acuda a la cita.
(Pohr fah-bohr ah-koo-dah ah lah see-tah)

Please open your mouth some more.
Por favor, abra más la boca.
(Pohr fah-bohr, ah-brah mahs lah boh-kah)

Please put this gown on.
Por favor, póngase está bata.
(Pohr fah-bohr, pohn-gah-seh ehs-tah bah-tah)

Please return as needed.
En caso necesario, puede regresar.
(Ehn kah-soh neh-seh-sah-ree-oh, poo-eh-deh reh-greh-sahr)

Please return in six months.
Por favor regrese en seis meses.
(Pohr fah-bohr reh-greh-seh ehn seh-ees meh-sehs)

Please sit down.
Siéntese, por favor.
(See-ehn-teh-seh, pohr fah-bohr)

Please!
¡Por favor!
(Pohr fah-bohr)

Please, bend your arm for about five minutes.
Por favor, doble el brazo por cinco minutos.
(Pohr fah-bohr, doh-bleh ehl brah-soh pohr seen-koh mee-noo-tohs)

Please, change clothes.
Por favor, cámbiese de ropa.
(Pohr fah-bohr, kahm-bee-eh-seh deh roh-pah)

Please, come back in a few minutes.
Por favor, regrese en unos minutos.
(Pohr fah-bohr, reh-greh-seh ehn oon-ohs mee-noo-tohs)

Please, cross your leg.
Por favor, cruce la pierna.
(Pohr fah-bohr, kroo-seh lah pee-ehr-nah)

Please, do not eat anything after midnight.
Por favor, no coma nada después de medianoche.
(Pohr fah-bohr, noh koh-mah nah-dah dehs-poo-ehs deh meh-dee-ah-noh-cheh)

Please, don't move.
Por favor, no se mueva.
(Pohr fah-bohr, noh seh moo-eh-bah)

Please, lie down.
Acuéstate, por favor.
(Ah-koo-ehs-tah-teh pohr fah-bohr)

Please, open your mouth some more.
Por favor, abra más la boca.
(Pohr fah-bohr, ah-brah mahs lah boh-kah)

Please, raise this arm.
Por favor, levante este brazo.
(Pohr fah-bohr, leh-bahn-teh ehs-teh brah-soh)

Please, raise your arm.
Por favor, levanta tu brazo.
(Pohr fah-bohr, leh-bahn-tah too brah-soh)

Please, repeat slowly!
¡Por favor, ¡repita despacio!
(Pohr fah-bohr, reh-pee-tah dehs-pah-see-oh)

Please, sign here.
Por favor, firme aquí.
(Pohr fah-bohr, feer-meh ah-kee)

Please, sign.
Por favor, firme.
(Pohr fah-bohr, feer-meh)

Please, sit down in the waiting room.
Por favor, siéntese en la sala de espera.
(Pohr fah-bohr, see-ehn-teh-seh ehn lah sah-lah deh ehs-peh-rah)

Please, sit up in the bed.
Por favor, siéntate en la cama.
(Pohr fah-bohr, see-ehn-tah-teh ehn lah kah-mah)

Please, stay/remain in bed.
Por favor, quédese en la cama.
(Pohr fah-bohr, keh-deh-seh ehn lah kah-mah)

Please, swallow.
Traga, por favor.
(Trah-gah pohr fah-bohr)

Please, tell the nurse to call me.
Por favor, dígale a la enfermera que
me llame.
*(Por fah-bohr, dee-gah-leh ah lah ehn-
fehr-meh-rah keh meh yah-meh)*

Please, wait a few minutes.
Por favor, espere unos minutos.
*(Pohr fah-bohr, ehs-peh-reh oo-nohs
mee-noo-tohs)*

Please, wait about thirty minutes.
Por favor, espere treinta minutos.
*(Pohr fah-bohr, ehs-peh-reh treh-een-
tah mee-noo-tohs)*

Please, walk.
Camina, por favor.
(Kah-mee-nah, pohr fah-bohr)

Point!
¡Apunte!/Señale!
(Ah-poon-teh/Seh-nyah-leh)

Point to your nose.
Apunte a la nariz.
(Ah-poon-teh ah lah nah-rees)

Point when it hurts.
Señale cuando duela/donde le duela.
*(Seh-nyah-leh koo-ahn-doh doo-eh-
lah/[dohn-deh leh doo-eh-lah])*

Practice with the brush; make sure you
go around all the teeth.
Practique con el cepillo; asegure de
cepillar alrededor de todos los
dientes.
*(Prahk-tee-keh kohn ehl seh-pee-yoh;
ah-seh-goo-reh deh seh-pee-yahr ahl-
reh-deh-dohr deh toh-dohs lohs dee-
ehn-tehs)*

Prepare discharge planning.
Prepare el plan para dar de alta.
*(Preh-pah-reh ehl plahn pah-rah dahr
deh ahl-tah)*

Press hard!
¡Presione fuerte!
(Preh-see-oh-neh foo-ehr-teh)

Problems like ulcers, high blood
pressure, and inability to enjoy life
and the world.
Problemas como úlceras, alta presión
y incapacidad de gozar la vida y el
mundo.
*(Proh-bleh-mahs koh-moh ool-seh-
rahs, ahl-tah preh-see-ohn, eh een-
kah-pah-see-dahd deh goh-sahr lah
bee-dah ee ehl moon-doh)*

Pronounce, please.
Pronouncien, por favor.
(Proh-noon-see-ehn, pohr fah-bohr)

Pull the cord in the bathroom.
Jale el cordón en el baño.
*(Hah-leh ehl kohr-dohn ehn ehl bah-
nyoh)*

Pull the knee to the chest.
Estira la rodilla al pecho.
*(Ehs-tee-rah lah roh-dee-yah ahl peh-
choh)*

Pull up your hips.
Levante la cadera.
(Leh-bahn-teh lah kah-deh-rah)

Pull your knee to your chest.
Estira la rodilla hacia el pecho.
*(Ehs-tee-rah lah roh-dee-yah ah-see-ah
ehl peh-choh)*

Pull!
¡Jale!
(Hah-leh)

Put the spoon in your mouth.
Ponga la cuchara en la boca.
*(Pohn-gah lah koo-chah-rah ehn lah
boh-kah)*

Push down with your feet against my
hands.
Empuje los pies contra mis manos.
*(Ehm-poo-heh lohs pee-ehs kohn-trah
mees mah-nohs)*

Push!
¡Empuje!
(Ehm-poo-heh)

Raise your head.
Levanta tu cabeza.
(Leh-bahn-tah too kah-beh-sah)

Reach out with your arm.
Alarge el brazo.
(Ah-lahr-geh ehl brah-soh)

Reaction to transfusions?
¿Reacción a transfusiones?
(Reh-ahk-see-ohn ah trahns-foo-see-ohn-ehs)

Read, please.
Lea, por favor.
(Leh-ah, pohr fah-bohr)

Recall?
¿Recuerda?
(Reh-koo-ehr-dah)

Relax your arm.
Relaje el brazo.
(Reh-lah-heh ehl brah-soh)

Relax your leg.
Relaje la pierna.
(Reh-lah-heh lah pee-ehr-nah)

Relax your muscle.
Relaja tu músculo.
(Reh-lah-hah too moos-koo-loh)

Relax!
¡Relaje!/Descanse!
(Reh-lah-heh/Dehs-kahn-seh)

Relax, calm down.
Relájese, cálmese.
(Reh-lah-heh-seh, kahl-meh-seh)

Relax, it will not hurt!
Relájese, ¡no le va a doler!
(Reh-lah-heh-seh, noh leh bah ah doh-lehr)

Remember that you are to urinate and
  put it in the container.
Recuerde que debe orinar y poner la
  orina en el recipiente.
*(Reh-koo-ehr-deh keh deh-beh oh-ree-
  nahr ee poh-nehr lah oh-ree-nah
  ehn ehl reh-see-pee-ehn-teh)*

Remember that you will do this for
  twenty-four hours.
Recuerde que hara esto por
  veinticuatro horas.
*(Reh-koo-ehr-deh keh ah-rah ehs-toh
  pohr beh-een-tee-koo-ah-troh oh-
  rahs)*

Remember the following precautions.
Recuerde las siguientes precauciones.
*(Reh-koo-ehr-deh lahs see-ghee-ehn-
  tehs preh-kah-oo-see-oh-nehs)*

Remember to bring them back.
Acuérdese de regresarlos/traerlos.
*(Ah-koo-ehr-deh-seh deh reh-greh-
  sahr-lohs/trah-ehr-lohs)*

Remove all throw rugs in the hall way.
Quite todas las carpetas del pasillo.
*(Kee-teh toh-dahs lahs kahr-peh-tahs
  dehl pah-see-yoh)*

Repeat one, two, three.
Repite uno, dos, tres.
(Reh-pee-teh oo-noh, dohs, trehs)

Repeat the word "99."
Repite la palabra "noventa y nueve."
*(Reh-pee-teh lah pah-lah-brah "noh-
  behn-tah ee noo-eh-beh")*

Repeat, please.
Repitan, por favor.
(Reh-pee-tahn, pohr fah-bohr)

Replantation.
Reimplantación.
(Reh-eem-plahn-tah-see-ohn)

Rest now.
Descanse ahora.
(Dehs-kahn-seh ah-oh-rah)

Rest.
Descanse.
(Des-kahn-seh)

Return in ten days.
Regrese en diez días.
(Reh-greh-seh ehn dee-ehs dee-ahs)

Right now it is throbbing like a bad toothache!
¡Ahora está punzando, como un mal dolor de muelas!
(Ah-oh-rah ehs-tah poon-sahn-doh, koh-moh oon mahl doh-lohr deh moo-eh-lahs)

Rinse your mouth.
Enjuague su boca.
(Ehn-hoo-ah-geh soo boh-kah)

Rotate it.
Gíralo/Dale vuelta/Rotalo.
(Hee-rah-loh/Dah-leh boo-ehl-tah/Roh-tah-loh)

Rotate your arm.
Rota tu brazo.
(Roh-tah too brah-soh)

Route.
Via/Ruta.
(Bee-ah/roo-tah)

Run!
¡Corra!
(Koh-rah)

Say "ah."
Dí "ah."
(Dee "ah")

Say it again.
Dígalo otra vez/Repita.
(Dee-gah-loh oh-trah behs/Reh-pee-tah)

Say your name.
Dí tu nombre.
(Dee too nohm-breh)

See you later!
¡Hasta luego!
(Ahs-tah loo-eh-goh)

See your doctor before you refill the prescription.
Vea al doctor antes de surtir la receta.
(Beh-ah ahl dohk-tohr ahn-tehs deh soohr-teer lah reh-seh-tah)

Select your foods after breakfast.
Seleccione las comidas después del desayuno.
(Seh-lehk-see-oh-neh lahs koh-mee-dahs dehs-poo-ehs del deh-sah-yoo-noh)

Select your foods from the menu.
Seleccione las comidas del menú.
(Seh-lehk-see-oh-neh lahs koh-mee-dahs dehl meh-nuh)

Sexually active homosexual and bisexual males or females.
Homosexuales activos y hombres o mujeres bisexuales.
(Oh-moh-sehx-oo-ah-lehs ahk-tee-bohs ee ohm-brehs oh moo-heh-rehs bee-sehx-oo-ah-lehs)

Share your feelings with your wife and one friend.
Comparta sus sentimientos con su esposa y un amigo.
(Kohm-pahr-tah soos sehn-tee-mee-ehn-tohs kohn soo ehs-poh-sah ee oon ah-mee-goh)

She assigns a dosage schedule in the computer.
Ella asigna el horario de dosis en la computadora.
(Eh-yah ah-seeg-nah ehl oh-rah-ree-oh deh doh-sees ehn lah kohm-poo-tah-doh-rah)

She is happy.
Ella está contenta.
(Eh-yah ehs-tah kohn-tehn-tah)

She is sad.
Ella está triste.
(Eh-yah ehs-tah trees-teh).

Shock?
¿Toques?
(Toh-kehs)

Should I drive?
¿Debo de manejar?
(Deh-boh deh mah-neh-hahr)

Show me your tongue!
¡Muéstreme la lengua!
(Moo-ehs-treh-meh lah lehn-goo-ah)

Sign here, please.
Firme aquí, por favor.
(Feer-meh ah-kee, pohr fah-bohr)

Since when?
¿Desde cuándo?
(Dehs-deh koo-ahn-doh)

Sit!
¡Siéntese!
(See-ehn-teh-seh)

Sit down!
¡Siéntese!
(See-ehn-teh-seh)

Sit down, please.
Siéntese, por favor.
(See-ehn-teh-seh pohr fah-bohr)

Sit here and wait.
Siéntese aquí y espere.
(See-ehn-teh-seh ah-kee ee ehs-peh-reh)

Sit in the chair.
Siéntese en la silla.
(See-ehn-teh-seh ehn lah see-yah)

Sit up!
¡Siéntese!
(See-ehn-teh-seh)

Sit upright!
¡Siéntate derecho!
(See-ehn-tah-teh deh-reh-choh)

Six to eleven (6 to 11) servings of
    starches:
Seis a once porciones de almidones:
*(Seh-ees ah ohn-seh pohr-see-ohn-ehs
    deh ahl-mee-doh-nehs)*

Sleep at least six hours daily.
Duerma por lo menos seis horas
    diarias.
*(Doo-ehr-mah pohr loh meh-nohs seh-
    ees oh-rahs dee-ah-ree-ahs)*

Sleep at least eight hours.
Duerma al menos ocho horas.
*(Doo-ehr-mah ahl meh-nohs oh-choh
    oh-rahs)*

Slowly, please.
Despacio, por favor.
(Dehs-pah-see-oh, pohr fah-bohr)

Smile.
Sonrié.
(Sohn-ree-eh)

So far. . .
Hasta ahora. . .
(Ahs-tah ah-oh-rah)

Social Security?
¿Seguro Social?
(Seh-goo-roh Soh-see-ahl)

Some develop: tiredness, fever, loss of
    appetite, weight loss, diarrhea, night
    sweats.
Algunos desarrollan: cansansio,
    fiebre, falta de apetito, pérdida
    de peso, diarrea, sudor
    nocturno.
*(Ahl-goo-nohs deh-sah-roh-yahn kahn-
    sahn-see-oh, fee-eh-breh, fahl-tah
    deh ah-peh-tee-toh, pehr-dee-dah
    deh peh-soh, dee-ah-reh-ah, soo-
    dohr nohk-toor-noh)*

Some people cannot tolerate gas-
    producing foods and should avoid
    eating them.
Algunas personas no toleran comidas
    que producen gas y deben de
    evitar comerlas.
*(Ahl-goo-nahs pehr-soh-nahs noh toh-
    leh-rahn koh-mee-dahs keh proh-
    doo-sehn gahs ee deh-behn deh
    eh-bee-tahr koh-mehr-lahs)*

Someone will take you to your hospital
    room.
Alguien lo llevará a su cuarto.
*(Ahl-ghee-ehn loh yeh-bah-rah ah soo
    koo-ahr-toh)*

Sore throat. . .
Dolor de garganta. . .
(Doh-lohr deh gahr-gahn-tah.)

Sorry, no toothpicks.
Lo siento, no hay palillos.
*(Loh see-ehn-toh, noh ah-ee pah-lee-
    yohs)*

Spanish is important.
El español es importante.
*(Ehl ehs-pah-nyohl ehs eem-pohr-
    tahn-teh)*

Speak!
¡Hable!
(Ah-bleh)

Speak slowly please.
Hable despacio, por favor.
*(Ah-bleh dehs-pah-see-oh, pohr fah-
bohr)*

Squeeze my hand.
Apriete mi mano.
(Ah-pree-eh-teh mee mah-noh)

Squeeze the fingers of each of my
hands.
Apriete cada uno de los dedos de mi
mano.
*(Ah-pree-eh-teh kah-dah oo-noh deh
lohs deh-dohs deh mee mah-noh)*

Stand straight!
¡Párese derecho(a)!
(Pah-reh-seh deh-reh-choh[-chah])

Stand up!
¡Levántate!
(Leh-bahn-tah-teh!)

Start at the beginning.
Empieze al principio.
(Ehm-pee-eh-seh ahl preen-see-pee-oh)

Stay as you are!
¡Quédese como está!
(Keh-deh-seh koh-moh ehs-tah)

Stay away!
¡Hágase a un lado!
(Ah-gah-seh ah oon lah-doh)

Stay like this for a while.
Quédese así por un rato.
(Keh-deh-seh ah-see pohr oon rah-toh)

Stay sitting here.
Quédese sentado aquí.
(Keh-deh-seh sehn-tah-doh ah-kee)

Stay still!
¡Quédese quieto!
(Keh-deh-seh kee-eh-toh)

Sterilize the bottles.
Esterilice las botellas/los biberones.
*(Ehs-teh-ree-lee-seh lahs boh-teh-
yahs/lohs bee-beh-roh-nehs)*

Stick out the tongue.
Saca la lengua.
(Sah-kah lah lehn-goo-ah)

Stop breathing.
No respire.
(Noh rehs-pee-reh)

Stop!
¡Párese/Detente/Deténgase!
*(Pah-reh-seh/Deh-tehn-teh/Deh-tehn-
gah-seh)*

Straighten the knee.
Endereza la rodilla.
(Ehn-deh-reh-sah lah roh-dee-yah)

Straighten your leg.
Endereza tu pierna.
(Ehn-deh-reh-sah too pee-ehr-nah)

Strain down.
Empuja.
(Ehm-poo-hah)

Such as?
¿Tal como?
(Tahl koh-moh)

Sure.
Seguro.
(Seh-goo-roh)

Swallow!
¡Trague!
(Trah-gheh)

Swallow, please.
Traga, por favor.
(Trah-gah, pohr fah-bohr)

Swelling of the ankles?
¿Hinchazón en los tobillos?
*(Een-chah-sohn ehn lohs toh-bee-
yohs)*

Take thirty minutes every day to
examine your feelings.
Tome treinta minutos diariamente
para examinar sus sentimientos.
*(Toh-meh treh-een-tah mee-noo-tohs
dee-ah-ree-ah-mehn-teh pah-rah
ehx-ah-mee-nahr soos sehn-tee-mee-
ehn-tohs.)*

Take a bath every day.
Báñese todos los días.
(Bah-nyeh-seh toh-dohs lohs dee-ahs)

Take a bath.
Báñese.
(Bah-nyeh-seh)

Take a deep breath, hold it.
Respire hondo, detenlo.
(Rehs-pee-reh ohn-doh, deh-tehn-loh)

Take a deep breath.
Respire hondo/profundo.
(Rehs-pee-reh ohn-doh/proh-foon-doh)

Take a deep breath; let it go.
Respira hondo; déjalo ir.
*(Rehs-pee-rah ohn-doh; deh-hah-loh
eer)*

Take all the medicine in the
prescription.
Tome toda la medicina indicada en
la receta.
*(Toh-meh toh-dah lah meh-dee-see-
nah een-dee-kah-dah ehn lah reh-
seh-tah)*

Take care of yourself!
¡Cuídese mucho!
(Koo-ee-deh-seh moo-choh)

Take him for vaccinations at two
months.
Llévelo a vacunar a los dos meses.
*(Yeh-beh-loh ah bah-koo-nahr ah lohs
dohs meh-sehs)*

Take it with a full glass of water.
Tómela con un vaso lleno de agua.
*(Toh-meh-lah kohn oon bah-soh yeh-
noh deh ah-goo-ah)*

Take on an empty stomach.
Tómela con el estómago vacío.
*(Toh-meh-lah kohn ehl ehs-toh-mah-
goh bah-see-oh)*

Take one hour before eating.
Tómela una hora antes de comer.
*(Toh-meh-lah oo-nah oh-rah ahn-tehs
deh koh-mehr)*

Take the elevator to the sixth floor.
Tome el elevador al sexto piso.
*(Toh-meh ehl eh-leh-bah-dohr ahl
sehx-toh pee-soh)*

Take the medicine with food.
Tome la medicina con comida.
*(Toh-meh lah meh-dee-see-nah kohn
koh-mee-dah)*

Take the medicine with juice.
Tome la medicina con jugo.
*(Toh-meh lah meh-dee-see-nah kohn
hoo-goh)*

Take the medicines daily.
Tome las medicinas diariamente.
*(Toh-meh lahs meh-dee-see-nahs dee-
ah-ree-ah-mehn-teh)*

Take the temperature rectally.
Tome la temperatura por el recto.
*(Toh-meh lah tehm-peh-rah-too-rah
pohr ehl rehk-toh)*

Take these pills after your meal.
Tómese estas pastillas después de la
cena.
*(Toh-meh-seh ehs-tahs pahs-tee-yahs
dehs-poo-ehs deh lah seh-nah)*

Take this antibiotic to prevent
infections and this analgesic for
pain.
Tome este antibiótico para evitar
infecciones y este analgésico para
el dolor.
*(Toh-meh ehs-teh ahn-tee-bee-oh-tee-
koh pah-rah eh-bee-tahr een-fehk-
see-oh-nehs ee ehs-teh
ah-nahl-heh-see-koh pah-rah ehl
doh-lohr)*

Take two aspirins.
Tome dos aspirinas.
(Toh-meh dohs ahs-pee-ree-nahs)

Take your hospital card.
Lleve su tarjeta del hospital.
*(Yeh-beh soo tahr-heh-tah dehl ohs-
pee-tahl)*

Take your medical file.
Lleve su archivo.
(Yeh-beh soo ahr-chee-boh)

Take your shoe(s) off.
Quítate tu/los zapato(s).
(Kee-tah-teh too/lohs sah-pah-toh(s))

Take your socks off.
Quítate los calcetines.
(Kee-tah-teh lohs kahl-seh-tee-nehs)

Talk!
¡Hable!
(Ah-bleh)

Telephone number?
¿Número de teléfono?
(Noo-meh-roh deh teh-leh-foh-noh)

Tell me!
¡Dígame!
(Dee-gah-meh)

Tell me if it hurts more when I press or when I let go.
Dígame si le duele más al presionar o al retirar la mano.
(Dee-gah-meh see leh doo-eh-leh mahs ahl preh-see-oh-nahr oh ahl reh-tee-rahr lah mah-noh)

Tell me if it hurts.
Dime si duele.
(Dee-meh see doo-eh-leh)

Tell me if there is pain/Tell me if this hurts.
Dime si duele.
(Dee-meh see doo-eh-leh)

Tell me what brought you here?
¿Dígame qué lo trajo aquí?
(Dee-gah-meh keh loh trah-hoh ah-kee)

Tell me what foods.
Dígame qué alimentos.
(Dee-gah-meh keh ah-lee-mehn-tohs)

Tell me when it feels numb.
Avíseme cuando sienta dormido.
(Ah-bee-seh-meh koo-ahn-doh see-ehn-tah dohr-mee-doh)

Tell me when you feel a contraction.
Dígame cuando sienta una contracción.
(Dee-gah-meh koo-ahn-doh see-ehn-tah oo-nah kohn-trahk-see-ohn)

Tell me when!
¡Dígame cuándo!
(Dee-gah-meh koo-ahn-doh)

Tell me where it hurts.
Dígame dónde le duele.
(Dee-gah-meh dohn-deh leh doo-eh-leh)

Tell me why you are here?
¿Dígame porque está aquí?
(Dee-gah-meh pohr keh ehs-tah ah-kee)

Tell me your name.
Dígame su nombre.
(Dee-gah-meh soo nohm-breh)

Tell me, have you ever had a heart attack?
¿Dígame, a tenido alguna vez un ataque cardíaco?
(Dee-gah-meh, ah teh-nee-doh ahl-goo-nah behs oon ah-tah-keh kahr-dee-ah-koh)

Tell me, where did the pain start?
Dígame, ¿dónde comenzó el dolor?
(Dee-gah-meh, dohn-deh koh-mehn-soh ehl doh-lohr)

Thank you!
¡Gracias!
(Grah-see-ahs)

Thank you, doctor.
Gracias, doctor.
(Grah-see-ahs, dohk-tohr)

Thank you for talking to me.
Gracias por hablar conmigo.
(Grah-see-ahs pohr ah-blahr kohn-mee-goh)

Thank you for the information.
Gracias por la información.
(Grah-see-ahs pohr lah een-fohr-mah-see-ohn)

Thank you very much!
¡Muchas gracias!
(Moo-chahs grah-see-ahs)

That bracelet is hers.
Aquella pulsera es de ella.
(Ah-keh-yah pool-seh-rah ehs deh eh-yah)

That gown is yours.
Aquella bata es suya.
(Ah-keh-yah bah-tah ehs soo-yah)

That is all!
¡Es todo!
(Ehs toh-doh)

That is for sure!
¡Délo por seguro!
(Deh-loh pohr seh-goo-roh)

That is plaque.
Esa es la placa.
(Eh-sah ehs lah plah-kah)

The aide cooks breakfast.
La ayudante cocina el desayuno.
(Lah ah-yoo-dahn-teh koh-see-nah ehl deh-sah-yoo-noh))

The anesthesiologist will visit you in the afternoon.
El anestesiólogo la visitará en la tarde.
(Ehl ah-nehs-teh-see-oh-loh-goh lah bee-see-tah-rah ehn lah tahr-deh)

The bed has one blanket.
La cama tiene una frazada/colcha.
(Lah kah-mah tee-eh-neh oo-nah frah-sah-dah/kohl-chah)

The bell will sound.
La campana sonará.
(Lah kahm-pah-nah soh-nah-rah)

The bottle will be kept in a bucket with ice.
La botella se mantendrá en una tina con hielo.
(Lah boh-teh-yah seh mahn-tehn-drah ehn oo-nah tee-nah kohn ee-eh-loh)

The building has beige brick.
El edificio tiene ladrillo crema.
(Ehl eh-dee-fee-see-oh tee-eh-neh lah-dree-yoh kreh-mah)

The clerical staff is very important.
Las secretarias son muy importantes.
(Lahs seh-kreh-tah-ree-ahs sohn moo-ee eem-pohr-tahn-tehs)

The clinic is in another building.
La clínica está en otro edificio.
(Lah klee-nee-kah ehs-tah ehn oh-troh eh-dee-fee-see-oh)

The computer says that you have an appointment.
La computadora dice que tiene una cita.
(Lah kohm-poo-tah-doh-rah dee-seh keh tee-eh-neh oh-nah see-tah)

The consent has to be signed by the patient.
El consentimiento debe ser firmado por el paciente.
(Ehl kohn-sehn-tee-mee-ehn-toh deh-beh sehr feer-mah-doh pohr ehl pah-see-ehn-teh)

The cover is hot.
La cubierta está caliente.
(Lah koo-bee-ehr-tah ehs-tah kah-lee-ehn-teh)

The doctor asks the patient.
El doctor le pregunta al paciente.
(Ehl dohk-tohr leh preh-goon-tah ahl pah-see-ehn-teh)

The doctor has to prescribe it.
El doctor/La doctora debe de recetarla.
(Ehl dohk-tohr/Lah dohk-tohr(ah) deh-beh deh reh-seh-tahr-lah)

The doctor will give you something for the pain.
El doctor le dará algo para el dolor.
(Ehl dohk-tohr leh dah-rah ahl-goh pah-rah ehl doh-lohr)

The doctor will see you in the Emergency Room.
Lo verá el doctor en el cuarto de emergencia.
(Loh beh-rah ehl dohk-tohr ehn ehl koo-ahr-toh deh eh-mehr-hehn-see-ah)

The doctor will see you there.
El doctor lo verá ahí.
(Ehl dohk-tohr loh beh-rah ah-ee)

The elevators are slow.
Los elevadores son lentos.
(Lohs eh-leh-bah-doh-rehs sohn lehn-tohs)

The elevators work twenty-four hours.
Los elevadores trabajan veinticuatro horas.
(Lohs eh-leh-bah-doh-rehs trah-bah-hahn beh-een-tee-koo-ah-troh oh-rahs)

The exam is difficult.
El examen es difícil.
(Ehl ehx-ah-mehn ehs dee-fee-seel)

The failure in the exams represents a disappointment for my family.
La falla en los exámenes representa una desilusión para mi familia.
(Lah fah-yah ehn lohs ehx-ah-meh-nehs reh-preh-sehn-tah oo-nah deh-see-loo-see-ohn pah-rah mee fah-mee-lee-ah)

The flow rate should be at ¹/₂ liter.
El flujo debe de ser de medio litro.
(Ehl floo-hoh deh-beh sehr deh meh-dee-oh lee-troh)

The following information is included in the label.
La siguiente información se incluye en la etiqueta.
(Lah see-ghee-ehn-teh een-fohr-mah-see-ohn seh een-kloo-yeh ehn lah eh-tee-keh-tah)

The following should be included in your diet every day: two to four servings of milk.
Lo siguiente se debe incluir en la dieta todos los días: dos a cuatro porciones de leche.
(Loh see-ghee-ehn-teh seh deh-beh een-kloo-eer ehn soo dee-eh-tah toh-dohs lohs dee-ahs: dohs ah koo-ah-troh pohr-see-ohn-ehs deh leh-cheh)

The fork, spoon and knife are wrapped in the napkin.
El tenedor, cuchara y cuchillo están envueltos en la servilleta.
(Ehl teh-neh-dohr, koo-chah-rah ee koo-chee-yoh ehs-tahn ehn-boo-ehl-tohs ehn lah sehr-bee-yeh-tah)

The hospital bills for some professional fees; otherwise, the professional fees are not included in the hospital's bill.
El hospital cobra por servicios profesionales que no están incluidos en la cuenta del hospital.
(Ehl ohs-pee-tahl koh-brah pohr sehr-bee-see-ohs proh-feh-see-oh-nah-lehs keh noh ehs-tahn een-kloo-ee-dohs ehn lah koo-ehn-tah dehl ohs-pee-tahl)

The hospital is not responsible.
El hospital no se hace responsable.
(Ehl ohs-pee-tahl noh seh ah-seh rehs-pohn-sah-bleh)

The hours of operation of the inpatient pharmacy are Monday through Friday, seven AM to one AM.
El horario de la farmacia para pacientes internados es de lunes a viernes de las siete de la mañana a la una de la mañana.
(Ehl oh-rah-ree-oh deh lah fahr-mah-see-ah pah-rah pah-see-ehn-tehs een-tehr-nah-dohs ehs deh loo-nehs ah bee-ehr-nehs deh lahs see-eh-teh deh lah mah-nyah-nah ah lah oo-nah deh lah mah-nyah-nah)

The inpatient pharmacy is open.
La farmacia para pacientes internados está abierta.
(Lah fahr-mah-see-ah pah-rah pah-see-ehn-tehs een-tehr-nah-dohs ehs-tah ah-bee-ehr-tah)

The kids left their skates on the stairs and I fell over them.
Los niños dejaron los patines en las escaleras y me tropecé.
(Lohs nee-nyohs deh-hah-rohn lohs pah-tee-nehs ehn lahs ehs-kah-leh-rahs ee meh troh-peh-seh)

The line is on the wall.
La línea está en la pared.
(Lah lee-nee-ah ehs-tah ehn lah pah-rehd)

The majority of patients have a life span of about eighteen to twenty-four months.
La mayoría de los pacientes tienen una sobrevivencia aproximada de dieciocho a veinticuatro meses.
(Lah mah-yoh-ree-ah deh lohs pah-see-ehn-tehs tee-eh-nehn oo-nah soh-breh-bee-behn-see-ah ah-prohx-ee-mah-dah deh dee-eh-see-oh-choh ah beh-een-tee-koo-ah-troh meh-sehs)

The meals are served at eleven thirty AM.
Los alimentos se sirven a las once y media.
(Lohs ah-lee-mehn-tohs seh seer-behn ah lahs ohn-seh ee meh-dee-ah)

The meals are served at five PM.
Los alimentos se sirven a las cinco de la tarde.
(Lohs ah-lee-mehn-tohs seh seer-behn ah lahs seen-koh deh lah tahr-deh)

The meals are served at seven AM.
Los alimentos se sirven a las siete de la mañana.
(Lohs ah-lee-mehn-tohs seh seer-behn ah lahs see-eh-teh deh lah mah-nyah-nah)

The measurement is difficult.
La medida es difícil.
(Lah meh-dee-dah ehs dee-fee-seel).

The next day, the bottle will be sent to the laboratory.
Al siguiente día, la botella se mandará al laboratorio.
(Ahl see-ghee-ehn-teh dee-ah, lah boh-teh-yah seh mahn-dah-rah ahl lah-boh-rah-toh-ree-oh)

The nurse explains the procedure and hospital routine.
La enfermera le explica el procedimiento y la rutina del hospital.
(Lah ehn-fehr-meh-rah leh ehx-plee-kah ehl proh-seh-dee-mee-ehn-toh ee lah roo-tee-nah dehl ohs-pee-tahl)

The nurse orders the medication from the pharmacy.
La enfermera ordena la medicina de la farmacia.
(Lah ehn-fehr-meh-rah ohr-deh-nah lah meh-dee-see-nah deh lah fahr-mah-see-ah)

The nurse said that you can't speak very well.
La enfermera dice que no puede hablar bien.
(Lah ehn-fehr-meh-rah dee-seh keh noh poo-eh-deh ah-blahr bee-ehn)

The nurse wants to talk to you.
La enfermera quiere hablarle.
(Lah ehn-fehr-meh-rah kee-eh-reh ah-blahr-leh)

The nurse will ask how you feel.
La enfermera le preguntará cómo se siente.
(Lah ehn-fehr-meh-rah leh preh-goon-tah-rah koh-moh seh see-ehn-teh)

The nurse will complete the assessment.
La enfermera completará la evaluación.
(Lah ehn-fehr-meh-rah kohm-pleh-tah-rah lah eh-bah-loo-ah-see-ohn)

The one who is six years old.
El que tiene seis años.
(Ehl keh tee-eh-neh seh-ees ah-nyohs)

The only way we can see plaque is by using a solution that stains the teeth.
La única manera de ver la placa es al usar una solución que mancha los dientes.
(Lah oo-nee-kah mah-neh-rah deh behr lah plah-kah ehs ahl oo-sahr oo-nah soh-loo-see-ohn keh mahn-chah lohs dee-ehn-tehs)

The owner. . .
Dueño/Amo. . .
(Doo-eh-nyoh/Ah-moh)

The pain has gotten worse.
El dolor ha empeorado.
(Ehl doh-lohr ah ehm-peh-ohr-ah-doh)

The pain is constant.
El dolor es constante.
(Ehl doh-lohr ehs kohns-tahn-teh)

The pain is cutting.
El dolor es cortante.
(Ehl doh-lohr ehs kohr-tahn-teh)

The pain is localized, sharp.
El dolor está fijo, agudo.
(Ehl doh-lohr ehs-tah fee-hoh, ah-goo-doh)

The pain is on the side.
El dolor está en el lado/costado.
(Ehl doh-lohr ehs-tah ehn ehl lah-doh/kohs-tah-doh)

The pain is sharp.
El dolor es agudo.
(Ehl doh-lohr ehs ah-goo-doh)

The pain is throbbing.
El dolor es punzante.
(Ehl doh-lohr ehs poon-sahn-teh)

The pain is worse.
El dolor es peor.
(Ehl doh-lohr ehs peh-ohr)

The pain started two hours ago.
El dolor comenzó hace dos horas.
(Ehl doh-lohr koh-mehn-soh ah-seh dohs oh-rahs)

The pain starts here (beneath the sternum) and goes to my jaw.
El dolor comienza aquí (abajo del esternón) y se va a la mandíbula.
(Ehl doh-lohr koh-mee-ehn-sah ah-kee [ah-bah-hoh dehl ehs-tehr-nohn] ee seh bah ah lah mahn-dee-boo-lah)

The pain starts here and travels down my left arm.
El dolor comienza aquí y se recorre por el brazo izquierdo.
(Ehl doh-lohr koh-mee-ehn-sah ah-kee ee seh reh-koh-reh pohr ehl brah-soh ees-kee-ehr-doh)

The patient asks:
El paciente pregunta:
(Ehl pah-see-ehn-teh preh-goon-tah)

The patient is happy.
El paciente está contento.
(Ehl pah-see-ehn-teh ehs-tah kohn-tehn-toh)

The patient responds by blinking.
El Paciente responde parpareando.
(Ehl pah-see-ehn-teh rehs-pohn-deh pahr-pah-reh-ahn-doh)

The pharmacist assists with patient education.
El farmacéutico/La farmacéutica asiste con la educación del paciente.
(Ehl fahr-mah-seh-oo-tee-koh/Lah fahr-mah-seh-oo-tee-kah ah-sees-teh kohn lah eh-doo-kah-see-ohn dehl pah-see-ehn-teh)

The pharmacist interprets the physician's order.
El farmacéutico interpreta la orden del doctor.
(Ehl fahr-mah-seh-oo-tee-koh een-tehr-preh-tah lah ohr-dehn dehl dohk-tohr)

The pharmacy is open Monday through Friday.
La farmacia está abierta de lunes a viernes.
(Lah fahr-mah-see-ah ehs-tah ah-bee-ehr-tah deh loo-nehs ah bee-ehr-nehs)

The pharmacy provides services as an integral part of total patient care.
La farmacia provee servicios como parte integral del cuidado total del paciente.
(Lah fahr-mah-see-ah proh-beh-eh sehr-bee-see-ohs koh-moh pahr-teh een-teh-grahl dehl koo-ee-dah-doh toh-tahl dehl pah-see-ehn-teh)

The pharmacy staff deliver and pick up orders every hour from the floors.
Los empleados de la farmacia recogen y surten órdenes cada hora en los pisos.
(Lohs ehm-pleh-ah-dohs deh lah fahr-mah-see-ah reh-koh-hehn ee soohr-tehn ohr-deh-nehs kah-dah oh-rah ehn lohs pee-sohs)

The plates are plastic.
Los platos son de plástico.
(Lohs plah-tohs sohn deh plahs-tee-koh)

The prescription will be ready at _____.
La receta estará lista a las _____.
(Lah reh-seh-tah ehs-tah-rah lees-tah ah lahs _____)

The procedure is difficult.
El procedimiento es difícil.
(Ehl proh-seh-dee-mee-ehn-toh ehs dee-fee-seel)

The rails lower down.
El barandal se baja.
(Ehl bah-rahn-dahl seh bah-hah)

The rings are mine.
Los anillos son míos.
(Lohs ah-nee-yohs sohn mee-ohs)

The salt and pepper are in these packets.
La sal y la pimienta están en estos paquetes.
(Lah sahl ee lah pee-mee-ehn-tah ehs-tahn ehn ehs-tohs pah-keh-tehs)

The secretary will help.
La secretaria lo ayudará.
(Lah seh-kreh-tah-ree-ah loh ah-yoo-dah-rah)

The staff delivers and picks up orders every hour from the floors.
Los empleados recogen y surten órdenes cada hora en los pisos.
(Los ehm-pleh-ah-dohs reh-koh-hehn ee soor-tehn ohr-deh-nehs kah-dah oh-rah ehn lohs pee-sohs)

The stairs are at the end of the hallway.
Las escaleras están al fin del pasillo.
(Lahs ehs-kah-leh-rahs ehs-tahn ahl feehn dehl pah-see-yoh)

The stairs will take you to a walkway.
Las escaleras lo llevarán a un pasillo sobre la calle.
(Lahs ehs-kah-leh-rahs loh yeh-bah-rahn ah oon pah-see-yoh soh-breh lah kah-yeh)

The Surgery floor is in the hospital towers.
El piso de cirugía está en las torres del hospital.
(Ehl pee-soh deh see-roo-hee-ah ehs-tah ehn lahs toh-rehs dehl ohs-pee-tahl)

The television has four channels.
El televisor tiene cuatro canales.
(Ehl teh-leh-bee-sohr tee-eh-neh koo-ah-troh kah-nah-lehs)

The water is in the glass/pitcher.
El agua está en el vaso/la jarra.
(Ehl ah-goo-ah ehs-tah ehn ehl bah-soh/lah hah-rah)

The water is warm.
El agua está tibia.
(Ehl ah-goo-ah ehs-tah tee-bee-ah)

Then they will take blood samples.
Luego le van a tomar muestras de sangre.
(Loo-eh-goh leh bahn ah toh-mahr moo-ehs-trahs deh sahn-greh)

Then, turn to the left.
Luego voltee a la izquierda.
(Loo-eh-goh bohl-teh-eh ah lah ees-kee-ehr-dah)

There are a few things that you have to keep in mind.
Hay varias cosas que debe recordar.
(Ah-ee bah-ree-ahs koh-sahs keh deh-beh reh-kohr-dahr)

There are a lot of patients.
Hay muchos pacientes.
(Ah-ee moo-chohs pah-see-ehn-tehs)

There are bathrooms for guests in the corner.
Hay baños para las visitas en la esquina.
(Ah-ee bah-nyohs pah-rah lahs bee-see-tahs ehn lah ehs-kee-nah)

There are many diets available to patients.
Hay muchas dietas para los pacientes.
(Ah-ee moo-chahs dee-eh-tahs pah-rah lohs pah-see-ehn-tehs)

There is a front desk.
Hay un escritorio al frente.
(Ah-ee oon ehs-kree-toh-ree-oh ahl frehn-teh)

There is a shower.
Hay una ducha/regadera.
(Ah-ee oo-nah doo-chah/reh-gah-deh-rah)

There is a straw.
Hay un popote.
(Ah-ee oon poh-poh-teh)

There is also a bathtub/tub.
También hay una bañera/tina.
(Tahm-bee-ehn ah-ee oo-nah bah-nyeh-rah/tee-nah)

There is an educational channel.
Hay un canal educativo.
(Ah-ee oon kah-nahl eh-doo-kah-tee-boh)

There is an emergency light.
Hay una luz para emergencias.
(Ah-ee oo-nah loos pah-rah eh-mehr-hehn-see-ahs)

There will be a separate charge for professional services, such as physician services.
Habrá gastos en separado por servicios profesionales tales como servicios médicos.
(Ah-brah gahs-tohs ehn seh-pah-rah-doh pohr sehr-bee-see-ohs proh-feh-see-oh-nah-lehs tah-lehs koh-moh sehr-bee-see-ohs meh-dee-kohs)

These books are mine.
Estos libros son míos.
(Ehs-tohs lee-brohs sohn mee-ohs)

These buttons move the bed up/down.
Estos botones mueven la cama arriba/abajo.
(Ehs-tohs boh-toh-nehs moo-eh-behn lah kah-mah ah-ree-bah/ah-bah-hoh)

These meats can be substituted.
Estas carnes se pueden substituir.
(Ehs-tahs kahr-nehs seh poo-eh-dehn soobs-tee-too-eer)

They are around the corner.
Están alrededor de la esquina.
(Ehs-tahn ahl-reh-deh-dohr deh lah ehs-kee-nah)

They are happy.
Ellos están contentos.
(Eh-yohs ehs-tahn kohn-tehn-tohs)

They are men.
Ellos son hombres.
(Eh-yohs sohn ohm-brehs)

They are Mrs. Luna's.
Son de la señora Luna.
(Sohn de lah seh-nyoh-rah Loo-nah)

They are sad.
Ellas están tristes.
(Eh-yahs ehs-tahn trees-tehs)

They are the ones that first greet the patient.
Ellas son las primeras personas que saludan al paciente.
(Eh-yahs sohn lahs pree-meh-rahs pehr-soh-nahs keh sahl-oo-dahn ahl pah-see-ehn-teh)

They can help clean.
Pueden ayudar a limpiar.
(Poo-eh-dehn ah-yoo-dahr ah leem-pee-ahr)

They can't break.
No se pueden romper.
(Noh seh poo-eh-dehn rohm-pehr)

They will let you talk to your family.
Le permitirán hablar con su familia.
(Leh pehr-mee-tee-rahn ah-blahr kohn soo fah-mee-lee-ah)

Think about what makes you depressed.
Piense qué le causa depresión.
(Pee-ehn-seh keh leh kah-oo-sah deh-preh-see-ohn)

This button lowers (raises) the headboard.
Este botón baja (sube) la cabecera de la cama.
(Ehs-teh boh-tohn bah-hah [soo-beh] lah kah-beh-seh-rah deh lah kah-mah)

This chair turns into a bed.
Esta silla se hace cama.
(Ehs-tah see-yah seh ah-seh kah-mah)

This is a handout that deals with the hospital's guidelines.
Este es un folleto que trata de las reglas del hospital.
(Ehs-teh ehs oon foh-yeh-toh keh trah-tah deh lahs reh-glahs dehl ohs-pee-tahl)

This is a large place.
Este es un lugar grande.
(Ehs-teh ehs oon loo-gahr grahn-deh)

This is a new formula.
Esta es una fórmula nueva.
(Ehs-tah ehs oo-nah fohr-moo-lah noo-eh-bah)

This is a sedative.
Este es un sedante.
(Ehs-teh ehs oon seh-dahn-teh)

This is an antacid.
Este es un antiácido.
(Ehs-teh ehs oon ahn-tee-ah-see-doh)

This is an employee.
Este es un empleado.
(Ehs-teh ehs oon ehm-pleh-ah-doh)

This is done quickly.
Esto se hace rápido.
(Ehs-toh seh ah-seh rah-pee-doh)

This is my first time here.
Esta es mi primera vez aquí.
(Ehs-tah ehs mee pree-mehr-ah behs ah-kee)

This is the call bell.
Esta es la campana/el timbre.
(Ehs-tah ehs lah kahm-pah-nah/teem-breh)

This is the call buzzer.
Este es el timbre.
(Ehs-teh ehs ehl teem-breh)

This is the clinic.
Esta es la clínica.
(Ehs-tah ehs lah klee-nee-kah)

This is the lobby.
Esta es la sala de espera.
(Ehs-tah ehs lah sah-lah deh ehs-peh-rah)

This is the radio.
Este es el radio.
(Ehs-teh ehs ehl rah-dee-oh)

This is the service area.
Esta es el área de servicio.
(Ehs-tah ehs ehl ah-reh-ah deh sehr-bee-see-oh)

This is the tray.
Está es la bandeja/charola.
(Ehs-tah ehs lah bahn-deh-hah/chah-roh-lah)

This is to help your teeth become stronger and if cavities are present it will help slow the process.
Esto ayudará a hacer que los dientes sean más fuertes y si tiene cavidades, ayudará a retardar el proceso.
(Ehs-toh ah-yoo-dahr-ah ah ah-sehr keh lohs dee-ehn-tehs seh-ahn mahs foo-ehr-tehs ee see tee-ehn-eh kah-bee-dah-dehs, ah-yoo-dahr-ah ah reh-tahr-dahr ehl proh-seh-soh)

This is your room.
Este es el cuarto.
(Ehs-teh ehs ehl koo-ahr-toh)

This medicine is a pain killer.
Esta medicina quita/alivia el dolor.
(Ehs-tah meh-dee-see-nah kee-tah/ah-lee-bee-ah ehl doh-lohr)

This pencil is red.
Este lápiz es rojo.
(Ehs-teh lah-pees ehs roh-hoh)

This prescription may not be refilled.
Esta receta no se puede surtir de nuevo.
(Ehs-tah reh-seh-tah noh seh poo-eh-deh soor-teer deh noo-eh-boh)

This will feel cold.
Esto se sentirá frío.
(Ehs-toh seh sehn-tee-rah free-oh)

This will take you to the end of the hall.
Esta la llevará al final del pasillo.
(Ehs-tah lah yeh-bah-rah ahl feen-ahl dehl pah-see-yoh)

Three times a day.
Tres veces al día.
(Trehs beh-sehs ahl dee-ah)

Tighten your muscle!
¡Apriete el músculo!
(Ah-pree-eh-teh ehl moos-koo-loh)

Tighten!
¡Aprieta!
(Ah-pree-eh-tah)

Today I am here to examine the baby.
Estoy aquí hoy para examinar al bebé.
(Ehs-toh-ee ah-kee oh-ee pah-rah ehx-ah-mee-nahr ahl beh-beh)

Today is Monday.
Hoy es lunes.
(Oh-ee ehs loo-nehs)

Tomorrow they will give you a special test.
Mañana le harán un análisis especial.
(Mah-nyah-nah leh ah-rahn oon ah-nah-lee-sees ehs-peh-see-ahl)

Tomorrow, at seven AM, go to the lab and have your blood drawn.
Mañana a las siete vaya al laboratorio para tomar una muestra de sangre.
(Mah-nyah-nah ah lahs see-eh-teh bah-yah ahl lah-boh-rah-toh-ree-oh pah-rah toh-mahr oo-nah moo-ehs-trah deh sahn-greh)

Tomorrow, bring a specimen of your stool in this container.
Mañana, traiga una muestra de su excremento en este frasco.
(Mah-nyah-nah, trah-ee-gah oo-nah moo-ehs-trah deh soo ehx-kreh-mehn-toh ehn ehs-teh frahs-koh)

Tomorrow you are going to have your surgery.
Mañana le van a hacer la cirugía.
(Mah-nyah-nah leh bahn ah ah-sehr lah see-roo-hee-ah)

Will your husband be here?
¿Estará aquí su esposo?
(Ehs-tah-rah ah-kee soo ehs-poh-soh)

Tonight, eat lightly.
Esta noche coma ligero.
(Ehs-tah noh-cheh koh-mah lee-heh-roh)

Total number of pills?
¿Número total de pastillas?
(Noo-meh-roh toh-tahl deh pahs-tee-yahs)

Touch your face with your hand.
Toque la cara con la mano.
(Toh-keh lah kah-rah kohn lah mah-noh)

Transportation is here.
El transporte está aquí.
(Ehl trahns-pohr-teh ehs-tah ah-kee)

Transportation will take you back to your room.
Transportación lo regresará a su cuarto.
(Trahns-pohr-tah-see-ohn loh reh-greh-sah-rah ah soo koo-ahr-toh)

Treat everyone with affection.
Trate a todos con afecto.
(Trah-teh ah toh-dohs kohn ah-fehk-toh)

Try again!
¡Pruebe otra vez!
(Proo-eh-beh oh-trah behs)

Try to ask about the surgery.
Procure pedir informes sobre la cirugía.
(Proh-koo-reh peh-deer een-fohr-mehs soh-breh lah see-roo-hee-ah)

Try to calm down.
Trate de calmarse.
(Trah-teh deh kahl-mahr-seh)

Try to have a bowel movement every day.
Procure hacer del baño diariamente.
(Proh-koo-reh ah-sehr dehl bah-nyoh dee-ah-ree-ah-mehn-teh)

Turn!
¡Voltée!
(Bohl-teh-eh)

Turn it to the left.
Voltéalo hacia la izquierda.
(Bohl-teh-ah-loh ah-see-ah lah ees-kee-ehr-dah)

Turn it to the right.
Voltéalo hacia la derecha.
(Bohl-teh-ah-loh ah-see-ah lah deh-reh-chah)

Turn left.
Voltéa a la izquierda.
(Bohl-teh-ah ah lah ees-kee-ehr-dah)

Turn on your side.
Voltéese de lado.
(Bohl-teh-eh-seh deh lah-doh)

Turn right/to the right.
Voltée a la derecha.
(Bohl-teh-ah-teh ah lah deh-reh-chah)

Turn the forearm.
Voltéa el antebrazo.
(Bohl-teh-ah ehl ahn-teh-brah-soh)

Turn your head to the left.
Voltéa la cabeza a la izquierda.
(Bohl-teh-ah lah kah-beh-sah ah lah ees-kee-ehr-dah)

Turn your head to the right.
Voltéa la cabeza a la derecha.
(Bohl-teh-ah lah kah-beh-sah uh lah deh-reh-chah)

Twice a day.
Dos veces al día.
(Dohs beh-sehs ahl dee-ah)

Twist your upper extremities.
Tuerce las extremidades superiores.
(Too-ehr-seh lahs ehx-treh-mee-dah-dehs soo-peh-ree-oh-rehs)

Twist your waist.
Tuerce la cintura.
(Too-ehr-seh lah seen-too-rah)

Ulcerations?
¿Ulceraciones?
(Ool-seh-rah-see-oh-nehs)

Unusual bleeding or discharge.
Sangrado o flujo profuso.
(Sahn-grah-doh oh floo-hoh proh-foo-soh)

Upper extremities:
Extremidades superiores:
(Ehx-treh-mee-dah-dehs soo-peh-ree-oh-rehs)

Use comfortable clothes and shoes.
Use ropa y zapatos cómodos.
(Oo-seh roh-pah ee sah-pah-tohs koh-moh-dohs)

Use commands and phrases when performing physical examinations.
Use comandos/ordenes y frases utiles cuando performe/prepare el examen físico.
(Oo-seh koh-mahn-dohs/ohr-dehn-ehs ee frah-sehs oo-tee-lehs koo-ahn-doh pehr-fohr-meh/preh-pah-reh ehl ehx-ah-mehn fee-see-koh)

Use contraceptive measures.
Use medidas contraceptivas.
(Oo-seh meh-dee-dahs kohn-trah-sehp-tee-bahs)

Use dental floss.
Use hilo dental.
(Oo-seh ee-loh dehn-tahl)

Use the house shoes, the floor is cold.
Use las pantunflas/chanclas, el piso está frío.
(Oo-seh lahs pahn-toon-flahs/chahn-klahs, ehl pee-soh ehs-tah free-oh)

Use the nursing process to develop a plan of care.
Use el proceso de enfermería para desarrollar un plan de cuidado.
(Oo-seh ehl proh-seh-soh deh ehn-fehr-meh-ree-ah pah-rah deh-sah-roh-yahr oon plahn deh koo-ee-dah-doh)

Use thumbs and forefingers to guide the floss.
Use el dedo gordo y el índice para guiar el hilo.
(Oo-seh ehl deh-doh gohr-doh ee ehl een-dee-seh pah-rah ghee-ahr ehl ee-loh)

Using a circular motion, brush one to two teeth at a time.
Usando movimiento circular, cepille uno o dos dientes a la vez.
(Oo-sahn-doh moh-bee-mee-ehn-toh seer-koo-lahr, seh-pee-yeh oo-noh oh dohs dee-ehn-tehs ah lah behs)

Very good!
¡Muy bien!
(Moo-ee bee-ehn)

Vials, pills, capsules, liquids and IV fluids are available in the pharmacy.
Botellas, pastillas, cápsulas, líquidos y sueros se encuentran en la farmacia.
(Boh-teh-yahs, pahs-tee-yahs, kahp-soo-lahs, lee-kee-dohs ee soo-eh-rohs seh ehn-koo-ehn-trahn ehn lah fahr-mah-see-ah)

Visiting hours are from nine in the morning to nine at night.
Las horas de visita son de las nueve de la mañana a las nueve de la noche.
(Lahs oh-rahs deh bee-see-tah sohn deh lahs noo-eh-beh deh lah mah-nyah-nah ah lahs noo-eh-beh deh lah noh-cheh)

Visiting hours are from two to eight PM.
Las horas de visita son de las dos a las ocho de la noche.
(Lahs oh-rahs deh bee-see-tah sohn deh lahs dohs ah lahs oh-choh deh lah noh-cheh)

Void a little, then put urine in this cup.
Orine un poco, luego ponga la orina en esta taza.
(Oh-ree-neh oon poh-koh, loo-eh-goh pohn-gah lah oh-ree-nah ehn ehs-tah tah-sah)

Volume?
¿Volumen?
(Boh-loo-mehn)

Wait in the lobby.
Espere en el vestíbulo.
(Ehs-peh-reh ehn ehl behs-tee-boo-loh)

Wait several minutes!
¡Espera varios minutos!
(Ehs-peh-rah bah-ree-ohs mee-noo-tohs)

Wait your turn.
Espere su turno.
(Ehs-peh-reh soo toor-noh)

Wait!
¡Espere!
(Ehs-peh-reh)

Wake up!
¡Despierte!
(Dehs-pee-ehr-teh)

Walk six paces.
Camine seis pasos.
(Kah-mee-neh seh-ees pah-sohs)

Walk straight ahead!
¡Camine derecho!
(Kah-mee-neh deh-reh-choh)

Walk two blocks.
Camine dos cuadras.
(Kah-mee-neh dohs koo-ah-drahs)

Walk!
¡Camine!
(Kah-mee-neh)

Walk, please.
Camina, por favor.
(Kah-mee-nah, pohr fah-bohr)

Was he premature?
¿Fué prematuro?
(Foo-eh preh-mah-too-roh)

Was he/she conscious?
¿Estaba conciente?
(Ehs-tah-bah kohn-see-ehn-teh)

Was the car burning?
¿Estaba el carro en llamas?
(Ehs-tah-bah ehl kah-roh ehn yah-mahs)

Was the delivery normal?
¿Fué normal el parto?
(Foo-eh nohr-mahl ehl pahr-toh)

Was the victim alive/dead?
¿Estaba la víctima con vida/muerta?
(Ehs-tah-bah lah beek-tee-mah kohn bee-dah/moo-ehr-tah)

Was the victim on the road?
¿Estaba la víctima en el camino?
(Ehs-tah-bah lah beek-tee-mah ehn ehl kah-mee-noh)

Was the victim unconscious?
¿Estaba la víctima inconsciente?
(Ehs-tah-bah lah beek-tee-mah een-kohn-see-ehn-teh)

Wash his hands before eating.
Lávele las manos antes de comer.
(Lah-beh-leh lahs mah-nohs ahn-tehs deh koh-mehr)

Wash well all fruits and vegetables.
Láve bien todas las frutas y verduras.
(Lah-beh bee-ehn toh-dahs lahs froo-tahs ee behr-doo-rahs)

Wash your face!
¡Lávese la cara!
(Lah-beh-seh lah kah-rah)

Watch for the arrow.
Fíjese en la flecha.
(Fee-hehseh ehn lah fleh-chah)

Watch his growth and development.
Vigile su crecimiento y desarrollo.
(Bee-hee-leh soo kreh-see-mee-ehn-toh ee deh-sah-roh-yoh)

Watch his navel.
Vigile su ombligo.
(Bee-hee-leh soo ohm-blee-goh)

Watch his urine and his bowel movements.
Vigile su orina y sus evacuaciones.
(Bee-hee-leh sooh oh-ree-nah ee soos eh-bah-koo-ah-see-oh-nehs)

Watch if he has abnormal movements.
Vigile si presenta movimientos anormales.
(Bee-hee-leh see preh-sehn-tah moh-bee-mee-ehn-tohs ah-nohr-mah-lehs)

Watch if he sleeps quietly.
Vigile si su sueño es tranquilo.
(Bee-hee-leh see soo soo-eh-nyoh ehs trahn-kee-loh)

Watch that his nose is clear.
Vigile que su nariz esté libre.
(Bee-hee-leh keh soo nah-rees ehs-teh lee-breh)

Watch that your wound doesn't get infected.
Vigile que su herida no se infecte.
(Bee-hee-leh keh soo eh-ree-dah noh seh een-fehk-teh)

Watch your bleeding.
Vigile su sangrado.
(Bee-hee-leh soo sahn-grah-doh)

We also have deserts.
También tenemos postres.
(Tahm-bee-ehn teh-neh-mohs pohs-trehs)

We are available twenty-four hours per day.
Damos servicio veinticuatro horas por día.
(Dah-mohs sehr-bee-see-oh beh-een-tee-koo-ah-troh oh-rahs pohr dee-ah)

We are going in the ambulance.
Vamos en la ambulancia.
(Bah-mohs ehn lah ahm-boo-lahn-see-ah)

We are going to pull.
Vamos a jalar.
(Bah-mohs ah hah-lahr)

We are going to pull the sheet at the count of three.
Vamos a jalar la sábana al contar tres.
(Bah-mohs ah hah-lahr lah sah-bah-nah ahl kohn-tahr trehs)

We are going to the hospital.
Vamos al hospital.
(Bah-mohs ahl ohs-pee-tahl)

We are going to x-rays.
Vamos a rayos X.
(Bah-mohs ah rah-yohs eh-kiss)

We are here!
¡Ya llegamos/Estamos aquí!
(Yah yeh-gah-mohs/Ehs-tah-mohs ah-kee)

We can control the patient's pain.
Podemos controlar el dolor del paciente.
(Poh-deh-mohs kohn-troh-lahr ehl doh-lohr dehl pah-see-ehn-teh ee mahn-tehn-ehr-loh koh-moh-doh)

We can keep the patient comfortable.
Podemos mantener cómodo al paciente.
(Poh-deh-mohs mahn-teh-nehr koh-moh-doh ahl pah-see-ehn-teh)

We can walk down together.
Podremos caminar juntos.
(Poh-dreh-mohs kah-mee-nahr hoon-tohs)

We don't serve drinks like Cokes or any canned drinks.
No servimos refrescos como Coca-Cola o bebidas envasadas.
(Noh sehr-bee-mohs reh-frehs-kohs koh-moh Koh-kah-Koh-lah oh beh-bee-dahs ehn-bah-sah-dahs)

We have cereals.
Tenemos cereales.
(Teh-neh-mohs seh-reh-ah-lehs)

We have meats.
Tenemos carnes.
(Teh-neh-mohs kahr-nehs)

We have medical and surgical treatment.
Tenemos tratamiento médico y quirúrgico.
(Teh-neh-mohs trah-tah-mee-ehn-toh meh-dee-koh ee kee-roor-hee-koh)

We have to go far.
Tenemos que ir lejos.
(Teh-neh-mohs keh eer leh-hohs)

We inject a radioactive dye into the blood vessels and view the flow of blood through the vessels.
Se inyecta un medio de contraste en los vasos sanguíneos y se valora el flujo de la sangre por las venas.
(Seh een-yehk-tah oon meh-dee-oh deh kohn-trahs-teh ehn lohs bah-sohs sahn-ghee-neh-ohs ee seh bah-lor-ah ehl floo-hoh deh lah sahn-greh pohr lahs beh-nahs)

We need to bring you back.
Necesitamos que regrese.
(Neh-seh-see-tah-mohs keh reh-greh-seh)

We need to count them.
Tenemos que contarlas.
(Teh-neh-mohs keh kohn-tahr-lahs)

We send the menu to the kitchen.
Mandamos el menú a la cocina.
(Mahn-dah-mohs ehl meh-noo ah lah koh-see-nah)

We serve lunch at twelve noon.
Servimos la comida al mediodía.
(Sehr-bee-mohs lah koh-mee-dah ahl meh-dee-oh-dee-ah)

We will begin with the use of angiography.
Comenzaremos con el estudio de angiografía.
(Koh-mehn-sah-reh-mohs kohn ehl ehs-too-dee-oh deh ahn-ghee-oh-grah-fee-ah)

We will start with diagnostic studies to assess how severe your problem might be.
Empezaremos con estudios para evaluar la gravedad de su problema.
(Ehm-peh-sah-reh-mohs kohn ehs-too-dee-ohs pah-rah eh-bah-loo-ahr lah grah-beh-dahd deh soo proh-bleh-mah)

We will x-ray the abdomen again.
Vamos a tomar otras radiografías del abdomen.
(Bah-mohs ah toh-mahr oh-trahs rah-dee-oh-grah-fee-ahs dehl ahb-doh-mehn)

Wear this bracelet all the time.
Use esta pulsera todo el tiempo.
(Oo-seh ehs-tah pool-seh-rah toh-doh ehl tee-ehm-poh)

Well, I just changed jobs.
Bueno, apenas cambié de trabajo.
(Boo-eh-noh ah-peh-nahs kahm-bee-eh deh trah-bah-hoh)

Well, I do have a tingling feeling in my left left foot. It must have gone to sleep.
Pues, tengo picazón en el pie izquierdo. Se me durmió.
(Poo-ehs, tehn-goh pee-kah-sohn ehn ehl pee-eh ees-kee-ehr-doh. Seh meh duhr-mee-oh)

Well, it is possible.
Pues, es posible.
(Poo-ehs, ehs poh-see-bleh)

Well, you are going home tomorrow, but you must return to my office in eight days so I can remove your sutures.
Bueno, mañana se va a su casa, pero debe regresar a mi oficina en ocho días para retirar los puntos de sutura.
(Boo-ch noh, mah-nyah-nah seh bah ah soo kah-sah, peh-roh deh-beh reh-greh-sahr ah mee oh-fee-see-nah ehn oh-choh dee-ahs pah-rah reh-tee-rahr lohs poon-tohs deh soo-too-rah)

Were you hit by a car?
¿Le golpeó un carro?
(Leh gohl-peh-oh oon kah-roh)

Were you hospitalized?
¿Lo hospitalizaron?
(Loh ohs-pee-tah-lee-sah-rohn)

Were you knocked down, did you fall, or were you thrown?
¿Se golpeó, se cayó o lo lanzó el impacto?
(Seh gohl-peh-oh, seh kah-yoh, oh loh lahn-soh ehl eem-pahk-toh)

Were you thrown forward/backward?
¿Fué lanzado hacia adelante/hacia atrás?
(Foo-eh lahn-sah-doh ah-see-ah ah-dehl-ahn-teh/ah-see-ah ah-trahs)

Were you thrown from the car?
¿Fué lanzado fuera del carro?
(Foo-eh lahn-sah-doh foo-eh-rah dehl kah-roh)

What?
¿Qué/Qué tal?
(Keh/Keh tahl)

What a beautiful day!
¡Qué día tan más hermoso!
(Keh dee-ah tahn mahs ehr-moh-soh)

What are some of the diseases affecting persons with AIDS?
¿Cuáles son las enfermedades que aparecen en personas infectadas con SIDA?
(Koo-ah-lehs sohn lahs ehn-fehr-meh-dah-dehs keh ah-pah-reh-sehn ehn pehr-soh-nahs een-fehk-tah-dahs kohn see-dah)

What are the months of the year?
¿Cuáles son los meses del año?
(Koo-ah-lehs sohn lohs meh-sehs dehl ah-nyoh)

What are the symptoms?
¿Cuáles son los síntomas?
(Koo-ah-lehs sohn lohs seen-toh-mahs)

What brought you to the hospital?
¿Qué lo trajo al hospital?
(Keh loh trah-hoh ahl ohs-pee-tahl)

What can be done to prevent AIDS?
¿Qué se puede hacer para prevenir el SIDA?
(Keh seh poo-eh-deh ah-sehr pah-rah preh-beh-neer ehl see-dah)

What can I help you with?
¿En que puedo ayudarlo?
(Ehn keh poo-eh-doh ah-yoo-dahr-loh)

What caused the accident?
¿Qué causó el accidente?
(Keh kah-oo-soh ehl ahk-see-dehn-teh)

What caused the pain?
¿Qué causó el dolor?
(Keh kah-oo-soh ehl doh-lohr)

What causes AIDS?
¿Qué causa el SIDA?
(Keh kah-oo-sah ehl see-dah)

What color?
¿De qué color?
(Deh keh koh-lohr)

What day, what month?
¿Qué día, qué mes?
(Keh dee-ah, keh mehs)

What did you do that caused the pain?
¿Qué hacía cuando apareció el dolor?
(Keh ah-see-ah koo-ahn-doh ah-pah-reh-see-oh ehl doh-lohr?)

What did you eat?
¿Qué comió?
(Keh koh-mee-oh)

What did you eat for breakfast?
¿Qué comió en el desayuno?
(Keh koh-mee-oh ehn ehl deh-sah-yoo-noh)

What do you do?
¿Qué hace usted?
(Keh ah-seh oos-tehd)

What do you feel?
¿Qué siente?
(Keh see-ehn-teh)

What drugs/medicine do you use?
¿Qué drogas/medicamento usa?
(Keh droh-gahs/meh-dee-kah-mehn-toh oo-sah)

What foods do you dislike?
¿Qué alimentos le disgustan?
(Keh ah-lee-mehn-tohs leh dees-goos-tahn)

What foods do you like?
¿Qué alimentos le gustan?
(Keh ah-lee-mehn-tohs leh goos-tahn)

What formula does he take?
¿Qué fórmula toma?
(Keh fohr-moo-lah toh-mah)

What grade are you in?
¿En qué año estás?
(Ehn keh ah-nyoh ehs-tahs)

What happened here?
¿Qué pasa aquí?
(Keh pah-sah ah-kee)

What happened to him?
¿Qué le pasó?
(Keh leh pah-soh)

What happens?
¿Qué pasa?
(Keh pah-sah)

What hospital do you go to?
¿A qué hospital va?
(Ah keh ohs-pee-tahl bah)

What house chores do you do?
¿Qué quehaceres haces?
(Keh keh-ah-seh-rehs ah-sehs)

What is bothering you the most?
¿Qué es lo que más le molesta?
(Keh ehs loh keh mahs leh moh-lehs-tah)

What is going on?
¿Qué le pasa?
(Keh leh pah-sah)

What is hurting you?
¿Qué le duele?
(Keh leh doo-eh-leh)

What is it?
¿Qué es?
(Keh ehs)

What is that?
¿Qué es eso?
(Kueh ehs eh-soh)

What is the address?
¿Cuál es la dirección?
(Koo-ahl ehs lah dee-rehk-see-ohn)

What is the main reason you are here
today?
¿Cuál es la razón principal por que
está aqui?
*(Koo-ahl ehs lah rah-sohn preen-see-
pahl pohr keh ehs-tah ah kee)*

What is the matter?
¿Qué le pasa/sucede?
(Keh leh pah-sah/soo-seh-deh)

What is the name?
¿Cuál es el nombre?
(Koo-ahl ehs ehl nohm-breh)

What is the name of the company?
¿Cómo se llama la compañía?
*(Koh-moh seh yah-mah lah kohm-
pah-nyee-ah)*

What is the name of the insurance?
¿Cuál es el nombre del seguro?
*(Koo-ahl ehs ehl nohm-breh dehl seh-
goo-roh)*

What is the name of the school?
¿Cómo se llama la escuela?
*(Koh-moh seh yah-mah lah ehs-koo-
eh-lah)*

What is the name of the street?
¿Cuál es el nombre de la calle?
*(Koo-ahl ehs ehl nohm-breh deh lah
kah-yeh)*

What is the number of your house?
¿Qué número tiene su casa?
*(Keh noo-meh-roh tee-eh-neh soo kah-
sah)*

What is the pain like?
¿Qué tipo de dolor tiene?
(Keh tee-poh deh doh-lohr tee-eh-neh)

What is the phone number?
¿Cuál es el número de teléfono?
*(Koo-ahl ehs ehl noo-meh-roh deh teh-
leh-foh-noh)*

What is the street name?
¿Cuál es el número de la calle?
*(Koo-ahl ehs ehl noo-meh-roh deh lah
kah-yeh)*

What is the worst problem?
¿Cuál es su peor problema?
*(Koo-ahl ehs soo peh-ohr proh-bleh-
mah)*

What is the year you were born?
¿En que año nació?
(Ehn keh ah-nyoh nah-see-oh)

What is the zip code?
¿Cual es su código postal?
*(Koo-ahl ehs soo koh-dee-goh pohs-
tahl)*

What is that?
¿Qué es eso?
(Keh ehs eh-soh)

What is this?
¿Qué es esto?
(Keh ehs ehs-toh)

What is wrong?
¿Qué pasa?
(Keh pah-sah)

What is your address?
¿Cuál es su dirección?
(Koo-ahl ehs soo dee-rehk-see-ohn)

What is your
birthdate?/year?/month?/day?
¿Cuál es la fecha de
nacimiento/año/mes/día?
*(Koo-ahl ehs lah feh-chah deh nah-
see-mee-ehn-toh/ah-nyoh/mehs/dee-
ah)*

What is your brother's name?
¿Cómo se llama su hermano?
(Koh-moh seh yah-mah soo ehr-mah-noh)

What is your husband's name?
¿Cómo se llama su esposo?
(Koh-moh seh yah-mah soo ehs-poh-soh)

What is your last name?
¿Cuál es su apellido?
(Koo-ahl ehs soo ah-peh-yee-doh)

What is your name?
¿Cómo se llama?
(Koh-moh seh yah-mah)

What is your occupation?
¿Qué clase de trabajo tiene?
(Keh klah-seh deh trah-bah-hoh tee-eh-neh)

What is your phone number?
¿Cuál es su número de teléfono?
(Koo-ahl ehs soo noo-meh-roh deh teh-leh-foh-noh)

What is your religion?
¿Cuál es su religión?
(Koo-ahl ehs soo reh-lee-hee-ohn)

What is your Social Security number?
¿Cuál es su número de seguro social?
(Koo-ahl ehs soo noo-meh-roh deh seh-goo-roh soh-see-ahl)

What is your wife's name?
¿Como se llama su esposa?
(Koh-moh seh yah-mah soo ehs-poh-sah)

What kind of accident?
¿Qué tipo de accidente?
(Keh tee-poh deh ahk-see-dehn-teh)

What kind of coffee?
¿Qué clase de café?
(Keh klah-seh deh kah-feh)

What kind of drinks?
¿Qué clase de bebidas?
(Keh klah-seh deh beh-bee-dahs)

What kind of grades do you make?
¿Qué calificaciones sacas?
(Keh kah-lee-fee-kah-see-ohn-ehs sah-kahs)

What kind of juices?
¿Qué clase de jugos?
(Keh klah-seh deh hoo-gohs)

What kind of surgery?
¿Qué clase de operaciones?
(Keh klah-seh deh oh-peh-rah-see-ohn-ehs)

What kind of weapons have you used?
¿Qué clase de armas a usado?
(Keh klah-seh deh ahr-mahs ah oo-sah-doh)

What kind of work do you do?
¿Qué clase de trabajo hace?
(Keh klah-seh deh trah-bah-hoh ah-seh)

What kind?
¿Qué clase?
(Keh klah-seh)

What kinds of problems?
¿Qué clase de problemas?
(Keh klah-seh deh proh-bleh-mahs)

What makes the pain better?
¿Qué hace mejorar el dolor?
(Keh ah-seh meh-hoh-rahr ehl doh-lohr)

What medical problem do you have?
¿Qué problema médico tiene?
(Keh proh-bleh-mah meh-dee-koh tee-eh-neh)

What medicines do you take?
¿Qué medicinas toma?
(Keh meh-dee-see-nahs toh-mah)

What other discomfort do you have?
¿Qué otra molestia tiene?
(Keh oh-trah moh-lehs-tee-ah tee-eh-neh)

What problems do you have?
¿Qué problemas tiene?
(Keh proh-bleh-mahs tee-eh-neh)

What subject do you like best?
¿Qué materia te gusta más?
(Keh mah-teh-ree-ah teh goos-tah mahs)

What symptoms do you have?
¿Qué síntomas tiene?
(Keh seen-toh-mahs tee-eh-neh)

What time is it?
¿Qué hora es?
(Keh oh-rah ehs)

What triggered your depression?
¿Qué precipitó su depresión?
(Keh preh-see-pee-toh soo deh-preh-see-ohn)

What was the color of the urine?
¿Cuál era el color de la orina?
(Koo-ahl eh-rah ehl koh-lohr deh lah oh-ree-nah)

What were you doing?
¿Qué estaba haciendo?
(Keh ehs-tah-bah ah-see-ehn-doh)

What work do you do?
¿Que trabajo hace usted?
(Keh trah-bah-hoh ah-seh oos-ted)

What would you like to eat first?
¿Qué quiere comer primero?
(Keh kee-eh-reh koh-mehr pree-meh-roh)

What's going on?
¿Qué pasa?
(Keh pah-sah)

What's happening?
¿Qué le pasa?
(Keh leh pah-sah)

What's the matter?
¿Qué pasa?
(Keh pah-sah)

Wheat bread and cereals.
Pan de trigo y cereales.
(Pahn deh tree-goh ee seh-reh-ah-lehs)

When?
¿Cuándo?
(Koo-ahn-doh)

When did this happen?
¿Cuándo le pasó esto?
(Koo-ahn-doh leh pah-soh ehs-toh)

When did you notice the skin rash?
¿Cuándo se dió cuenta de la piel rosada?
(Koo-ahn-doh seh dee-oh koo-ehn-tah deh lah pee-ehl roh-sah dah)

When did you see the dentist last?
¿Cuándo vió al dentista la última vez?
(Koo-ahn-doh bee-oh ahl dehn-tees-tah lah ool-tee-mah behs)

When I tell you, hold your breath.
Cuándo le avise, no respire.
(Koo-ahn-doh leh ah-bee-seh, noh rehs-pee-reh)

When is your due date?
¿Cuándo se alivia?
(Koo-ahn-doh seh ah-lee-bee-ah)

When was he/she born?
¿Cuándo nació?
(Koo-ahn-doh nah-see-oh)

When was the last one?
¿Cuándo fue el último?
(Koo-ahn-doh foo-eh ehl ool-tee-moh)

When was the last time?
¿Cuándo fue la última vez?
(Koo-ahn-doh foo-eh lah ool-tee-mah behs)

When was the last time he had a bowel movement?
¿Cuándo fue la última vez que evacuó/hizo del baño?
(Koo-ahn-doh foo-eh lah ool-tee-mah behs keh eh-bah-koo-oh/ee-soh dehl bah-nyoh)

When was the last time that you took medicine?
¿Cuándo fue la última vez que tomó medicina?
(Koo-ahn-doh foo-eh lah ool-tee-mah behs keh toh-moh meh-dee-see-nah)

When was the last time you ate?
¿Cuándo fue la última vez que
 comió?
*(Koo-ahn-doh foo-eh lah ool-tee-mah
 behs keh koh-mee-oh)*

When was the last time you used the
 toilet?
¿Cuándo fue la última vez que hizo
 del baño/que obró?
*(Koo-ahn-doh foo-eh lah ool-tee-mah
 behs keh ee-soh dehl bah-nyoh/keh
 oh-broh)*

When was the last time you were here?
¿Cuándo fue la última vez que
 estubo aquí?
*(Koo-ahn-doh foo-eh lah ool-tee-mah
 behs keh ehs-too-boh ah-kee)*

When was your last normal period?
¿Cuándo tuvo su última
 menstruación normal?
*(Koo-ahn-doh too-boh soo ool-tee-mah
 mehns-troo-ah-see-ohn nohr-mahl)*

When you feel depressed go for a walk.
Cuándo se deprima salga de paseo.
*(Koo-ahn-doh seh deh-pree-mah sahl-
 gah deh pah-seh-oh)*

When you get there, turn right.
Cuándo llegue ahí, dé vuelta a la
 derecha.
*(Koo-ahn-doh yeh-gheh ah-ee, deh
 boo-ehl-tah ah lah deh-reh-chah)*

When you have pain, do you get
 nauseated?
¿Cuándo tiene dolor, le da náuseas?
*(Koo-ahn-doh tee-eh-neh doh-lohr, leh
 dahn nah-oo-seh-ahs)*

When you let go.
Cuando retira la mano.
*(koo-ahn-doh reh-tee-rah lah mah-
 noh)*

Where?
¿Dónde?
(Dohn-deh)

Where are they?
¿Dónde están?
(Dohn-deh ehs-tahn)

Where are you from?
¿De dónde es usted?
(Deh dohn-deh ehs oos-tehd)

Where can I reach your mother or
 father?
¿Dónde puedo localizar a su mamá o
 su papá?
*(Dohn-deh poo-eh-doh loh-kah-lee-
 sahr ah soo mah-mah oh soo pah-
 pah)*

Where do I need to go?
¿Adónde necesito ir?
(Ah-dohn-deh neh-seh-see-toh eer)

Where do you live?
¿Dónde vive?
(Dohn-deh bee-beh)

Where do you work?
¿Dónde trabaja?
(Dohn-deh trah-bah-hah)

Where does it hurt?
¿Dónde le duele?
(Don-deh leh doo-eh-leh)

Where is it?
¿Dónde está?
(Dohn-deh ehs-tah)

Where is your husband?
¿Dónde está su esposo?
(Dohn-deh ehs-tah soo ehs-poh-soh)

Where were you born?
¿Dónde nació usted?
(Dohn-deh nah-see-oh oos-tehd)

Where were you going?
¿Adónde iba?
(Ah-dohn-deh ee-bah)

Where were you hit?
¿Dónde se golpeó?
(Dohn-deh seh gohl-peh-oh)

Which?
¿Cuál?
(Koo-ahl)

Which book do you want?
¿Qué libro quieres?
(Keh lee-broh kee-eh-rehs)

Which kind?
¿Qué clase?
(Keh klah-seh)

Which of the books do you want?
¿Cuál de los libros quieres?
(Koo-ahl deh lohs lee-brohs kee-eh-rehs)

Which ones?
¿Cuáles?
(Koo-ah-lehs)

Who?
¿Quién?
(Kee-ehn)

Who? (all)
¿Quiénes?
(Kee-ehn-ehs)

Who can take care of the children?
¿Quién puede cuidar a los niños?
(Kee-ehn poo-eh-deh koo-ee-dahr ah lohs nee-nyohs)

Who can we call in case of an emergency?
¿A quién le llamamos en caso de emergencia?
(Ah kee-ehn leh yah-mah-mohs ehn kah-soh deh eh-mehr-hehn-see-ah)

Who do you talk to?
¿Con quién hablas?
(Kohn kee-ehn ah-blahs)

Who helps you at home?
¿Quién le ayuda en casa?
(Kee-ehn leh ah-yoo-dah ehn kah-sah)

Who helps you?
¿Quién te ayuda?
(Kee-ehn teh ah-yoo-dah)

Who is at risk of getting AIDS?
¿Quién está en riesgo de contraer el SIDA?
(Kee-ehn ehs-tah ehn ree-ehs-goh deh kohn-trah-ehr ehl see-dah)

Who is going to pay the hospital?
¿Quién va a pagar el hospital?
(Kee-ehn bah ah pah-gahr ehl ohs-pee-tahl)

Who moved him/her?
¿Quién lo/la movió?
(Kee-ehn loh/lah moh-bee-oh)

Who saw the accident?
¿Quién vió el accidente?
(Kee-ehn bee-oh ehl ahk-see-dehn-teh)

Who takes care of you at home?
¿Quién lo cuida en casa?
(Kee-ehn loh koo-ee-dah ehn kah-sah)

Who takes you to school?
¿Quién te lleva a la escuela?
(Kee-ehn teh yeh-bah ah lah ehs-koo-eh-lah)

Whose books are these?
¿De quién son estos libros?
(Deh kee-ehn sohn ehs-tohs lee-brohs)

Whose car is it?
¿De quién es el carro?
(Deh kee-ehn ehs ehl kah-roh)

Whose card is it?
¿De quién es la tarjeta?
(Deh kee-ehn ehs lah tahr-heh-tah)

Whose pen is it?
¿De quién es la pluma?
(Deh kee-ehn ehs lah ploo-mah)

Whose x-rays are these?
¿De quién son estos rayos X/estas radiografías?
(Deh kee-ehn sohn ehs-tohs rah-yohs eh-kiss/ehs-tahs rah-dee-oh-grah-fee-ahs)

Why?
¿Por qué?
(Pohr keh)

Why do you make me do things?
¿Por qué me haces hacer cosas?
(Pohr-keh meh ah-sehs ah-sehr koh-sahs)

Why not?
¿Por qué no?
(Pohr keh noh)

Will it pay for the hospital?
¿Paga por la hospitalización?
(Pah-gah pohr lah ohs-pee-tah-lee-sah-see-ohn)

Will you need help?
¿Necesitará ayuda?
(Neh-seh-see-tah-rah ah-yoo-dah)

Will you need to see a social worker?
¿Necesitará ver a la trabajadora social?
(Neh-seh-see-tah-rah behr ah lah trah-bah-hah-doh-rah soh-see-ahl)

Wind eighteen inches of floss around one middle finger.
Enrede dieciocho pulgadas de hilo alrededor del tercer dedo.
(Ehn-reh-deh dee-eh-see-oh-choh pool-gah-dahs deh ee-loh ahl-reh-deh-dohr dehl tehr-sehr deh-doh)

Wind the rest around the middle finger of the other hand.
Enrede el resto alrededor del dedo medio de la otra mano.
(Ehn-reh-deh ehl rehs-toh ahl-reh-deh-dohr dehl deh-doh meh-dee-oh deh lah oh-trah mah-noh)

With how many people?
¿Con cuántas personas?
(Kohn koo-ahn-tahs pehr-soh-nahs)

Work phone number?
¿Teléfono del trabajo?
(Teh-leh-foh-noh dehl trah-bah-hoh)

Wrinkle your nose.
Arruga la nariz.
(Ah-roo-gah lah nah-rees)

Write, please.
Escriban, por favor.
(Ehs-kree-bahn, pohr fah-bohr)

Yes.
Sí.
(See)

Yes, a little.
Sí, un poco.
(See, oon poh-koh)

Yes, go to the end of the hall.
Sí, vaya al final del pasillo.
(See, bah-yah ahl fee-nahl dehl pah-see-yoh)

Yes, I speak English.
Sí, yo hablo inglés.
(See, yoh ah-bloh een-glehs)

Yes, I speak Spanish.
Sí, hablo español.
(See, ah-bloh ehs-pah-nyohl)

Yes, in the afternoon.
Sí, por la tarde.
(See, pohr lah tahr-deh)

Yes, last week.
Sí, la semana pasada.
(See, lah seh-mah-nah pah-sah-dah)

Yes, my dad.
Sí, mi papá.
(See, mee pah-pah)

Yes, please wait.
Sí, espere por favor.
(See, ehs-peh-reh pohr fah-bohr)

You are giving us permission to treat you.
Nos dá usted permiso de tratarla.
(Nohs dah oos-ted pehr-mee-soh deh trah-tahr-lah)

You are not answering my questions.
No contesta mis preguntas.
(Noh kohn-tehs-tah mees preh-goon-tahs)

You are not going?
¿Usted no va?
(Oos-tehd noh bah)

You are welcome.
De nada.
(Deh nah-dah)

You ate well.
Comió bien.
(Koh-mee-oh bee-ehn)

You can also ask for snacks.
También puede pedir aperitivos.
(Tahm-bee-ehn poo-eh-deh peh-deer ah-peh-ree-tee-bohs)

You can breathe.
Puede respirar.
(Poo-eh-deh rehs-pee-rahr)

You can breathe now.
Ya puede respirar.
(Yah poo-eh-deh rehs-pee-rahr)

You can bring your family here.
Puede traer a su familia aquí.
(Poo-eh-deh trah-ehr ah soo fah-mee-lee-ah ah-kee)

You can buy canned drinks in the cafeteria.
Puede comprar bebidas envasadas en la cafetería.
(Poo-eh-deh kohm-prahr beh-bee-dahs ehn-bah-sah-dahs ehn lah kah-feh-teh-ree-ah)

You can call collect.
Puede llamar por cobrar.
(Poo-eh-deh yah-mahr pohr koh-brahr)

You can cross at the walkway.
Puede cruzar por el pasillo sobre la calle.
(Poo-eh-deh kroo-sahr pohr ehl puh-see-yoh soh-breh lah kah-yeh)

You can drink water.
Puede tomar agua.
(Poo-eh-deh toh-mahr ah-goo-ah)

You can eat in your room or in the visitors room.
Puede comer en su cuarto o en el cuarto para visitas.
(Poo-eh-deh koh-mehr ehn soo koo-ahr-toh oh ehn ehl koo-ahr-toh pah-rah bee-see-tahs)

You can feed him/her solid foods.
Puede darle alimentos sólidos.
(Poo-eh-deh dahr-leh ah-lee-mehn-tohs soh-lee-dohs)

You can go back to work in one week.
Puede regresar al trabajo en una semana.
(Poo-eh-deh reh-greh-sahr ahl trah-bah-hoh ehn oo-nah seh-mah-nah)

You can have flowers.
Puede tener flores.
(Poo-eh-deh teh-nehr floh-rehs)

You can make local phone calls.
Puede hacer llamadas locales.
(Poo-eh-deh ah-sehr yah-mah-dahs loh-kah-lehs)

You can order coffee here.
Puede ordenar café aquí.
(Poo-eh-deh ohr-deh-nahr kah-feh ah-kee)

You can order one or two portions.
Puede ordenar una o dos porciones.
(Poo-eh-deh ohr-deh-nahr oo-nah oh dohs pohr-see-oh-nehs)

You can pay on terms.
Puede pagar a plazos.
(Poo-eh-deh pah-gahr ah plah-sohs)

You can put cards on the shelf.
Puede poner tarjetas en el estante.
(Poo-eh-deh poh-nehr tahr-heh-tahs ehn ehl ehs-tahn-teh)

You can raise the feet.
Puede levantar los pies.
(Poo-eh-deh leh-bahn-tahr lohs pee-ehs)

You can raise the head.
Puede levantar la cabeza.
(Poo-eh-deh leh-bahn-tahr lah kah-beh-sah)

You can refill _____ times.
Puede surtir _____ veces.
(Poo-eh-deh soor-teer _____ beh-sehs)

You can smoke on the patio.
Puede fumar en el patio.
(Poo-eh-deh foo-mahr ehn ehl pah-tee-oh)

You can tape pictures to the wall.
Puede pegar retratos en la pared.
(Poo-eh-deh peh-gahr reh-trah-tohs ehn lah pah-rehd)

You can walk on crutches.
Puede caminar con muletas.
(Poo-eh-deh kah-mee-nahr kohn moo-leh-tahs)

You can write an "X?"
Puede escribir una "X?"
(Poo-eh-deh ehs-kree-beer oo-nah eh-kiss)

You cannot hang anything from the ceiling.
No puede colgar nada del techo.
(Noh poo-eh-deh kohl-gahr nah-dah dehl teh-choh)

You cannot hang anything from the door.
No puede colgar nada en la puerta.
(Noh poo-eh-deh kohl-gahr nah-dah ehn lah poo-ehr-tah)

You cannot open the windows.
No puede abrir las ventanas.
(Noh poo-eh-deh ah-breer lahs behn-tah-nahs)

You cannot smoke here.
No puede fumar aquí.
(Noh poo-eh-deh foo-mahr ah-kee)

You cannot smoke in your room.
No puede fumar en el cuarto.
(Noh poo-eh-deh foo-mahr ehn ehl koo-ahr-toh)

You can't miss them!
¡No tiene pierde!
(Noh tee-eh-neh pee-ehr-deh)

You do not know the case.
Usted no sabe el caso.
(Oos-tehd noh sah-beh ehl kah-soh)

You do not know the plan?
¿Usted no sabe el plan?
(Oos-tehd noh sah-beh ehl plahn)

You don't have to pay cash.
No tiene que pagar al contado.
(Noh tee-eh-neh keh pah-gahr ahl kohn-tah-doh)

You enjoyed working on your house yesterday.
Disfrutó el trabajar en su casa ayer.
(Dees-froo-toh ehl trah-bah-hahr ehn soo kah-sah ah-yehr)

You have a private bathroom.
Tiene un baño/inodoro privado.
(Tee-eh-neh oon bah-nyoh/ee-noh-doh-roh pree-bah-doh)

You have bruises and white patches/spots.
Tiene moretones y manchas blancas.
(Tee-eh-neh moh-reh-toh-nehs ee mahn-chahs blahn-kahs)

You have false teeth.
Tiene dentaduras postizas.
(Tee-eh-neh dehn-tah-doo-rahs pohs-tee-sahs)

You have to choose three meals a day.
Tiene que escojer tres comidas diarias.
(Tee-eh-neh keh ehs-koh-hehr trehs koh-mee-dahs dee-ah-ree-ahs)

You have to cross the street.
Tiene que cruzar la calle.
(Tee-eh-neh keh kroo-sahr lah kah-yeh)

You have to give permission for treatment.
Tiene que dar permiso para el tratamiento.
(Tee-eh-neh keh dahr pehr-mee-soh pah-rah ehl trah-tah-mee-ehn-toh)

You have to go to the floor directly.
Debe de ir al piso directamente.
(Deh-beh deh eer ahl pee-soh dee-rehk-tah-mehn-teh)

You have to wait your turn.
Tendrá que esperar su turno.
(Tehn-drah keh ehs-peh-rahr soo tuhr-noh)

Your husband will be cared for by the doctor, nurse, social worker, and the priest.
Cuidará a su esposo el doctor, la enfermera, la trabajadora social y el sacerdote.
(Koo-ee-dah-rah ah soo ehs-poh-soh ehl dohk-tohr, lah en-fer-mer-ah, lah trah-bah-hah-doh-rah soh-see-ahl, ee ehl sah-sehr-doh-teh)

You may be here about four hours.
Estara aquí cerca de cuatro horas.
(Ehs-tah-rah ah-kee sehr-kah deh koo-ah-troh oh-rahs)

You must go to the hospital.
Debe ir al hospital.
(Deh-beh eer ahl ohs-pee-tahl)

You must pay a deposit.
Debe pagar un depósito.
(Deh-beh pah-gahr oon deh poh-see-toh)

You must tell us your needs.
Debe decirnos que necesita.
(Deh-beh deh-seer-nohs keh neh-seh-see-tah)

You need to be admitted.
Necesita internarse al hospital.
(Neh-seh-see-tah een-tehr-nahr-seh ahl ohs-pee-tahl)

You need to brush your teeth better.
Necesita cepillar mejor sus dientes.
(Neh-seh-see-tah seh-pee-yahr meh-hohr soos dee-ehn-tehs)

You need to drink water.
Necesita tomar agua.
(Neh-seh-see-tah toh-mahr ah-goo-ah)

You need to return.
Necesita regresar.
(Neh-seh-see-tah reh-greh-sahr)

You need to sign this form.
Debe firmar está forma.
(Deh-beh feer-mahr ehs-tah fohr-mah)

You need two witnesses if consent is via telephone or if patient cannot sign his name and only makes a mark.
Necesita dos testigos si el consentimiento se dá por teléfono o si el paciente no puede firmar su nombre y solo hace una marca.
(Neh-seh-see-tah dohs tehs-tee-gohs see ehl kohn-sehn-tee-mee-ehn-toh seh dah pohr teh-leh-foh-noh oh see ehl pah-see-ehn-teh noh poo-eh-deh feer-mahr soo nohm-breh ee soh-loh ah-seh oo-nah mahr-kah)

You will be all right!
¡Estará bien!
(Ehs-tah-rah bee-ehn)

You will feel pain like a pin prick.
Sentirá dolor como una picadura.
(Sehn-tee-rah doh-lohr koh-moh oo-nah pee-kah-doo-rah)

You will get help.
Se le ayudará.
(Sch lch ah-yoo-dah-rah)

You will have to rest at at least seven days.
Tendrá que guardar reposo al menos siete días.
(Tehn-drah keh goo-ahr-dahr reh-poh-soh ahl meh-nohs see-eh-teh dee-ahs)

You will have to wait.
Tendrá que esperar.
(Tehn-drah keh ehs-peh-rahr)

You will need a cast.
Necesitará un yeso.
(Neh-seh-see-tah-rah oon yeh-soh)

You will need help.
Necesitará ayuda.
(Neh-seh-see-tah-rah ah-yoo-dah)

You will need to brush a little better in these areas.
Necesitará cepillarse mejor en estas áreas.
(Neh-seh-see-tah-rah seh-pee-yahr-seh meh-hohr ehn ehs-tahs ah-reh-ahs)

You will pass the cafeteria.
Pasará la cafetería.
(Pah-sah-rah lah kah-feh-teh-ree-ah)

You will see the sign on the wall.
Verá el letrero en la pared.
(Beh-rah ehl leh-treh-roh ehn lah pah-rehd)

Your appetite is good?
¿Tiene buen apetito?
(Tee-eh-neh boo-ehn ah-peh-tee-toh)

Your clothes go in the closet.
Su ropa va en el
  closet/ropero/armario.
*(Soo roh-pah bah ehn ehl kloh-
  seht/roh-peh-roh/ahr-mah-ree-oh)*

Your diet should be low in fats and hot
  sauces.
Su dieta debe ser baja en grasas y
  picantes.
*(Soo dee-eh-tah deh-beh sehr bah-hah
  ehn grah-sahs ee pee-kahn-tehs)*

Your family can bring your clothes
  tomorrow.
Su familia le puede traer su ropa
  mañana.
*(Soo fah-mee-lee-ah leh poo-eh-deh
  trah-ehr soo roh-pah mah-nyah-
  nah)*

Your leg is broken.
Tiene la pierna quebrada/fracturada.
*(Tee-eh-neh lah pee-ehr-nah keh-brah-
  dah/frahk-too-rah-dah)*

Your lips should not be dry.
Tus labios no deben estar secos.
*(Toohs lah-bee-ohs noh deh-behn ehs-
  tahr seh-kohs)*

Your skin color looks good.
El color de su piel es normal.
*(Ehl koh-lohr deh soo pee-ehl ehs
  nohr-mahl)*

Your towels are in the bathroom.
Sus toallas están en el baño.
*(Soos too-ah-yahs ehs-tahn ehn ehl
  bah-nyoh)*

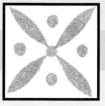

Word Index

Índice de Palabras

A	a	*(ah)*
a	un	*(oon)*
a/an	un	*(oon)*
abdomen	abdomen	*(ahb-doh-mehn)*
abnormal	anormal	*(ah-nohr-mahl)*
about	acerca de/por/acerca	*(ah-sehr-kah deh/pohr/ah-sehr-kah)*
above	arriba/sobre	*(ah-rree-bah/soh-breh)*
absence	ausencia	*(ah-oo-sehn-see-ah)*
abuse	abuso	*(ah-boo-soh)*
accent	acento	*(ah-sehn-toh)*
accept	aceptar	*(ah-sehp-tahr)*
acceptable	aceptable	*(ah-sehp-tah-bleh)*
accident	accidente	*(ahk-see-dehn-teh)*
according	según	*(seh-goon)*
acetic	acético	*(ah-seh-tee-koh)*
acid	ácido	*(ah-see-doh)*
acne	acne	*(ahk-neh)*
acoustic	acústico	*(ah-koos-tee-koh)*
acquired	adquirida	*(ahd-kee-ree-dah)*
activities	actividades	*(ahk-tee-bee-dah-dehs)*
additive	aditivo	*(ah-dee-tee-boh)*
address	dirección	*(dee-rehk-see-ohn)*
adenoid	adenoide	*(ah-deh-noh-ee-deh)*
adhesive	adhesivo	*(ah-deh-see-boh)*
administration	administracion	*(ahd-meh-nees-trah-see-ohn)*
admitting	admitiendo	*(ahd-meh-tee-ehn-doh)*
adrenalism	adrenalismo	*(ah-dreh-nah-lees-moh)*
adults	adultos	*(ah-dool-tohs)*
after	después de	*(dehs-poo-ehs deh)*
again	otra vez	*(oh-trah behs)*
against	contra	*(kohn-trah)*
age	edad	*(eh-dahd)*
aggressive	agresivo	*(ah-greh-see-boh)*
agree	acordar	*(ah-kohr-dahr)*

403

air	aire	*(ah-ee-reh)*
airway	vía aérea	*(bee-ah ah-eh-reh-ah)*
albino	albino	*(ahl-bee-noh)*
alcohol	alcohol	*(ahl-kohl)*
alcoholic	alcohólico	*(ahl-koh-lee-koh)*
alcoholic/beverages	alcohólicas/bebidas	*(ahl-koh-lee-kahs/beh-bee-dahs)*
alert	avisele	*(ah-bee-seh-leh)*
alignment	alineación	*(ah-lee-neh-ah-see-ohn)*
all right	bien	*(bee-ehn)*
all/everything	todo	*(toh-doh)*
allergies	alergias	*(ah-lehr-hee-ahs)*
allergy	alérgico	*(ah-lehr-hee-koh)*
allergy	alergia	*(ah-lehr-hee-ah)*
alone	solo	*(soh-loh)*
alphabet	abecedario	*(ah-beh-seh-dah-ree-oh)*
also	también	*(tahm-bee-ehn)*
always	siempre	*(see-ehm-preh)*
amber	ambar	*(ahm-bahr)*
amber	ámbar	*(ahm-bahr)*
amber	ambarino	*(ahm-bah-ree-noh)*
ambulance	ambulancia	*(ahm-boo-lahn-see-ah)*
amebic	amébico	*(ah-meh-bee-koh)*
ammonia	amonia/amoníaco	*(ah-moh-nee-ah/ah-moh-nee-ah-koh)*
among/between	entre	*(ehn-treh)*
amputation	amputación	*(ahm-poo-tah-see-ohn)*
amputee	amputado	*(ahm-poo-tah-doh)*
amygdala	amígdala	*(ah-meeg-dah-lah)*
an	un/una	*(oon/oo-nah)*
analgesic	analgésicos	*(ah-nahl-heh-see-kohs)*
analysis	análisis	*(ah-nah-lee-sees)*
analyze	analizar	*(ah-nah-lee-sahr)*
anaphylactic shock	choque anafilático	*(choh-keh ah-nah-fee-lah-tee-koh)*
anatomic position	posición anatómica	*(poh-see-see-ohn ah-nah-toh-mee-kah)*
and	y	*(ee)*
anemia	anemia	*(ah-neh-mee-ah)*
anesthesia	anestesia	*(ah-nehs-teh-see-ah)*
aneurysm	aneurisma	*(ah-neh-oo-rees-mah)*
anger	enojo	*(eh-noh-hoh)*
angina	angina	*(ahn-hee-nah)*
angioma	angioma	*(ahn-hee-oh-mah)*
angle	ángulo	*(ahn-goo-loh)*
angulation	angulación	*(ahn-goo-lah-see-ohn)*
ant	hormiga	*(ohr-mee-gah)*
antacid	antiácidos	*(ahn-tee-ah-see-dohs)*
antemetic	antiemético	*(ahn-tee-eh-meh-tee-koh)*
antianxiety	contra la ansiedad	*(kohn-trah lah ahn-see-eh-dahd)*
antianxiety	ansiolíticos	*(ahn-see-oh-lee-tee-kohs)*
antiarrhythmic	antiarritmias	*(ahn-tee-ah-reeht-mee-ahs)*

antibiotic(s)	antibiótico(s)	*(ahn-tee-bee-oh-tee-koh[s])*
antibodies	anticuerpos	*(ahn-tee-koo-ehr-pohs)*
anticoagulant	anticoagulante	*(ahn-tee-koh-ah-goo-lahn-teh)*
anticonvulsant	anticonvulsivo	*(ahn-tee-kohn-bool-see-boh)*
antidiarrheal	antidiarrea	*(ahn-tee-dee-ah-rreh-ah)*
antiemetic	antiemético	*(ahn-tee-eh-meh-tee-koh)*
antiepileptic	antiepiléptico	*(ahn-tee-eh-pee-lehp-tee-koh)*
antihistamine	antihistamínico	*(ahn-tee-ees-tah-mee-nee-koh)*
antiviral	antivirus	*(ahn-tee-bee-roos)*
anxiety	ansiedad	*(ahn-see-eh-dahd)*
anxious	ansioso	*(ahn-see-oh-soh)*
any	alguno	*(ahl-goo-noh)*
aorta	aorta	*(ah-ohr-tah)*
apothecary	apotecarios	*(ah-poh-teh-kah-ree-ohs)*
appendicitis	apendicitis	*(ah-pehn-dee-see-tees)*
appetizers	bocadillos	*(boh-kah-dee-yoh)*
appetizing	apetitosas	*(ah-peh-tee-toh-sahs)*
apple	manzana	*(mahn-sah-nah)*
approaches	se dirige	*(seh dee-ree-heh)*
April	abril	*(ah-breel)*
around	alrededor de	*(ahl-rreh-deh-dohr deh)*
arrest	arresto	*(ah-rehs-toh)*
arrow	flecha	*(fleh-chah)*
arteriogram	arteriograma	*(ahr-teh-ree-oh-grah-mah)*
arteriosclerosis	arterioesclerosis	*(ahr-teh-ree-oh-ehs-kleh-roh-sees)*
arthritis	artritis	*(ahr-tree-tees)*
articles	artículos	*(ahr-tee-koo-lohs)*
as	por/como	*(pohr/koh-moh)*
ask	preguntar	*(preh-goon-tahr)*
asparagus	espárragos	*(ehs-pah-rah-gohs)*
aspirin	aspirina	*(ahs-pee-ree-nah)*
assessment	avalúo	*(ah-bah-loo-oh)*
assist them	ayudeles	*(ah-yoo-deh-lehs)*
asthma	asma	*(as-mah)*
at	a	*(ah)*
at the	al	*(ahl)*
attention	atención	*(ah-tehn-see-ohn)*
August	agosto	*(ah-gohs-toh)*
aunt	tía	*(tee-ah)*
author	autor	*(ah-oo-tohr)*
available	disponibile	*(dees-poh-nee-bleh)*
avenue	avenida	*(ah-beh-nee-dah)*
avocados	aguacates	*(ah-goo-ah-kah-tehs)*
B	b	*(beh)*
baby	bebé	*(beh-beh)*
baby tooth	diente de leche	*(dee-ehn-teh deh leh-cheh)*
back	espalda	*(ehs-pahl-dah)*
bacon	tocino	*(toh-see-noh)*
bacteria	bacteria	*(bahk-teh-ree-ah)*

bad	mal	*(mahl)*
baked	asadas	*(ah-sah-dahs)*
baked chicken	pollo asado	*(poh-yoh ah-sah-doh)*
baked potatoes	papas asadas	*(pah-pahs ah-sah-dahs)*
balanced	balanceada	*(bah-lahn-seh-ah-dah)*
bananas	plátanos	*(plah-tah-nohs)*
barbaric	bárbaro	*(bahr-bah-roh)*
barbiturates	barbitúricos	*(bahr-bee-too-ree-kohs)*
basin	lavabo	*(lah-bah-doh)*
bath/bathroom	baño	*(bah-nyoh)*
beans	frijoles/habas	*(free-hoh-lehs/ah-bahs)*
beans (pinto)	frijol pinto	*(free-hohl peen-toh)*
because	porque	*(pohr-keh)*
bed	cama	*(kah-mah)*
bed cover	colcha	*(kohl-chah)*
bed rails	barandal	*(bah-rahn-dahl)*
bedpan	bacín	*(bah-seen)*
bedroom	recamara	*(reh-kah-mah-rah)*
bedspread	colcha	*(kohl-chah)*
beef	carne de res	*(kahr-neh deh rehs)*
beef/cattle	res	*(rehs)*
beets	betavel	*(beh-tah-behl)*
before	antes de	*(ahn-tehs deh)*
beginning	principio	*(preen-see-pee-oh)*
behavior	conducta	*(kohn-dook-tah)*
behind	detrás de	*(deh-trahs deh)*
bell(s)	campana(s)	*(kahm-pah-nah[s])*
below	abajo	*(ah-bah-hoh)*
bend	doblar	*(doh-blahr)*
beneath/under	debajo de	*(deh-bah-hoh deh)*
benign	benigno	*(beh-neeg-noh)*
bereavement	desamparo	*(dehs-ahm-pah-roh)*
besides	además de	*(ah-deh-mahs deh)*
better	mejor	*(meh-hohr)*
between	entre	*(ehn-treh)*
big	grande	*(grahn-deh)*
birth control	control de fertilidad	*(kohn-trohl deh fehr-tee-lee-dahd)*
birthmark	lunares	*(loo-nah-rehs)*
biscuits	bisquetes/bizcocho	*(bees-keh-tehs/bees-koh-choh)*
bit	poco	*(poh-koh)*
bite	muerda	*(moo-ehr-dah)*
black	negro	*(neh-groh)*
bladder	vejiga	*(beh-hee-gah)*
blanket	frazada/covertor	*(frah-sah-dah/koh-behr-tohr)*
bleeding	sangrado	*(sahn-grah-doh)*
blocks	cuadras	*(koo-ah-drahs)*
blond	rubio	*(roo-bee-oh)*
blood	sangre	*(sahn-greh)*
blood bank	banco de sangre	*(bahn-koh deh sahn-greh)*
blood count	biometría hemática	*(bee-oh-meh-tree-ah eh-mah-tee-kah)*

blood flow	circulación sanguínea	*(seer-koo-lah-see-ohn sahn-ghee-neh-ah)*
blood stream	arroyo de la sangre	*(ah-roh-yoh deh lah sahn-greh)*
blouse	blusa	*(bloo-sah)*
blue	azul	*(ah-sool)*
bluish	azuloso(a)	*(ah-soo-loh-soh[sah])*
body	cuerpo	*(koo-ehr-poh)*
boil	hervir	*(ehr-beer)*
boiled	hervidos	*(ehr-bee-dohs)*
bone	hueso	*(oo-eh-soh)*
book	libro	*(lee-broh)*
bookcase	armario/estante	*(ahr-mah-ree-oh/ehs-tahn-teh)*
books	libros	*(lee-brohs)*
boredom	fastidio	*(fahs-tee-dee-oh)*
boric acid	ácido bórico	*(ah-see-doh boh-ree-koh)*
bottle	botella	*(boh-teh-yah)*
bowel	intestino	*(een-tehs-tee-noh)*
boy(s)	niño(s)/muchacho(s)	*(nee-nyoh[s]/moo-chah-choh[s])*
braces	abrazaderas	*(ah-brah-sah-deh-rahs)*
bradycardia	bradicardia	*(brah-dee-kahr-dee-ah)*
brand names	marcas de productos	*(mahr-kahs deh proh-dook-tohs)*
bread(s)	pan(es)	*(pahn[-ehs])*
breaded	empanizado	*(ehm-pah-nee-sah-doh)*
breakfast	desayuno	*(deh-sah-yoo-noh)*
breast(chicken)	pechuga	*(peh-choo-gah)*
breast(woman)	pecho/seno	*(peh-choh/seh-noh)*
bridge	puente móvil	*(poo-ehn-teh moh-beel)*
broiled fish	pescado al horno	*(pehs-kah-doh ahl ohr-noh)*
broiled	asado	*(ah-sah-doh)*
broken bone	hueso roto	*(oo-eh-soh roh-toh)*
bronchitis	bronquitis	*(brohn-kee-tees)*
brother	hermano	*(ehr-mah-noh)*
brother-in-law	cuñado	*(koo-nyah-doh)*
brown (hair)	pelo café	*(peh-loh kah-feh)*
brown (skin tone)	moreno	*(moh-reh-noh)*
bruises/echymosis	moretones/equimosis	*(moh-reh-toh-nehs/eh-kee-moh-sees)*
build	construir	*(kohn-stroo-eer)*
building	edificio	*(eh-dee-fee-see-oh)*
burns	quemaduras	*(keh-mah-doo-rahs)*
burp	repetir/eructar	*(reh-peh-teer/eh-rook-tahr)*
burritos	burritos	*(boo-ree-tohs)*
butter	mantequilla	*(mahn-teh-kee-yah)*
button(s)	botón(es)	*(boh-tohn[-ehs])*
buzzing	zumbido	*(soom-bee-doh)*
by	por	*(pohr)*
by mouth	por la boca	*(pohr lah boh-kah)*
C	c	*(seh)*
cabbage	col/repollo	*(kohl/reh-poh-yoh)*
cabinet	gabinete	*(gah-bee-neh-teh)*
cafeteria	cafeteriá	*(kah-feh-teh-ree-ah)*

caffeine	cafeína	*(kah-feh-ee-nah)*
cake	pastel	*(pahs-tehl)*
call (for/name)	llamar	*(yah-mahr)*
call-bell	campana/timbre	*(kahm-pah-nah/teem-breh)*
callus	callo	*(kah-yoh)*
calm	calma	*(kahl-mah)*
can opener	abrelatas	*(ah-breh-lah-tahs)*
can	poder	*(poh-dehr)*
Canada	Canadá	*(kah-nah-dah)*
cancer	cáncer	*(kahn-sehr)*
candy	dulces	*(dool-sehs)*
canes	bastones	*(bahs-toh-nehs)*
canteloupe	melón	*(meh-lohn)*
capsule	cápsula	*(kahp-soo-lah)*
car	carro	*(kah-roh)*
carbonated drinks	bebidas gaseosas	*(beh-bee-dahs gah-seh-oh-sahs)*
card	tarjeta	*(tahr-heh-tah)*
cardiac	cardíaco	*(kahr-dee-ah-koh)*
cardiopulmonary	cardiopulmonar	*(kahr-dee-oh-pool-moh-nahr)*
care	cuidado	*(koo-ee-dah-doh)*
caries	caries	*(kah-ree-ehs)*
carotid	carótida	*(kah-roh-tee-dah)*
carpet	alfombra	*(ahl-fohm-brah)*
carrots	zanahorias	*(sah-nah-oh-ree-ahs)*
cast	yeso	*(yeh-soh)*
cataract	catarata	*(kah-tah-rah-tah)*
categories	categorias	*(kah-teh-goh-ree-ahs)*
cause	causa	*(kah-oo-sah)*
cavity	cavidad	*(kah-bee-dahd)*
ceiling	techo	*(teh-choh)*
celery	apio	*(ah-pee-oh)*
cell(s)	célula(s)	*(seh-loo-lah[s])*
cells (white)	glóbulos blancos	*(gloh-boo-lohs blahn-kohs)*
cement	cemento	*(seh-mehn-toh)*
centimeter	centímetro	*(sehn-tee-meh-troh)*
cereal (cooked)	cereal/cocido	*(seh-reh-ahl/koh-see-doh)*
cereal (dry)	cereal/seco	*(seh-reh-ahl/seh-koh)*
certain anxiety	cierta ansiedad	*(see-ehr-tah ahn-see-eh-dahd)*
Ch	Che	*(cheh)*
chair	silla	*(see-yah)*
chancre	chancro	*(chahn-kroh)*
change	cambiar	*(kahm-bee-ahr)*
change (money)	cambio	*(kahm-bee-oh)*
channel	canal	*(kah-nahl)*
chaplain/priest	capellán/sacerdote/cura	*(kah-peh-yahn/sah-sehr-doh-teh/koo-rah)*
chapter	capítulo	*(kah-pee-too-loh)*
characteristics	características	*(kahr-ahk-teh-rees-tee-kahs)*
chat	charlar	*(chahr-lahr)*
check	revise	*(reh-bee-seh)*

cheek	mejilla	*(meh-hee-yah)*
chemotherapy	quimioterapia	*(kee-mee-oh-teh-rah-pee-ah)*
cherries	cerezas	*(seh-reh-sahs)*
chest	pecho	*(peh-choh)*
chest pain	dolor de pecho	*(doh-lohr deh peh-choh)*
chicken	pollo	*(poh-yoh)*
child	niño(a)	*(nee-nyoh[-nyah])*
children	niños/hijos	*(nee-nyohs/ee-hohs)*
chocolate	chocolate	*(choh-koh-lah-teh)*
choking	ahogar	*(ah-oh-gahr)*
cholesterol	colesterol	*(koh-lehs-teh-rohl)*
chops	chuletas	*(choo-leh-tahs)*
cianotic	cianótico/violáceo	*(see-ah-noh-tee-koh/bee-oh-lah-*
		se-oh)
cirrhosis	cirrosis	*(see-rroh-sees)*
classification	clasificación	*(klah-see-fee-kah-see-ohn)*
classified	clasificado	*(klah-see-fee-kah-doh)*
classify	clasifique	*(klah-see-fee-keh)*
claustrophobia	claustrofobia	*(klah-oos-troh-foh-bee-ah)*
clavicle	clavícula	*(klah-bee-koo-lah)*
clean	limpiar	*(leem-pee-ahr)*
clear	claro/ambar	*(klah-roh/ahm-bahr)*
clinic	clínica	*(klee-nee-kah)*
clinical	clínico	*(klee-nee-koh)*
clock	reloj	*(reh-lohj)*
close	cerrar	*(seh-rrahr)*
closed reduction	reducción cerrada	*(reh-dook-see-ohn seh-rah-dah)*
clothes	ropa	*(roh-pah)*
coagulated	coagulado(a)	*(koh-ah-goo-lah-doh[-dah])*
coagulation	coagulación	*(koh-ah-goo-lah-see-ohn)*
coat	abrigo	*(ah-bree-goh)*
cocaine	cocaína	*(koh-kah-ee-nah)*
coffee	café	*(kah-feh)*
coffee pot	cafetera	*(kah-feh-teh-rah)*
cognitive	cognoscitivo	*(kohg-noh-see-tee-boh)*
cold	frío	*(free-oh)*
cold water	agua fría	*(ah-goo-ah free-ah)*
colic	cólico	*(koh-lee-koh)*
collection	coleccionar	*(koh-lehk-see-ohn-ahr)*
Colles' fracture	fractura de Colles	*(frahk-too-rah deh Koh-yehs)*
colonel	coronel	*(koh-rohn-ehl)*
coma	coma	*(koh-mah)*
comatose	comatoso	*(koh-mah-toh-soh)*
comb	peine	*(peh-ee-neh)*
come	venir	*(beh-neer)*
commands	mandatos	*(mahn-dah-tohs)*
comminuted fractures	fracturas conminutas	*(frahk-too-rahs kohn-mee-noo-tahs)*
common-law	concubina	*(kohn-koo-bee-nah)*
common	común	*(koh-moon)*

communicate	comunicar	*(koh-moo-nee-kahr)*
communication	comunicación	*(koh-moo-nee-kah-see-ohn)*
community	comunidad	*(koh-moo-nee-dahd)*
complain	quejar/quejarse	*(keh-hahr/keh-hahr-seh)*
complete dentures	dentadura completa	*(dehn-tah-doo-rah kohm-pleh-tah)*
complication(s)	complicacione(s)	*(kohm-plee-kah-see-ohn-eh[s])*
complications (major)	complicaciones mayores	*(kohm-plee-kah-see-oh-nes mah-yoh-rehs)*
compound fractures	fracturas compuestas	*(frahk-too-rahs kohm-poo-ehs-tahs)*
compromise	compromiso	*(kohm-proh-mee-soh)*
computer	computadora	*(kohm-poo-tah-doh-rah)*
concepts	conceptos	*(kohn-sehp-tohs)*
concubine/ common-law	concubina	*(kohn-koo-bee-nah)*
condiments	condimentos	*(kohn-dee-mehn-tohs)*
conditioning	acondicionado	*(ah-kohn-dee-see-oh-nah-doh)*
conduct	conducir	*(kohn-doo-seer)*
confirm	confirmar	*(kohn-feer-mahr)*
confuse	confundir	*(kohn-foon-deer)*
consciousness	conocimiento	*(koh-noh-see-mee-ehn-toh)*
constipation	constipación/ estreñimiento	*(kohns-tee-pah-see-ohn/ehs-treh-nyee-mee-ehn-toh)*
consultant	consultante	*(kohn-sool-tahn-teh)*
content	contenido	*(kohn-teh-nee-doh)*
continued	continuado	*(kohn-tee-noo-ah-doh)*
continuity	continuidad	*(kohn-tee-noo-ee-dahd)*
contraceptives	contraceptivos	*(kohn-trah-sehp-tee-bohs)*
contractions	contracciones	*(kohn-trahk-see-ohn-ehs)*
contrast	contraste	*(kohn-trahs-teh)*
control	control	*(kohn-trohl)*
convenient	conveniente	*(kohn-beh-nee-ehn-teh)*
cook	cocinar	*(koh-see-nahr)*
cookies	galletas	*(gah-yeh-tahs)*
coping	sobrellevando	*(soh-breh-yeh-bahn-doh)*
copper	cobre	*(koh-breh)*
corn	maíz/elote	*(mah-ees/eh-loh-teh)*
corn bread	pan de maíz	*(pahn deh mah-ees)*
corner	esquina	*(ehs-kee-nah)*
corn-flakes	hojitas de maíz	*(oh-hee-tahs deh mah-ees)*
cortisone	cortisona	*(kohr-tee-sohn-ah)*
cosmetic	cosmético	*(kohs-meh-tee-koh)*
cottage cheese	requesón	*(reh-keh-sohn)*
cough	tos	*(tohs)*
cousin	primo(a)	*(pree-moh[-mah])*
cousins	primos(as)	*(pree-mohs[-mahs])*
cover	cubrir	*(koo-breer)*
crab	cangrejos	*(kahn-greh-hohs)*
crackers	galletas saladas	*(gah-yeh-tahs sah-lah-dahs)*
cream	crema	*(kreh-mah)*
cream of wheat	crema de trigo	*(kreh-mah deh tree-goh)*

crisis	crisis	*(kree-sees)*
crisis intervention	intervención de la crisis	*(een-tehr-behn-see-ohn deh lah kree-sees)*
cross	cruzar	*(kroo-sahr)*
crowns	coronas	*(koh-roh-nahs)*
crutches	muletas	*(moo-leh-tahs)*
cry	llorar	*(yoh-rahr)*
cubic centimeter	centímetro cúbico	*(sehn-tee-meh-troh koo-bee-koh)*
cubic	cúbico	*(koo-bee-koh)*
cucumbers	pepinos	*(peh-pee-nohs)*
cup	taza	*(tah-sah)*
cure	curar	*(koo-rahr)*
custard	flan	*(flahn)*
customary	acostumbra	*(ah-kohs-toom-brah)*
cut down	redusca	*(reh-doos-kah)*
cut	cortar	*(kohr-tahr)*
D	d	*(deh)*
dad	papá	*(pah-pah)*
dark	negro	*(neh-groh)*
daughter	hija	*(ee-hah)*
days	dias	*(dee-ahs)*
deal with	tratar	*(trah-tahr)*
debris	restos	*(rehs-tohs)*
decaffeinated	decafeinado	*(deh-kah-feh-ee-nah-doh)*
December	diciembre	*(dee-see-ehm-breh)*
decent	decente	*(deh-sehn-teh)*
decide that	decide que	*(deh-see-deh keh)*
decongestants	descongestionantes	*(dehs-kohn-hehs-tee-oh-nahn-tehs)*
defense	defensa	*(deh fehn-sah)*
deficiency	deficiencia	*(deh-fee-see-ehn-see-ah)*
dehydrated	deshidratado	*(deh-see-drah-tah-doh)*
dehydration	deshidratación	*(deh-see-drah-tah-see-ohn)*
delirious	delirio	*(deh-lee-ree-oh)*
demented	demente	*(deh-mehn-teh)*
dementia	demencia	*(deh-mehn-see-ah)*
dental floss	hilo dental	*(ee-loh dehn-tahl)*
dental plaque	placa	*(plah-kah)*
dental surgeon	cirujano dentista	*(see-roo-hah-noh dehn-tees-tah)*
dental	dental	*(dehn-tahl)*
dentist	dentista	*(dehn-tees-tah)*
dentrific	dentrífico	*(dehn-tree-fee-koh)*
denture	dentadura	*(dehn-tah-doo-rah)*
deny	negar	*(neh-gahr)*
department	departamento	*(deh-pahr-tah-mehn-toh)*
dependence	dependencia	*(deh-pehn-dehn-see-ah)*
dependent	dependiente	*(deh-pehn-dee-ehn-teh)*
depressed	deprimido	*(deh-pree-mee-doh)*
deserve	merecer	*(meh-reh-sehr)*
desk	escritorio	*(ehs-kree-toh-ree-oh)*

desserts	postres	*(pohs-trehs)*
destroy	destruir	*(dehs-troo-eer)*
detect	descubra	*(dehs-koo-brah)*
detection	detección	*(deh-tehk-see-ohn)*
determine	determinar	*(deh-tehr-meh-nahr)*
develop	desarrollar	*(deh-sah-roh-yahr)*
development	desarrollo	*(deh-sah-rroh-yoh)*
diabetes	diabetes	*(dee-ah-beh-tehs)*
diabetic	diabético(a)	*(dee-ah-beh-tee-koh[-kah])*
diagnosis/diagnostic	diagnóstico	*(dee-ahg-nohs-tee-koh)*
diamonds	diamantes	*(dee-ah-mahn-tehs)*
diaper	pañal	*(pah-nyahl)*
diarrhea	diarrea	*(dee-ah-rreh-ah)*
die	morir	*(moh-reer)*
diet(s)	dieta(s)	*(dee-eh-tah[s])*
different	diferente	*(dee-feh-rehn-teh)*
difficulty	dificultad	*(dee-fee-kool-tahd)*
digitalis	digitálicos	*(dee-hee-tah-lee-kohs)*
diluent	diluente	*(dee-loo-ehn-teh)*
dinner	cena	*(seh-nah)*
direct	directo	*(dee-rehk-toh)*
directions	direcciones	*(dee-rehk-see-oh-nehs)*
disappear	desaparecer	*(deh-sah-pah-reh-sehr)*
discomfort	molestia	*(moh-lehs-tee-ah)*
discover	descubrir	*(dehs-koo-breer)*
dish	plato	*(plah-toh)*
dishwasher	lavaplatos	*(lah-bah-plah-tohs)*
disorder	desorden	*(deh-sohr-dehn)*
disorders	desórdenes	*(dehs-ohr-deh-nehs)*
division	división	*(dee-bee-see-ohn)*
dizzy	mareado	*(mah-reh-ah-doh)*
dizzy spell	desmayo/mareo	*(dehs-mah-yoh/mah-reh-oh)*
do	hace	*(ah-seh)*
doctor	doctor(a)/médico(a)	*(dohk-tohr[-toht-ah]/meh-dee-koh[-kah])*
doctor's office	oficina/consultorio	*(oh-fee-see-nah/kohn-sool-toh-ree-oh)*
door	puerta	*(poo-ehr-tah)*
dose	dosis	*(doh-sees)*
drapes	cortinas	*(kohr-tee-nahs)*
draw	tirar/dibujar/sacar	*(tee-rahr/dee-boo-hahr/sah-kahr)*
dress	vestir	*(behs-teer)*
dresser	aparador	*(ah-pah-rah-dohr)*
drink	beber/tomar	*(beh-behr/toh-mahr)*
driveway	entrada para autos	*(ehn-trah-dah pah-rah ahoo-tohs)*
drop	gota	*(goh-tah)*
drugs	drogas	*(droh-gahs)*
dry	seca	*(seh-kah)*
duck	pato	*(pah-toh)*
during	durante	*(doo-rahn-teh)*

E	e	*(eh)*
each	cada	*(kah-dah)*
early	temprano	*(tehm-prah-noh)*
East	este	*(ehs-teh)*
eat	comer	*(koh-mehr)*
eat breakfast	desayunar	*(deh-sah-yoo-nahr)*
echymosis	equimosis	*(eh-kee-moh-sees)*
eczema	eccema	*(ehk-seh-mah)*
eggplant	berenjena	*(beh-rehn-heh-nah)*
eggs	huevos	*(oo-eh-bohs)*
eight (AM)	las ocho	*(lahs oh-choh)*
eight	ocho	*(oh-choh)*
eighteen	diez y ocho	*(dee-ehs ee oh-choh)*
eighth	octavo(a)	*(ohk-tah-boh[-bah])*
eighty	ochenta	*(oh-chehn-tah)*
either/or	o/o	*(oh/oh)*
elder	anciana (feminine)	*(ahn-see-ah-nah)*
elderly	anciano	*(ahn-see-ah-noh)*
electrocardiogram	electrocardiograma	*(eh-lehk-troh-kahr-dee-oh-grah-mah)*
elevator	elevador	*(eh-leh-bah-dohr)*
eleven	once	*(ohn-seh)*
embolism	embolia	*(ehm-boh-lee-ah)*
embrace	abrazar	*(ah-brah-sahr)*
emerald	esmeralda	*(ehs-meh-rahl-dah)*
emergencies	emergencias	*(eh-mehr-hehn-see-ahs)*
emergency	emergencia	*(eh-mehr-hehn-see-ah)*
emergency room	cuarto de emergencia	*(koo-ahr-toh deh eh-mehr-hehn-see-ah)*
emetic	emético	*(ehm-eh-tee-koh)*
employ	emplear	*(ehm-pleh-ahr)*
enamel	esmalte	*(ehs-mahl-teh)*
enchiladas	enchiladas	*(ehn-chee-lah-dahs)*
end	al final	*(ahl fee-nahl)*
endoscopy	endoscopía	*(ehn-dohs-koh-pee-ah)*
enema	enema/sonda	*(eh-neh-mah/sohn-dah)*
English	inglés	*(een-glehs)*
enteritis	enteritis	*(ehn-teh-ree-tees)*
environment	ambiente familiar	*(ahm-bee-ehn-teh fah-mee-lee-ahr)*
epigastrium	epigastrio	*(eh-pee-gahs-tree-oh)*
epilepsy	epilepsia	*(eh-pee-lehp-see-ah)*
error	error	*(eh-rrohr)*
especially	especialmente	*(ehs-peh-see-ahl-mehn-teh)*
essence	esencia	*(eh-sehn-see-ah)*
essential	esencial	*(eh-sehn-see-ahl)*
etiology	etiología	*(eh-tee-oh-loh-hee-ah)*
euphoric	eufórico	*(eh-oo-foh-ree-koh)*
evaluation	evaluación	*(eh-bah-loo-ah-see-ohn)*
evaluation (psychosocial)	asesoría psicosocial	*(ah-seh-soh-ree-ah see-koh-soh-see-ahl)*

every	vez	*(behs)*
everything	todo	*(toh-doh)*
examinations	examenes	*(ehx-ah-meh-nehs)*
examine	examinarla	*(ehx-ah-mee-nahr-lah)*
excrement	excremento	*(ehx-kreh-mehn-toh)*
exercise	ejercicio	*(eh-hehr-see-see-oh)*
exit sign	salida	*(sah-lee-dah)*
explain	explicar	*(ehx-plee-kahr)*
expression	expresión(es)	*(ehx-preh-see-ohn[-ehs])*
external	externo	*(ehx-tehr-noh)*
extra	extra	*(ehx-trah)*
extract	extraer/sacar	*(ehx-trah-ehr/sah-kahr)*
extraction	extracción	*(ehx-trahk-see-ohn)*
exudate	exudado	*(ehx-oo-dah-doh)*
eye	ojo	*(oh-hoh)*
eyetooth	diente canino/ colmillo	*(dee-ehn-teh kah-nee-noh/kohl-mee-yoh)*
F	f	*(eh-feh)*
facial	facial	*(fah-see-ahl)*
factors	factores	*(fahk-toh-rehs)*
fail	fallar	*(fah-yahr)*
fajitas	fajitas	*(fah-hee-tahs)*
fall	otoño	*(oh-toh-nyoh)*
false	falso	*(fahl-soh)*
familiar	familiar	*(fah-mee-lee-ahr)*
family	familia	*(fah-mee-lee-ah)*
far	lejos de	*(leh-hohs deh)*
fasting	en ayunas	*(ehn ah-yoo-nahs)*
fat	grasa/obeso	*(grah-sah/oh-beh-soh)*
fatal	fatal	*(fah-tahl)*
father	padre	*(pah-dreh)*
father-in-law	suegro	*(soo-eh-groh)*
fear	miedo	*(mee-eh-doh)*
February	febrero	*(feh-breh-roh)*
feel	sentir	*(sehn-teer)*
fever	fiebre	*(fee-eh-breh)*
few	poco	*(poh-koh)*
fibroid	fibroide	*(fee-broh-ee-deh)*
fifteen	quince	*(keen-seh)*
fifth	quinto(a)	*(keen-toh[-tah])*
fifty	cincuenta	*(seen-koo-ehn-tah)*
fill	llenar	*(yeh-nahr)*
find	hallar/descubrir	*(ah-yahr/dehs-koo-breer)*
findings	hallazgos	*(ah-yahs-gohs)*
fire	lumbre	*(loom-breh)*
fire escape	escape de fuego	*(ehs-kah-peh deh foo-eh-goh)*
first	primero(a)	*(pree-meh-roh[-rah])*
fish	pescado	*(pehs-kah-doh)*
fistula	fístula	*(fees-too-lah)*

five	cinco	*(seen-koh)*
fix	componer	*(kohm-poh-nehr)*
fixation	fijación	*(fee-hah-see-ohn)*
flat	indiferente	*(een-dee-feh-rehn-teh)*
flexibility	flexibilidad	*(flehx-ee-bee-lee-dahd)*
floor	piso	*(pee-soh)*
flower vase	florero	*(floh-reh-roh)*
fluid	fluído	*(floo-ee-doh)*
fluoride	fluoruro	*(floh-roo-roh)*
following	siguiente	*(see-ghee-ehn-teh)*
foods	comidas	*(koh-mee-dahs)*
for	de/por/para	*(deh/pohr/pah-rah)*
for/by/therefore	por	*(pohr)*
fork	tenedor	*(teh-neh-dohr)*
form(s)	forma(s)	*(fohr-mah[s])*
formula	fórmula	*(fohr-moo-lah)*
forty	cuarenta	*(koo-ah-rehn-tah)*
four	cuatro	*(koo-ah-troh)*
fourteen	catorce	*(kah-tohr-seh)*
fourth	cuarto(a)	*(koo-ahr-toh[-tah])*
fracture (pelvic)	fractura pélvica	*(frahk-too-rah pehl-bee-kah)*
fractures	fracturas	*(frahk-too-rahs)*
fragments	fragmentos	*(frahg-mehn-tohs)*
freckles	pecas	*(peh-kahs)*
fremitus	frémito	*(freh-mee-toh)*
French fries	papas fritas	*(pah-pahs free-tahs)*
fresh	fresco	*(frehs-koh)*
Friday	viernes	*(bee-ehr-nehs)*
fried	fritos(as)	*(free-tohs[-tahs])*
fried chicken	pollo frito	*(poh-yoh free-toh)*
friend	amigo(a)	*(ah-mee-goh[-gah])*
friendship	amistad	*(ah-mees-tahd)*
from	de	*(deh)*
frontal	frontal	*(frohn-tahl)*
frozen	helado/congelado	*(eh-lah-doh/kohn-heh-lah-doh)*
fruit	fruta	*(froo-tah)*
fuchsia	fiucha	*(fee-oo-chah)*
function	función	*(foon-see-ohn)*
fundamental	fundamental	*(foon-dah-mehn-tahl)*
fungus	hongos	*(ohn-gohs)*
G	g	*(jeh)*
gallbladder	vesícula biliar/hiel	*(beh-see-koo-lah bee-lee-ahr/ee-ehl)*
gallon	galón	*(gah-lohn)*
gangrene	gangrena	*(gahn-greh-nah)*
garage	garaje	*(gah-rah-heh)*
gastroenteritis	gastroenteritis	*(gahs-troh-ehn-teh-ree-tees)*
gel/gelatin	gelatina	*(geh lah-tee-nah)*
general	general	*(heh-neh-rahl)*
generic	genérico	*(heh-neh-ree-koh)*

genial	genial	*(heh-nee-ahl)*
get	consiga	*(kohn-see-gah)*
gingivitis	gingivitis	*(heen-hee-bee-tees)*
girl(s)	niña(s)/muchacha(s)	*(nee-nyah[s]/moo-chah-chah[s])*
glass	vidrio/vaso/cristal	*(bee-dree-oh/bah-soh/krees-tahl)*
glaucoma	glaucoma	*(glah-oo-koh-mah)*
globule	glóbulo	*(gloh-boo-loh)*
gloves	guantes	*(goo-ahn-tehs)*
glycosuria	glucosuria	*(gloo-koh-soo-ree-ah)*
go	acuda/vé	*(ah-koo-dah/beh)*
goals	metas	*(meh-tahs)*
godfather	padrino	*(pah-dree-noh)*
godmother	madrina	*(mah-dree-nah)*
godparents	padrinos	*(pah-dree-nohs)*
gold	dorado	*(doh-rah-doh)*
good	bueno(a)	*(boo-eh-noh[-nah])*
gout	gota	*(goh-tah)*
gown	bata/vestido	*(bah-tah/behs-tee-doh)*
grains	granos	*(grah-nohs)*
grams	gramos	*(grah-mohs)*
grandchildren	nietos	*(nee-eh-tohs)*
grandfather	abuelo	*(ah-boo-eh-loh)*
grandmother	abuela	*(ah-boo-eh-lah)*
grandparents	abuelos	*(ah-boo-eh-lohs)*
grape(s)	uva(s)	*(oo-bah[s])*
grapefruit	toronja	*(toh-rohn-hah)*
grave	grave	*(grah-beh)*
gray	gris	*(grees)*
grayish	grisáseo	*(gree-sah-seh-oh)*
grayish-white	canoso	*(kah-noh-soh)*
green	verde	*(behr-deh)*
green beans	ejotes/habichuelas	*(eh-hoh-tehs/ah-bee-choo-eh-lahs)*
greetings	saludos	*(sah-loo-dohs)*
grief	pena	*(peh-nah)*
grieve	sufrir	*(soo-freer)*
growth	crecimiento	*(kreh-see-mee-ehn-toh)*
guide	guía	*(ghee-ah)*
guilt	culpa	*(kool-pah)*
gumboil	flemón/absceso	*(fleh-mohn/ahb-seh-soh)*
gynecologist	ginecólogo	*(hee-neh-koh-loh-goh)*
H	h	*(ah-cheh)*
habit	costumbre	*(kohs-toom-breh)*
hairbrush	cepillo de pelo	*(seh-pee-yoh deh peh-loh)*
hallway	pasillo	*(pah-see-yoh)*
ham	jamón	*(hah-mohn)*
hamburger	hamburguesa	*(ahm-boor-geh-sah)*
hand	mano(s)	*(mah-noh/mah-nohs)*
handshake	apretón de manos	*(ah-preh-tohn deh mah-nohs)*
handy	convenientes	*(kohn-beh-nee-ehn-tehs)*

hard-boiled	duros	*(doo-rohs)*
has	tiene	*(tee-eh-neh)*
hazard	peligro	*(peh-lee-groh)*
hazel	castaño	*(kahs-tah-nyoh)*
he/she/you	él/ella/usted	*(ehl/eh-yah/oos-tehd)*
headache	dolor de cabeza	*(doh-lohr deh kah-beh-sah)*
heal	sano	*(sah-noh)*
healing	curación	*(koo-rah-see-ohn)*
health	salud	*(sah-lood)*
health (mental)	salud mental	*(sah-lood mehn-tahl)*
heart(s)	corazón(corazones)	*(koh-rah-sohn/koh-rah-sohn-ehs)*
heater	calentador	*(kah-lehn-tah-dohr)*
heater (water)	calentador de agua	*(kah-lehn-tah-dohr deh ah-goo-ah)*
hello	hola	*(oh-lah)*
help	ayuda	*(ah-yoo-dah)*
helpful	conveniente	*(kohn-beh-nee-ehn-teh)*
helpful	útil/utiles	*(oo-teel/oo-tee-lehs)*
hematology	hematología	*(eh-mah-toh-loh-hee-ah)*
hematoma	hematoma	*(eh-mah-toh-mah)*
hemolysis	hemólisis	*(eh-moh-lee-sees)*
hemorrhage	hemorragia	*(eh-moh-rah-hee-ah)*
hepatitis	hepatitis	*(eh-pah-tee-tees)*
her	ella	*(eh-yah)*
here	aquí	*(ah-kee)*
hernia	hernia	*(ehr-nee-ah)*
high	alto	*(ahl-toh)*
him	él	*(ehl)*
himself	su	*(soo)*
hip	cadera	*(kah-deh-rah)*
his/hers/theirs	el suyo/la suya/los suyos/las suyas	*(ehl soo[yoh/lah soo-yah/lohs soo-yohs/lahs soo-yahs)*
hispanic(s)	hispano(s)	*(ees-pah-noh[s])*
history	historia	*(ees-toh-ree-ah)*
home	casa/hogar	*(kah-sah/oh-gahr)*
hope	esperanza	*(ehs-peh-rahn-sah)*
hose	medias	*(meh-dee-ahs)*
hospital(s)	hospital(es)	*(ohs-pee-tahl[-ehs])*
hostility	hostilidad	*(ohs-tee-lee-dahd)*
hot	calor	*(kah-lohr)*
hot dog	perro caliente/ emparedado de salchicha	*(peh-rroh kah-lee-ehn-teh/ehm-pah-reh-dah-doh deh sahl-chee-chah)*
hot sauce	salsa picante	*(sahl-sah pee-kahn-teh)*
hot water	agua caliente	*(ah-goo-ah kah-lee-ehn-teh)*
hour	hora	*(oh-rah)*
hours (visiting)	horas de visita	*(oh-rahs deh bee-see-tah)*
house	casa	*(kah-sah)*
household	caseras	*(kah-seh-rahs)*
how	cómo	*(koh-moh)*

however	pero	(peh-roh)
humanistic	humanístico	(oo-mah-nees-tee-koh)
hunt	cazar	(kah-sahr)
hurt	doler	(doh-lehr)
husband	esposo	(ehs-poh-soh)
hygienist	higienista	(ee-hee-eh-nees-tah)
hypertension	hipertensión	(ee-pehr-tehn-see-ohn)
hypertension (pulmonary)	hipertensión pulmonar	(ee-pehr-tehn-see-ohn pool-moh-nahr)
hyperthermia	hipertermia	(ee-pehr-tehr-mee-ah)
hypoglycemia	hipoglucemia	(ee-poh-gloo-seh-mee-ah)
I	i	(ee)
I	yo	(yoh)
ice	hielo	(ee-eh-loh)
ice cream	nieve/helado/ mantecado	(nee-eh-beh/eh-lah-doh/mahn-teh-kah-doh)
icteric	ictérico	(eek-teh-ree-koh)
idea	idea	(ee-deh-ah)
identification	identificación	(ee-dehn-tee-fee-kah-see-ohn)
identified	identificado	(ee-dehn-tee-fee-kah-doh)
if	si	(see)
ignorance	ignorancia	(eeg-noh-rahn-see-ah)
ignore	ignorar	(eeg-noh-rahr)
illness	enfermedad	(ehn-fehr-meh-dahd)
imaging	imagen	(ee-mah-hehn)
immunodeficiency	inmunodeficiencia	(een-moo-noh-deh-fee-see-ehn-see-ah)
implant	implante	(eem-plahn-teh)
implementation	implementación	(eem-pleh-mehn-tah-see-ohn)
implications	implicaciones	(eem-plee-kah-see-ohn-ehs)
important	importantes	(eem-pohr-tahn-tehs)
impression	impresión	(eem-preh-see-ohn)
in/on	en	(ehn)
in front of	enfrente de/delante de	(ehn-frehn-teh deh/deh-lahn-teh deh)
incidence	incidencia	(een-see-dehn-see-ah)
incision	incisión	(een-see-see-ohn)
independence	independencia	(een-deh-pehn-dehn-see-ah)
index	tarjeta	(tahr-heh-tah)
indigestion	indigestión	(een-dee-hehs-tee-ohn)
induce	inducir	(een-doo-seer)
infancy	infancia	(een-fahn-see-ah)
infection	infección	(een-fehk-see-ohn)
infections	infecciones	(een-fehk-see-ohn-ehs)
inflammation	inflamación	(een-flah-mah-see-ohn)
inhalant	inhalante	(een-ah-lahn-teh)
injection	inyección	(een-yehk-see-ohn)
insect	insecto	(een-sehk-toh)
instant	instantáneo	(eens-tahn-tah-neh-oh)

instructions	instrucciones	*(eens-trook-see-ohn ehs)*
instrument	instrumento	*(eens-troo-mehn-toh)*
insulin	insulina	*(een-soo-lee-nah)*
insurance	seguro	*(seh-goo-roh)*
integral	integral	*(een-teh-grahl)*
interaction	interacción	*(een-tehr-ahk-see-ohn)*
interest	interés	*(een-teh-rehs)*
internal	interior	*(een-teh-ree-ohr)*
interpersonal	interpersonal	*(een-tehr-pehr-soh-nahl)*
interrogation	interrogativo	*(een-teh-rroh-gah-tee-boh)*
interventions	intervenciones	*(een-tehr-behn-see-oh-nehs)*
intimate	íntimo	*(een-tee-moh)*
intramuscular	intramuscular	*(een-trah-moos-koo-lahr)*
intravenous	intravenoso	*(een-trah-beh-noh-soh)*
iodine	yodo	*(yoh-doh)*
irradiate	irradiar	*(ee-rrah-dee-ahr)*
irritable	irritable	*(ee-rree-tah-bleh)*
is/it	es/está	*(ehs/ehs-tah)*
it	lo	*(loh)*
J	j	*(hoh-tah)*
jacket	chaqueta	*(cha-keh-tah)*
jam	confitura	*(kohn-fee-too-rah)*
January	enero	*(eh-neh-roh)*
jelly	jalea	*(hah-leh-ah)*
jug (water)	jarra	*(hah-rrah)*
jugular	yugular	*(yoo-goo-lahr)*
juice(s)	jugo(s)	*(hoo-goh[s])*
juicy	jugosas	*(hoo-goh-sahs)*
July	julio	*(hoo-lee-oh)*
jump	saltar	*(sahl-tahr)*
June	junio	*(hoo-nee-oh)*
just	justo/sólo	*(hoos-toh/soh-loh)*
juvenile	juvenil	*(hoo-beh-neel)*
K	k	*(kah)*
keep	guardar/mantener	*(goo-ahr-dahr/mahn-teh-nehr)*
ketoacidosis	cetoacidosis	*(seh-toh-ah-see-doh-sees)*
key(s)	clave(s)	*(klah-beh[s])*
kilogram(s)	kilogramo(s)/kilo(s)	*(kee-loh-grah-moh[s]/kee-loh[s])*
kiss	besar	*(beh-sahr)*
kitchen	cocina	*(koh-see-nah)*
kleptomania	cleptomanía	*(klehp-toh-mah-nee-ah)*
knife	cuchillo	*(koo-chee-yoh)*
know	conocer/saber	*(koh-noh-sehr/sah-behr)*
L	l	*(eh-leh)*
laboratory	laboratorio	*(lah-boh-rah-toh-ree-oh)*
lamb	cordero	*(kohr-deh-roh)*
lamp	lámpara	*(lahm-pah-rah)*

lancet	lanceta	*(lahn-seh-tah)*
language	lenguaje	*(lehn-goo-ah-heh)*
laparoscopy	laparoscopía	*(lah-pah-rohs-koh-pee-ah)*
laryngitis	laringitis	*(lah-reen-hee-tees)*
lasagna	lasaña	*(lah-sah-nyah)*
last	última	*(ool-tee-mah)*
last name	apellido	*(ah-peh-yee-doh)*
laurel	laurel	*(lah-oo-rehl)*
lavage	lavabo	*(lah-bah-boh)*
laxative(s)	laxante(s)/purgante(s)	*(lahx-ahn-teh[s]/poor-gahn-teh[s])*
lay down	acostar	*(ah-kohs-tahr)*
lead	plomo	*(ploh-moh)*
leave	dejar	*(deh-hahr)*
left	izquierdo(a)	*(ees-kee-ehr-doh(-dah)*
leg	pierna	*(pee-ehr-nah)*
lemon	limón	*(lee-mohn)*
lesions	lesiones	*(leh-see-oh-nehs)*
less	menos	*(meh-nohs)*
let go	soltar	*(sohl-tahr)*
lettuce	lechuga	*(leh-choo-gah)*
leukocytes	leucocitos	*(leh-oo-koh-see-tohs)*
level	nivel	*(nee-vehl)*
lift	levantar/elevar	*(leh-bahn-tahr/eh-leh-bahr)*
ligament	ligamento	*(lee-gah-mehn-toh)*
light	luz	*(loos)*
light touch	caricia	*(kah-ree-see-ah)*
like	comparación	*(kohm-pah-rah-see-ohn)*
lima beans	habas	*(ah-bahs)*
lime	lima/limón	*(lee-mah/lee-mohn)*
limitations	limitaciones	*(lee-mee-tah-see-ohn-ehs)*
linen	lino	*(lee-noh)*
lingual	lingual	*(leen-goo-ahl)*
lipoatrophy	lipotrofia	*(lee-poh-troh-fee-ah)*
lipstick	lápiz de labios	*(lah-pees deh lah-bee-ohs)*
liquid	líquido(a)	*(lee-kee-doh[-dah])*
list	lista	*(lees-tah)*
liter	litro	*(lee-troh)*
lithium	litio	*(lee-tee-oh)*
little/few	poco	*(poh-koh)*
liver	hígado	*(ee-gah-doh)*
living room	sala	*(sah-lah)*
Ll	ll	*(eh-yeh doh-bleh eh-yeh)*
lobby	sala de espera/ vestíbulo	*(sah-lah deh ehs-peh-rah/behs-tee- boo-loh)*
loneliness	soledad	*(soh-leh-dahd)*
lose	perder	*(pehr-dehr)*
loss	pérdida	*(pehr-dee-dah)*
lotion	loción	*(loh-see-ohn)*
love	amor	*(ah-mohr)*

low	baja	*(bah-hah)*
low cholesterol	colesterol bajo/	*(koh-lehs-teh-rohl bah-hoh/poh-koh*
	poco colesterol	*koh-lehs-teh-rohl)*
low fat	poca grasa	*(poh-kah grah-sah)*
low sodium	baja en sal/poca sal	*(bah-hah ehn sahl/poh-kah sahl)*
lower	rebajar/baje	*(reh-bah-hahr/bah-heh)*
lubricant	lubricante	*(loo-bree-kahn-teh)*
lunch	comida	*(koh-mee-dah)*
lungs	pulmones	*(pool-moh-nehs)*
lupus	lupos	*(loo-pohs)*
M	m	*(eh-meh)*
macaroni	macarrón	*(mah-kah-rrohn)*
machine	máquina	*(mah-kee-nah)*
magazine	revista	*(reh-bees-tah)*
magnetic	magnético	*(mahg-neh-tee-koh)*
make	hacer/hagales	*(ah-sehr/ah-gah-lehs)*
malignant	maligno	*(mah-leeg-noh)*
man	hombre	*(ohm-breh)*
man/woman (young)	joven	*(hoh-behn)*
management	manejo	*(mah-neh-hoh)*
manifestation	manifestación	*(mahn-ee-fehs-tah-see-ohn)*
manipulation	manipulación	*(mahn-ee-poo-lah-see-ohn)*
manual	manual	*(mah-noo-ahl)*
many	muchas	*(moo-chahs)*
March	marzo	*(mahr-soh)*
marrow	médula	*(meh-doo-lah)*
marry	casar	*(kah-sahr)*
martyr	mártir	*(mahr-teer)*
mashed	majadas	*(mah-hah-dahs)*
material	material	*(mah-teh-ree-ahl)*
maternal	maternal	*(mah-tehr-nahl)*
mathematics	matemáticas	*(mah-teh-mah-tee-kahs)*
mattress	colchón	*(kohl-chohn)*
May	mayo	*(mah-yoh)*
may help	le puede ayudar	*(leh poo-eh-deh ah-yoo-dahr)*
may not be	no se pueden	*(noh seh poo-eh-dehn)*
mayonnaise	mayonesa	*(mah-yoh-neh-sah)*
me	mí	*(mee)*
meals	comidas	*(koh-mee-dahs)*
measures	medidas	*(meh-dee-dahs)*
meat	carne	*(kahr-neh)*
meats (red)	carnes rojas	*(kahr-nehs roh-hahs)*
mechanisms	mecanismos	*(meh-kah-nees-mohs)*
medical	médico	*(meh-dee-koh)*
medication(s)	medicamento(s)	*(meh-dee-kah-mehn-toh[s])*
medicine (nuclear)	medicina nuclear	*(meh-dee-see-nah noo-kleh-ahr)*
medicine(s)	medicina	*(meh-dee-see-nah)*
medulla	médula	*(meh-doo-lah)*

melon	melón	*(meh-lohn)*
member(s)	miembro(s)	*(mee-ehm-broh[s])*
memorize	memorizar	*(meh-moh-ree-sahr)*
memory	memoria	*(meh-moh-ree-ah)*
meningitis	meningitis	*(meh-neen-hee-tees)*
menudo	menudo	*(meh-noo-doh)*
menus	menus	*(meh-noos)*
meter	metro	*(meh-troh)*
methodology	metodología	*(meh-toh-doh-loh-hee-ah)*
metric	metricas	*(meh-tree-kahs)*
microwave	microondas	*(mee-kroh-ohn-dahs)*
migrate	emigrar	*(eh-mee-grahr)*
milk	leche	*(leh-cheh)*
milk (whole)	leche entera	*(leh-cheh ehn-teh-rah)*
milligram	miligramo	*(mee-lee-grah-moh)*
milliliter	mililitro	*(mee-lee-lee-troh)*
mine	el mío/la mía/los míos/las mías	*(ehl mee-oh/lah mee-ah/lohs mee-ohs/lahs mee-ahs)*
minerals	minerales	*(mee-neh-rah-lees)*
minimum	mínimo	*(mee-nee-moh)*
mirror	espejo	*(ehs-peh-hoh)*
miscellaneous	miscelánea	*(mee-seh-lah-neh-ah)*
Miss	señorita	*(seh-nyoh-ree-tah)*
mistrust	desconfianza	*(dehs-kohn-fee-ahn-sah)*
model	modelo	*(moh-deh-loh)*
modern	moderno	*(moh-dehr-noh)*
modifiers	modificadores	*(moh-dee-fee-kah-doh-rehs)*
molar	muela	*(moo-eh-lah)*
mole	verrugas	*(beh-roo-gahs)*
mom	mamá	*(mah-mah)*
Monday	lunes	*(loo-nehs)*
monitor	monitor	*(moh-nee-tohr)*
month(s)	mes(es)	*(mehs[-ehs])*
moral	moral	*(moh-rahl)*
more	mucho/más	*(moo-choh/mahs)*
morphine	morfina	*(mohr-fee-nah)*
mother	madre	*(mah-dreh)*
mother-in-law	suegra	*(soo-eh-grah)*
mouth	boca/oral	*(boh-kah/oh-rahl)*
move	mover/mueva	*(moh-behr/moo-eh-bah)*
Mr.	señor	*(seh-nyohr)*
Mrs.	señora	*(seh-nyoh-rah)*
mustard	mostaza	*(mohs-tah-sah)*
N	n	*(eh-neh)*
name(s)	nombre(s)	*(nohm-breh[s])*
napkin	servilleta	*(sehr-bee-yeh-tah)*
narcotics	narcóticos	*(nahr-koh-tee-kohs)*
nasal	nasal	*(nah-sahl)*
nature	naturaleza	*(nah-too-rah-leh-sah)*

nausea	náusea	(nah-oo-seh-ah)
navel	ombligo	(ohm-blee-goh)
near	cerca de	(sehr-kah deh)
need	necesita	(neh-seh-see-tah)
needle	aguja	(ah-goo-hah)
needs	necesidades	(neh-seh-see-dah-dehs)
neither/nor	ni/ni	(nee/nee)
neither	tampoco	(tahm-poh-koh)
neonatal	neonatal	(neh-oh-nah-tahl)
nephew	sobrino	(soh-bree-noh)
nephropathy	nefropatía	(neh-froh-pah-tee-ah)
nervous	nervioso	(nehr-bee-oh-soh)
neuropathy	neuropatía	(neh-oo-roh-pah-tee-ah)
neurotic	neurótico	(neh-oo-roh-tee-koh)
neutral	neutral	(neh-oo-trahl)
never	jamás/nunca	(hah-mahs/noon-kah)
next	siguiente	(see-ghee-ehn-teh)
nicotine	nicotina	(nee-koh-tee-nah)
niece	sobrina	(soh-bree-nah)
nightgown	camisa de dormir/ bata	(kah-mee-sah deh dohr-meer/bah-tah)
nine	nueve	(noo-eh-beh)
nineteen	diez y nueve	(dee-ehs ee noo-eh-beh)
ninety	noventa	(noh-behn-tah)
ninth	noveno(a)	(noh-beh-noh[-nah])
nitroglycerin	nitroglicerina	(nee-troh-glee-seh-ree-nah)
no one	nadie	(nah-dee-eh)
no salt	sin sal	(seen sahl)
no smoking	no se permite fumar	(noh seh pehr-mee-teh foo-mahr)
no	no	(noh)
nobody	nadie	(nah-dee-eh)
none	ninguno	(neen-goo-noh)
noon/midnight	las doce/las cero horas	(lahs doh-seh/lahs seh-roh oh-rahs)
normal	normal	(nohr-mahl)
North	norte	(nohr-teh)
nose	nariz	(nah-rees)
noses	narices	(nah-ree-sehs)
not	no	(noh)
not any	ninguno	(neen-goo-noh)
not ever	jamás/nunca	(hah-mahs/noon-kah)
not translated	no se traducen	(noh seh trah-doo-sehn)
note	note	(noh-teh)
nothing	nada	(nah-dah)
nouns	nombres	(nohm-brehs)
November	noviembre	(noh-bee-ehm-breh)
novocaine	novocaina	(noh-boh-kah-ee-nah)
now	ahora	(ah-oh-rah)
numb	adormecido	(ah-dohr-meh-see-doh)
number(s)	número(s)	(noo-meh-roh[s])

nurse	enfermero(a)	*(ehn-fehr-meh-roh[-rah])*
nutrition	nutrición	*(noo-tree-see-ohn)*
nutritional	alimenticios	*(ah-lee-mehn-tee-see-ohs)*
O	o	*(oh)*
oatmeal	avena	*(ah-beh-nah)*
obesity	obesidad	*(oh-beh-see-dahd)*
observe	observe	*(ohb-sehr-beh)*
obsession	obsesión	*(ohb-seh-see-ohn)*
obstruction	obstrucción	*(ohb-strook-see-ohn)*
occasion	ocasión	*(oh-kah-see-ohn)*
occipital	occipital	*(ohk-see-pee-tahl)*
occur	ocurrir	*(oh-koo-rreer)*
October	octubre	*(ohk-too-breh)*
odontalgia/tooth ache	odontalgia/dolor de muela	*(oh-dohn-tahl-hee-ah/doh-lohr deh moo-eh-lah)*
of	de	*(deh)*
office	oficina	*(oh-fee-see-nah)*
oil	aceite	*(ah-seh-ee-teh)*
ointment	unguento	*(oon-goo-ehn-toh)*
older	mayores	*(mah-yoh-rehs)*
olive	aceituna	*(ah-seh-ee-too-nah)*
on	en	*(ehn)*
oncologic	oncología	*(ohn-koh-loh-hee-ah)*
one	un/uno	*(oon/oo-noh)*
one(AM/PM)	la una/las trece horas)	*(lah oo-nah/lahs treh-seh oh-rahs)*
onions	cebolla	*(seh-boh-yah)*
only	solamente	*(soh-lah-mehn-teh)*
opaque	opaco	*(oh-pah-koh)*
open	abra	*(ah-brah)*
ophthalmic	oftálmico	*(ohf-tahl-mee-koh)*
opinion	opinión	*(oh-pee-nee-ohn)*
opportunistic	oportunista	*(oh-pohr-too-nees-tah)*
opportunity	oportunidad	*(oh-pohr-too-nee-dahd)*
optic	óptico	*(ohp-tee-koh)*
or	o	*(oh)*
oral	oral	*(oh-rahl)*
orange	naranja	*(nah-rahn-hah)*
orangy	anaranjado	*(ah-nah-rahn-hah-doh)*
order	solicitar	*(sohl-ee-see-tahr)*
orders	ordenes	*(ohr-deh-nehs)*
organ(s)	órgano(s)	*(ohr-gah-noh[s])*
other	otras	*(oh-trahs)*
otic	ótico	*(oh-tee-koh)*
ounces	onzas	*(ohn-sahs)*
ours	el nuestro/la nuestra/los nuestros/las nuestras	*(ehl noo-ehs-troh/lah noo-ehs-trah/lohs noo-ehs-trohs/lahs noo-ehs-trahs)*

personality	personalidad	*(pehr-soh-nah-lee-dahd)*
pharmacy	farmacia	*(fahr-mah-see-ah)*
phases	fases	*(fah-sehs)*
philosophy	filosofía	*(fee-loh-soh-fee-ah)*
phone	teléfono	*(teh-leh-foh-noh)*
phrases	frases	*(frah-sehs)*
physician(f)	médica/doctora	*(meh-dee-kah/dohk-toh-rah)*
physician(m)	médico/doctor	*(meh-dee-koh/dohk-tohr)*
physicians	los médicos	*(lohs meh-dee-kohs)*
physique	físico	*(fee-see-koh)*
pickles	pepino	*(peh-pee-noh)*
picture	retrato	*(reh-trah-toh)*
pie(s)	pastel(es)	*(pahs-tehl[-ehs])*
piece	pieza	*(pee-ehs-ah)*
pill	píldora	*(peel-doh-rah)*
pillow	almohada	*(ahl-moh-ah-dah)*
pillowcase	funda	*(foon-dah)*
pin prick	picadura	*(pee-kah-doo-rah)*
pineapple	piña	*(pee-nyah)*
pink	rosa	*(roh-sah)*
pinkish	rosado	*(roh-sah-doh)*
pity	lástima	*(lahs-tee-mah)*
pizza	pizza	*(pee-sah)*
place	lugar/poner/colocar	*(loo-gahr/poh-nehr/koh-loh-kahr)*
plan	plan	*(plahn)*
planning	planificación	*(plah-nee-fee-kah-see-ohn)*
plate	platón	*(plah-tohn)*
play	jugar	*(hoo-gahr)*
please	por favor	*(pohr fah-bohr)*
plum(s)	ciruelos(as)	*(see-roo-eh-lohs[-lahs])*
plural	plural	*(ploo-rahl)*
pneumonia	pulmonía/neumonía	*(pool-moh-nee-ah/neh-oo-moh-nee-ah)*
point	señalar/apunte	*(seh-nyah-lahr/ah-poon-teh)*
poisons	venenos	*(beh-neh-nohs)*
polydipsia	polidipsia	*(poh-lee-deep-see-ah)*
polyphagia	polifagia	*(poh-lee-fah-hee-ah)*
polyuria	poliuria	*(poh-lee-oo-ree-ah)*
porcelain	porcelana	*(pohr-seh-lah-nah)*
porch/patio	pórtico/patio	*(pohr-tee-koh/pah-tee-oh)*
pork	puerco	*(poo-ehr-koh)*
postoperative	postoperatorio	*(pohst-oh-peh-rah-toh-ree-oh)*
potatoes	papas	*(pah-pahs)*
potatoes (mashed)	puré de papas	*(poo-reh deh pah-pahs)*
potential	posibles	*(poh-see-blehs)*
pots/pans	trastes/vasijas	*(trahs-tehs/bah-see-hahs)*
pound	libra	*(lee-brah)*
practice	práctica	*(prahk-tee-kah)*
precaution	precaución	*(preh-kah-oo-see-ohn)*

pregnant	embarazada	*(ehm-bah-rah-sah-dah)*
preliminary	preliminar	*(preh-lee-mee-nahr)*
preoperative	preoperatorio	*(preh-oh-peh-rah-toh-ree-oh)*
preparation	preparación	*(preh-pah-rah-see-ohn)*
prepare (to)	preparar	*(preh-pah-rahr)*
prescribed	ordenado	*(ohr-deh-nah-doh)*
prescription	receta	*(reh-seh-tah)*
present day	moderno	*(moh-dehr-noh)*
prevention	prevención	*(preh-behn-see-ohn)*
preventive	preventivo	*(preh-behn-tee-boh)*
priest	sacerdote	*(sah-sehr-doh-teh)*
prison	cárcel	*(kahr-sehl)*
probable	probable	*(proh-bah-bleh)*
problem	problema(s)	*(proh-bleh-mah[s])*
procedure(s)	procedimiento(s)	*(proh-seh-dee-mee-ehn-toh[s])*
progression	progresión	*(proh-greh-see-ohn)*
prolonged	prolongada	*(proh-lohn-gah-dah)*
promise	prometer	*(proh-meh-tehr)*
pronounce	pronuncia	*(pro-noon-see-ah)*
pronunciation	pronunciación	*(proh-noon-see-ah-see-ohn)*
pronouns	pronombres	*(proh-nohm-brehs)*
provides	provee	*(proh-beh-eh)*
prune(s)	ciruela(s)	*(see-roo-eh-lah[s])*
pruritic	prurítico	*(proo-ree-tee-koh)*
psoriasis	soriasis	*(soh-ree-ah-sees)*
pubic	púbico	*(poo-bee-koh)*
pull	jale	*(hah-leh)*
pulse	pulso	*(pool-soh)*
puncture	pinchazo/picadura	*(peen-chah-soh/pee-kah-doo-rah)*
pure	puro	*(poo-roh)*
pureed	puré	*(poo-reh)*
purpose	propósito	*(proh-poh-see-toh)*
pyorrhea	piorrea	*(pee-oh-rreh-ah)*
Q	q	*(koo)*
quart	cuarto	*(koo-ahr-toh)*
question(s)	pregunta(s)	*(preh-goon-tah[s])*
quite attached	acostumbrados	*(ah-kohs-toom-brah-dohs)*
R	r	*(eh-reh)*
race	raza	*(rah-sah)*
racial	racial	*(rah-see-ahl)*
radio	radio	*(rah-dee-oh)*
radioactive	radioactivo	*(rah-dee-oh-ahk-tee-boh)*
radiologic	radiológico	*(rah-dee-oh-loh-hee-koh)*
radiotherapy	radioterapia	*(rah-dee-oh-teh-rah-pee-ah)*
railroad	tren	*(trehn)*
raisins	pasas	*(pah-sahs)*
rare	raro	*(rah-roh)*

raw	crudo	*(kroo-doh)*
raw	crudos	*(kroo-dohs)*
razor (shave)	máquina de afeitar	*(mah-kee-nah deh ah-feh-ee-tahr)*
razor	navaja	*(nah-bah-hah)*
reach	alcanzar	*(ahl-kahn-sahr)*
read	leer	*(leh-ehr)*
realign	realinear	*(reh-ah-lee-nee-ahr)*
reason	razón	*(rah-sohn)*
reassurance	asegurar	*(ah-seh-goo-rahr)*
receive	recivir	*(reh-see-beer)*
receptionist	recepcionista	*(reh-sehp-see-ohn-ees-tah)*
recognize	reconocer	*(reh-koh-noh-sehr)*
recommendations	recomendaciones	*(reh-koh-men-dah-see-ohn-es)*
recovery	recuperación	*(reh-koo-peh-rah-see-ohn)*
rectal	rectal	*(rehk-tahl)*
rectum	recto	*(rehk-toh)*
recuperating	recuperando	*(reh-koo-peh-rahn-doh)*
red	rojo	*(roh-hoh)*
reduction	reducción	*(reh-dook-see-ohn)*
reduction (open)	reducción abierta	*(reh-dook-see-ohn ah-bee-ehr-tah)*
refried	refritos	*(reh-free-tohs)*
refrigerator	refrigerador	*(reh-free-heh-rah-dohr)*
regular	regular	*(reh-goo-lahr)*
rehabilitation	rehabilitación	*(reh-ah-bee-lee-tah-see-ohn)*
relation	relación	*(reh-lah-see-ohn)*
relax	descansa/relaja	*(dehs-kahn-sah/reh-lah-hah)*
remain	quedese	*(keh-deh-seh)*
remember	recordar/acordarse	*(reh-kohr-dahr/ah-kohr-dahr-seh)*
repell	repeler	*(reh-peh-lehr)*
replantation	reimplantación	*(reh-eehm-plahn-tah-see-ohn)*
reports	reportes	*(reh-pohr-tehs)*
requirements	requerimiento	*(reh-keh-ree-mee-ehn-toh)*
residue	residuo	*(reh-see-doo-oh)*
resin	resina	*(reh-see-nah)*
resonance	resonancia	*(reh-sohn-ahn-see-ah)*
resources	recursos	*(reh-koor-sohs)*
respect	respeto	*(rehs-peh-toh)*
respond	responder	*(rehs-pohn-dehr)*
response	contestación	*(kohn-tehs-tah-see-ohn)*
responsibilities	responsabilidades	*(rehs-pohn-sah-bee-lee-dah-dehs)*
rest	reposo	*(reh-poh-soh)*
restless	inquieto	*(een-kee-eh-toh)*
restroom	cuarto de baño	*(koo-ahr-toh deh bah-nyoh)*
retardation (mental)	retraso mental	*(reh-trah-soh mehn-tahl)*
retinopathy	retinopatía	*(reh-tee-noh-pah-tee-ah)*
return	volver/regresar	*(bohl-behr/reh-greh-sahr)*
rheumatic fever	fiebre reumática	*(fee-eh-breh reh-oo-mah-tee-kah)*
rheumatic	reumático	*(reh-oo-mah-tee-koh)*
rib(s)	costilla(s)	*(kohs-tee-yah[s])*
rice	arroz	*(ah-rrohs)*

right	derecho(a)	*(deh-reh-choh[-chah])*
rigidity	rigidez	*(ree-hee-dehs)*
risk	riesgo	*(ree-ehs-goh)*
road	camino	*(kah-mee-noh)*
roast	rostizado	*(rohs-tee-sah-doh)*
roast-beef	rosbif	*(rohs-beef)*
rolls	panecillos	*(pah-neh-see-yohs)*
room	cuarto	*(koo-ahr-toh)*
room (operating)	cuarto de cirugía quirófano	*(koo-ahr-toh deh see-roo-hee-ah/kee-roh-fah-noh)*
room (x-ray)	cuarto de rayos X	*(koo-ahr-toh deh rah-yohs eh-kiss)*
roseola	roseola	*(roh-seh-oh-lah)*
rotation	rotación	*(roh-tah-see-ohn)*
route(s)	ruta(s)	*(roo-tah[s])*
routine	rutina	*(roo-tee-nah)*
rr	rr	*(doh-bleh eh-rreh)*
rub	frotar/restregar	*(froh-tahr/rehs-treh-gahr)*
rubella	rubéola	*(roo-beh-oh-lah)*
ruby	rubí	*(roo-bee)*
S	s	*(eh-seh)*
saccharin	sacarina	*(sah-kah-ree-nah)*
salad	ensalada	*(ehn-sah-lah-dah)*
saliva	saliva	*(sah-lee-bah)*
salt	sal	*(sahl)*
sample	muestra	*(moo-ehs-trah)*
sanitary	sanitario	*(sah-nee-tah-ree-oh)*
Saturday	sábado	*(sah-bah-doh)*
saucer	platillo	*(plah-tee-yoh)*
sausage	chorizo/salchicha	*(choh-ree-soh/sahl-chee-chah)*
science	ciencia	*(see-ehn-see-ah)*
scleral	escleral	*(ehs-kleh-rahl)*
scorpion	alacrán	*(ah-lah-krahn)*
scrambled	revueltos	*(reh-boo-ehl-tohs)*
scratch	raspón	*(rahs-pohn)*
scream	gritar	*(gree-tahr)*
sealant	placa protectora	*(plah-kah proh-tehk-toh-rah)*
season	estación	*(ehs-tah-see-ohn)*
sebaceous	sebásceo	*(seh-bah-seh-oh)*
second	segundo(a)	*(seh-goon-doh[-dah])*
secrete	secretar	*(seh-kreh-tahr)*
sedatives	sedativo/sedantes	*(seh-dah-tee-boh/seh-dahn-tehs)*
see	ver	*(behr)*
selected	selectas	*(seh-lehk-tahs)*
selection	selección	*(seh-lehk-see-ohn)*
sell	vender	*(behn-dehr)*
semi-solid	semisólido	*(seh-mee-soh-lee-doh)*
sensation	sensación	*(sehn-sah-see-ohn)*
sensitive	sensitivo	*(sehn-see-tee-boh)*
sentence	oración	*(oh-rah-see-ohn)*
September	septiembre	*(sehp-tee-ehm-breh)*

series	series	*(seh-ree-ehs)*
serology	serología	*(seh-roh-loh-hee-ah)*
serve	servimos	*(sehr-bee-mohs)*
served	servido	*(sehr-bee-doh)*
services	servicios	*(sehr-bee-see-ohs)*
setting	area	*(ah-reh-ah)*
seven	siete	*(see-eh-teh)*
seventeen	diez y siete	*(dee-ehs ee see-eh-teh)*
seventh	séptimo(a)	*(sehp-tee-moh[mah])*
seventy	setenta	*(seh-tehn-tah)*
several	varios	*(bah-ree-ohs)*
sex	sexo	*(sehx-oh)*
sexual	sexual	*(sehx-oo-ahl)*
she	ella	*(eh-yah)*
sheets	sábanas	*(sah-bah-nahs)*
shirt	camisa	*(kah-mee-sah)*
shoes	zapatos	*(sah-pah-tohs)*
shortening	manteca	*(mahn-teh-kah)*
should	debe	*(deh-beh)*
shower	baño/regadera/ducha	*(bah-nyoh/reh-gah-deh-rah/ doo-chah)*
shrimp	camarones	*(kah-mah-roh-nehs)*
sign	firme/letrero	*(feer-meh/leh-treh-roh)*
signs	signos/señales	*(seeg-nohs/seh-nyah-lehs)*
similar	similares	*(see-mee-lah-rehs)*
simple	sencillas	*(sehn-see-yahs)*
since	desde/como	*(dehs-deh/koh-moh)*
single	solo/uno	*(soh-loh/oo-noh)*
singular	singular	*(seen-goo-lahr)*
sister	hermana	*(ehr-mah-nah)*
sister-in-law	cuñada	*(koo-nyah-dah)*
Sit!	¡Siéntese!	*(see-ehn-teh-seh)*
sites	sitios	*(see-tee-ohs)*
situation	situación	*(see-too-ah-see-ohn)*
six	seis	*(seh-ees)*
sixteen	diez y seis	*(dee-ehs ee seh-ees)*
sixth	sexto(a)	*(sehx-toh[tah])*
sixty	sesenta	*(seh-sehn-tah)*
skeleton	esqueleto	*(ehs-keh-leh-toh)*
skirt	falda	*(fahl-dah)*
sleep	sueño	*(soo-eh-nyoh)*
small (age/fit)	pequeño/chico	*(peh-keh-nyoh/chee-koh)*
smile	sonríe/sonrisa	*(sohn-ree-eh/sohn-ree-sah)*
smoke	fumar	*(fooh-mahr)*
sneeze	estornudo	*(ehs-tohr-noo-doh)*
so	así qué	*(ah-see keh)*
social worker	trabajadora social	*(trah-bah-hah-doh-rah soh-see-ahl)*
social	social	*(soh-see-ahl)*
sociocultural	sociocultural	*(soh-see-oh-kool-too-rahl)*
socks	calcetines/calcetas	*(kahl-seh-tee-nehs/kahl-seh-tahs)*

sofa	sofá	*(soh-fah)*
soft	suave	*(soo-ah-beh)*
soldier	soldado	*(sohl-dah-doh)*
solid	sólido	*(soh-lee-doh)*
solution	solución	*(soh-loo-see-ohn)*
solvent	solvente	*(sohl-behn-teh)*
somatic	somático	*(soh-mah-tee-koh)*
somatization	somatización	*(soh-mah-tee-sah-see-ohn)*
some hearts	unos corazones	*(Oo-nohs koh-rah-soh-nehs)*
some pencils	unos lápices	*(oo-nohs lah-pee-sehs)*
some tables	unas mesas	*(Oo-nahs meh-sahs)*
some	algunos/unos	*(ahl-goo-nohs/oo-nohs)*
somebody	alguien	*(ahl-ghee-ehn)*
someone	alguien	*(ahl-ghee-ehn)*
something	algo	*(ahl-goh)*
sometimes	a veces/algunas veces	*(ah beh-sehs/ahl-goo-nahs beh-sehs)*
son	hijo	*(ee-hoh)*
soup(s)	caldo(s)/sopa(s)	*(kahl-doh[s]/soh-pah[s])*
South	sur	*(soor)*
spagetti	espageti	*(ehs-pah-geh-tee)*
Spanish	el español	*(ehl ehs-pah-nyohl)*
speak	hablar	*(ah-blahr)*
special	especiales	*(ehs-peh-see-ah-lehs)*
specimen	muestra	*(moo-ehs-trah)*
spectrum	espectro	*(ehs-pehk-troh)*
spices	especias	*(ehs-peh-see-ahs)*
spicy	condimentadas	*(kohn-dee-mehn-tah-dahs)*
spinach	espinaca	*(ehs-pee-nah-kah)*
spinal	espinal	*(ehs-pee-nahl)*
spirit	espíritu	*(ehs-pee-ree-too)*
spots	manchas	*(mahn-chahs)*
spots (white)	manchas blancas	*(mahn-chahs blahn-kahs)*
spread	untar/extender	*(oon-tahr/ehx-tehn-dehr)*
spring	primavera	*(pree-mah-beh-rah)*
stairs	escaleras	*(ehs-kah-leh-rahs)*
start	comenzar	*(koh-mehn-sahr)*
STAT	STAT	*(ehs-taht)*
station (nurses)	estación de enfermeras	*(ehs-tah-see-ohn deh ehn-fehr-meh-rahs)*
steak	bistec	*(bees-tehk)*
step	pisar	*(pee-sahr)*
stepdaughter	hijastra	*(ee-hahs-trah)*
stepfather	padrastro	*(pah-drahs-troh)*
stepmother	madrastra	*(mah-drahs-trah)*
stepson	hijastro	*(ee-hahs-troh)*
sterile	estéril	*(ehs-teh-reel)*
sternum	esternón	*(ehs-tehr-nohn)*
stethoscope	estetoscopio	*(ehs-teh-tohs-koh-pee-oh)*
stockings	medias	*(meh-dee-ahs)*

stove	estufa	*(ehs-too-fah)*
straight	derecho	*(deh-reh-choh)*
straw	popote	*(poh-poh-teh)*
strawberry	fresa	*(freh-sah)*
street/avenue	calle/avenida	*(kah-yeh/ah-beh-nee-dah)*
stress	tensión	*(tehn-see-ohn)*
stroke	ataque de apoplejía	*(ah-tah-keh deh ah-poh-pleh-hee-ah)*
studies	estudios	*(ehs-too-dee-ohs)*
stupor	estupor	*(ehs-too-pohr)*
subaxillary	subaxilar	*(soob-ahx-ee-lahr)*
subcutaneous	subcutáneo	*(soob-koo-tah-neh-oh)*
sublingual	sublingual	*(soob-leen-goo-ahl)*
subnormal	subnormal	*(soob-nohr-mahl)*
substernal	substernal	*(soobs-tehr-nahl)*
substitutes	substitutos	*(soobs-tee-too-tohs)*
successful	con éxito	*(kohn ehx-ee-toh)*
suffer	sufrir	*(soo-freer)*
sugar	azúcar	*(ah-soo-kahr)*
suit	traje	*(trah-heh)*
summer	verano	*(beh-rah-noh)*
Sunday	domingo	*(doh-meen-goh)*
supper	cena	*(seh-nah)*
suppository	supositorio	*(soo-poh-see-toh-ree-oh)*
surgeon	cirujano	*(see-roo-hah-noh)*
surgery	cirugía	*(see-roo-hee-ah)*
surgical	quirúrgico	*(kee-roor-hee-koh)*
surroundings	alrededor	*(ahl-reh-deh-dohr)*
sutures	suturas/puntos	*(soo-too-rahs/poon-tohs)*
sweater	chamarra/sueter	*(cha-mah-rrah/soo-eh-tehr)*
swelling	hinchazón	*(een-chah-sohn)*
swollen	hinchado	*(een-chah-doh)*
symbol	símbolo	*(seem-boh-loh)*
symptoms	síntomas	*(seen-toh-mahs)*
syncope	síncope	*(seen-koh-peh)*
syndrome	síndrome	*(seen-droh-meh)*
syringe	jeringa	*(heh-reen-gah)*
syrup	jarabe/zumo	*(hah-rah-beh/soo-moh)*
systemic	sistemático	*(sees-teh-mah-tee-koh)*
systole	sístole	*(sees-toh-leh)*
T	t	*(teh)*
table (overnight)	mesa de noche	*(meh-sah deh noh-cheh)*
table(s)	mesa(s)	*(meh-sah[s])*
tablespoon	cuchara/cucharada	*(koo-chah-rah/koo-chah-rah-dah)*
tablet	tableta	*(tah-bleh-tah)*
tacos	tacos	*(tah-kohs)*
take	tomar/llevar	*(toh-mahr/yeh-bahr)*
tamales	tamales	*(tah-mah-lehs)*
taste	gusto	*(goos-toh)*

tea	té	*(teh)*
teaspoon	cucharita/ cucharadita	*(koo-chah-ree-tah/koo-chah-rah-dee-tah)*
technician/technical	técnico	*(tehk-nee-koh)*
television	televisor	*(teh-leh-bee-sohr)*
temperature	temperatura	*(tehm-peh-rah-too-rah)*
temporal	temporal	*(tehm-poh-rahl)*
ten	diez	*(dee-ehs)*
tense	tenso	*(tehn-soh)*
tension	tensión	*(tehn-see-ohn)*
tenth	décimo(a)	*(deh-see-moh[mah])*
terminal	terminal	*(tehr-mee-nahl)*
terms	términos	*(tehr-mee-nohs)*
tests	pruebas	*(proo-eh-bahs)*
tetanus	tétanos	*(teh-tah-nohs)*
than	qué	*(keh)*
thank you	gracias	*(grah-see-ahs)*
that	aquél/aquéllo/ aquélla	*(ah-kehl/ah-keh-yoh/ah-keh-yah)*
that	eso/esa	*(eh-soh/eh-sah)*
that	qué	*(keh)*
that have	qué tienen	*(keh tee-eh-nehn)*
the	el/la	*(ehl/lah)*
their	su/sus	*(soo/soos)*
them	ustedes	*(oos-teh-dehs)*
theories	teorías	*(teh-oh-ree-ahs)*
therapeutic	terapéuticas	*(teh-rah-peh-oo-tee-kahs)*
therapy	terapia	*(teh-rah-pee-ah)*
there are	hay	*(ah-ee)*
therefore	por	*(pohr)*
thermometer	termómetro	*(tehr-moh-meh-troh)*
these	estos(as)	*(ehs-tohs[-tahs])*
they	ellos(as)	*(eh-yohs[-yahs])*
third	tercero(a)	*(tehr-seh-roh[-rah])*
thirteen	trece	*(treh-seh)*
thirty	treinta	*(treh-een-tah)*
this	este/esto(a)	*(ehs-teh/ehs-toh[-tah])*
those	aquéllos/aquéllas	*(ah-keh-yohs/ah-keh-yahs)*
those	esos/esas	*(eh-sohs/eh-sahs)*
three	tres	*(trehs)*
thrombus	coágulo	*(koh-ah-goo-loh)*
Thursday	jueves	*(hoo-eh-behs)*
thyroid	tiróide/tiroidea	*(tee-roh-ee-deh/tee-roh-ee-deh-ah)*
tie	corbata	*(kohr-bah-tah)*
tight	apretado	*(ah-preh-tah-doh)*
time	cada	*(kah-dah)*
tissue (muscle)	tejido	*(teh-hee-doh)*
tissues	tisues	*(tee-sooh[-ehs])*
tisue damage	daño del tejido	*(dah-nyoh dehl teh-hee-doh)*
to accept	aceptar	*(ah-sehp-tahr)*

to activate	activar	(ahk-tee-bahr)
to administer	administrar	(ahd-mee-nees-trahr)
to advise	aconsejar	(ah-kohn-seh-hahr)
to agree	acordar	(ah-kohr-dahr)
to appreciate	apreciar	(ah-preh-see-ahr)
to arrive	llegar	(yeh-gahr)
to ask	preguntar	(preh-goon-tahr)
to assess	asesorar/evaluar	(ah-seh-soh-rahr/eh-bah-loo-ahr)
to auscultate	auscultar	(ah-oos-kool-tahr)
to authorize	autorizar	(ahoo-toh-ree-sahr)
to avoid	evitar	(eh-bee-tahr)
to bathe	bañar	(bah-nyahr)
to be	estar/ser	(ehs-tahr/sehr)
to be able	poder	(poh-dehr)
to be afraid	temer	(teh-mehr)
to be available	disponible	(dees-poh-nee-bleh)
to be born	nacer	(nah-sehr)
to be supportive	apoyar	(ah-poh-yahr)
to beat/knock	golpear	(gohl-peh-ahr)
to become ill	enfermar	(ehn-fehr-mahr)
to believe	creer	(kreh-ehr)
to bleed	sangrar	(sahn-grahr)
to boil	hervir	(ehr-beer)
to bore	aburrir	(ah-boo-rreer)
to break	romper	(rohm-pehr)
to breathe	respirar	(rehs-pee-rahr)
to bring near	acercar	(ah-sehr-kahr)
to bring	traer	(trah-ehr)
to build	construir	(kohns-troo-eer)
to call	llamar	(yah-mahr)
to carry	llevar	(yeh-bahr)
to change	cambiar	(kahm-bee-ahr)
to clean	limpiar	(leem-pee-ahr)
to close	cerrar	(seh-rrahr)
to come	venir	(beh-neer)
to communicate	comunicar	(koh-moo-nee-kahr)
to complain	quejar	(keh-hahr)
to conduct	conducir	(kohn-doo-seer)
to confuse	confundir	(kohn-foon-deer)
to conserve	conservar	(kohn-sehr-bahr)
to control	controlar	(kohn-troh-lahr)
to cook	cocinar	(koh-see-nahr)
to cough	toser	(toh-sehr)
to cover	cubrir	(koo-breer)
to cross	cruzar	(kroo-sahr)
to cry	llorar	(yoh-rahr)
to cure	curar	(koo-rahr)
to cut	cortar	(kohr-tahr)
to deny	negar	(neh-gahr)
to deserve	merecer	(meh-reh-sehr)

to destroy	destruir	*(dehs-troo-eer)*
to dic	morir	*(moh-reer)*
to disappear	desaparecer	*(deh-sah-pah-reh-sehr)*
to discover/find	descubrir	*(dehs-koo-breer)*
to do/make	hacer	*(ah-sehr)*
to dress	vestír	*(behs-teer)*
to drink	beber/tomar	*(beh-behr/toh-mahr)*
to eat breakfast	desayunar	*(deh-sah-yoo-nahr)*
to eat	comer	*(koh-mehr)*
to embrace	abrazar	*(ah-brah-sahr)*
to employ	emplear	*(ehm-pleh-ahr)*
to evaluate	evaluar	*(eh-bah-loo-ahr)*
to examine	examinar	*(ex-ah-mee-nahr)*
to feel	sentír	*(sehn-teer)*
to fill	llenar/empastar/ rellenar	*(yeh-nahr/ehm-pahs-tahr/reh-yeh- nahr)*
to find	descubrir/hallar	*(dehs-koo-breer/ah-yahr)*
to finish	acabar	*(ah-kah-bahr)*
to fix	componer	*(kohm-poh-nehr)*
to fly	volar	*(boh-lahr)*
to follow	seguir	*(seh-gheer)*
to gain by	ganar	*(gah-nahr)*
to get acquainted	darse a conocer	*(dahr-seh ah koh-noh-sehr)*
to get better	mejorar	*(meh-hoh-rahr)*
to get up/raise	levantar	*(leh-bahn-tahr)*
to give	dar	*(dahr)*
to go by	pasar	*(pah-sahr)*
to go out	salir	*(sah-leer)*
to go to bed	acostarse	*(ah-kohs-tahr-seh)*
to go	ir	*(eer)*
to greet	saludar	*(sah-loo-dahr)*
to hang	colgar	*(kohl-gahr)*
to have	haber/tener	*(ah-behr/teh-nehr)*
to heal	sanar	*(sah-nahr)*
to hear me	oirme	*(oh-eer-meh)*
to hear/listen	escuchar/oír	*(ehs-koo-chahr/oh-eer)*
to hesitate	vacilar	*(bah-see-lahr)*
to hit	pegar	*(peh-gahr)*
to hunt	cazar	*(kah-sahr)*
to hurt	doler	*(doh-lehr)*
to inform	informar	*(een-fohr-mahr)*
to interpret	interpretar	*(een-tehr-preh-tahr)*
to joke/kid	bromear	*(broh-meh-ahr)*
to jump	saltar	*(sahl-tahr)*
to keep	guardar	*(goo-ahr-dahr)*
to kid	bromear	*(broh-meh-ahr)*
to kiss	besar	*(beh-sahr)*
to knock	golpear	*(gohl-peh-ahr)*
to know	conocer	*(koh-noh-sehr)*
to lay down	acostar/dormir	*(ah-kohs-tahr/dohr-meer)*

to leave	dejar	*(deh-hahr)*
to let go	soltar	*(sohl-tahr)*
to listen	oir	*(oh-eer)*
to live	vivir	*(bee-beer)*
to loose	perder	*(pehr-dehr)*
to make	hacer	*(ah-sehr)*
to marry	casar	*(kah-sahr)*
to name	nombrar	*(nohm-brahr)*
to need	necesitar	*(neh-seh-see-tahr)*
to operate	operar	*(oh-peh-rahr)*
to paint	pintar	*(peen-tahr)*
to palpate	palpar	*(pahl-pahr)*
to pay	pagar	*(pah-gahr)*
to play	jugar	*(hoo-gahr)*
to point	señalar	*(seh-nyah-lahr)*
to present	presentar	*(preh-sehn-tahr)*
to promise	prometer	*(proh-meh-tehr)*
to protect	protejer	*(proh-teh-hehr)*
to provoke	provocar	*(proh-boh-kahr)*
to raise	levantar	*(leh-bahn-tahr)*
to reach	alcanzar	*(ahl-kahn-sahr)*
to receive	recibir	*(reh-see-beer)*
to recognize	reconocer	*(reh-koh-noh-sehr)*
to reduce	reducir	*(reh-doo-seer)*
to remain	quedar	*(keh-dahr)*
to remember	acordar/recordar	*(ah-kohr-dahr/reh-kohr-dahr)*
to respond	responder	*(rehs-pohn-dehr)*
to return	regresar/volver	*(reh-greh-sahr/bohl-behr)*
to revise	revisar	*(reh-bee-sahr)*
to scream	gritar	*(gree-tahr)*
to see	ver	*(behr)*
to select	seleccionar	*(seh-lehk-see-oh-nahr)*
to sell	vender	*(behn-dehr)*
to separate	separar	*(seh-pah-rahr)*
to serve	servir	*(sehr-beer)*
to shake	temblar	*(tehm-blahr)*
to sit	sentar	*(sehn-tahr)*
to sleep	dormir	*(dohr-meer)*
to speak	hablar	*(ah-blahr)*
to start	comenzar	*(koh-mehn-sahr)*
to step	pisar	*(pee-sahr)*
to stop	parar	*(pah-rahr)*
to suffer	sufrir	*(soo-freer)*
to suspend	suspender	*(soos-pehn-dehr)*
to take out	sacar	*(sah-kahr)*
to take	tomar/llevar	*(toh-mahr/yeh-bahr)*
to talk to	hablar con	*(ah-blahr kohn)*
to talk	hablar	*(ah-blahr)*
to tell	decir	*(deh-seer)*
to thank for	agradecer	*(ah-grah-deh-sehr)*

to try	tratar	*(trah-tahr)*
to turn off	apagar	*(ah-pah-gahr)*
to turn	girar/voltear/dar vuelta	*(hee-rahr/bohl-teh-ahr/dahr boo-ehl-tah)*
to visit	visitar	*(bee-see-tahr)*
to vomit	vomitar	*(boh-mee-tahr)*
to wait	esperar	*(ehs-peh-rahr)*
to wake	despertar	*(dehs-pehr-tahr)*
to walk	caminar	*(kah-mee-nahr)*
to want	querer	*(keh-rehr)*
to wash	lavar	*(lah-bahr)*
to wish	desear	*(deh-seh-ahr)*
to work	trabajar	*(trah-bah-hahr)*
to write	escribir	*(ehs-kree-beer)*
to	a	*(ah)*
toast	pan tostado	*(pahn tohs-tah-doh)*
toilet	escusado	*(ehs-koo-sah-doh)*
tolerant	tolerante	*(toh-leh-rahn-teh)*
tomatoe	tomate	*(toh-mah-teh)*
tomorrow	mañana	*(mah-nyah-nah)*
tonsillitis	tonsilitis/amigdalitis	*(tohn-see-lee-tees/ah-meeg-dah-lee-tees)*
too much	mucho	*(moo-choh)*
toothache	dolor de muelas	*(doh-lohr deh moo-eh-lahs)*
toothbrush	cepillo de dientes	*(seh-pee-yoh deh dee-ehn-tehs)*
toothpaste	pasta de dientes	*(pahs-tah deh dee-ehn-tehs)*
toothpick	palillo	*(pah-lee-yoh)*
topical	topical/tópico	*(toh-pee-kahl/toh-pee-koh)*
torso	torso	*(tohr-soh)*
total	total	*(toh-tahl)*
toward	hacia	*(ah-see-ah)*
towel	toalla	*(too-ah-yah)*
tower	torre	*(toh-rreh)*
traction	tracción	*(trak-see-ohn)*
tranquilizer	tranquilizante	*(trahn-kee-lee-sahn-teh)*
transfusion	transfusión	*(trahns-foo-see-ohn)*
translate	traducir/interpretar	*(trah-doo-seer/een-tehr-preh-tahr)*
transparent	transparente	*(trahns-pah-rehn-teh)*
traumatic	traumático	*(trah-oo-mah-tee-koh)*
treatment	tratamiento	*(trah-tah-mee-ehn-toh)*
tree	árbol	*(ahr-bohl)*
trust	confianza	*(kohn-fee-ahn-sah)*
try	intentar/tratar	*(een-tehn-tahr/trah-tahr)*
tube(s)	tubo(s)	*(too-boh[s])*
Tuesday	martes	*(mahr-tehs)*
tumor	tumor	*(too-mohr)*
tuna	atún	*(ah-toon)*
turkey	pavo/guajolote	*(pah-boh/goo-ah-hoh-loh-teh)*
twelve (midnight)	veinticuatro horas	*(beh-een-tee-koo-ah-troh oh-rahs)*

twelve (noon)	doce	*(doh-seh)*
twelve	doce	*(doh-seh)*
twenty	veinte	*(beh-een-teh)*
two	dos	*(dohs)*
type(s)	tipo(s)	*(tee-poh[s])*
typewriter	máquina de escribir	*(mah-kee-nah deh ehs-kree-beer)*
U	u	*(oo)*
ulcer(s)	úlcera(s)	*(ool-seh-rah[s])*
ulnar	ulnar	*(ool-nahr)*
ultrasound	ultrasonido	*(ool-trah-soh-nee-doh)*
uncle	tío	*(tee-oh)*
under	debajo de	*(deh-bah-hoh deh)*
underwear	ropa interior	*(roh-pah een-teh-ree-ohr)*
union	unión	*(oo-nee-ohn)*
universal	universal	*(oo-nee-behr-sahl)*
until	hasta	*(ahs-tah)*
urea	urea	*(oo-reh-ah)*
uremia	uremia	*(oo-reh-mee-ah)*
ureteritis	uretritis	*(oo-reh-tree-tees)*
urinal	pato	*(pah-toh)*
urine	orina	*(oh-ree-nah)*
urticaria	urticaria	*(oor-tee-kah-ree-ah)*
use	usar	*(oo-sahr)*
used	usado	*(oo-sah-doh)*
useful	utiles	*(oo-tee-lehs)*
uterus	útero	*(oo-teh-roh)*
utilize	utilizar	*(oo-tee-lee-sahr)*
uvula	úvula	*(oo-boo-lah)*
V	v	*(oo-beh/beh)*
vaccinations	vacunas	*(bah-koo-nahs)*
vaginal	vaginal	*(bah-hee-nahl)*
vaginitis	vaginitis	*(bah-hee-nee-tees)*
vagus	vago	*(bah-goh)*
valve	válvula	*(bahl-boo-lah)*
vanilla	vainilla	*(bah-ee-nee-yah)*
vapor	vapor	*(bah-pohr)*
varicocele	varicocele	*(bah-ree-koh-seh-leh)*
variety	variedad	*(bah-ree-eh-dahd)*
vegetables	vegetales	*(beh-heh-tah-lehs)*
vein	vena	*(beh-nah)*
venereal	venéreo	*(beh-neh-reh-oh)*
ventilation	ventilación	*(behn-tee-lah-see-ohn)*
verbs	verbos	*(behr-bohs)*
vermouth	vermut	*(behr-moot)*
vertebrate	vertebrado	*(behr-teh-brah-doh)*
vertigo	vértigo	*(behr-tee-goh)*
vestibule	vestíbulo	*(behs-tee-boo-loh)*
veterinary	veterinaria	*(beh-teh-ree-nah-ree-ah)*

worker	trabajador	*(trah-bah-hah-dohr)*
wound	herida	*(eh-ree-dah)*
writing	escribiendo	*(ehs-kree-bee-ehn-doh)*

X	x	*(eh-kiss)*
xiphoid	xifoide	*(see-foh-ee-deh)*
x-rays	rayos-x	*(rah-yohs eh-kiss)*

Y	y	*(ee-gree-eh-gah)*
year	año	*(ah-nyoh)*
yellow	amarillo	*(ah-mah-ree-yoh)*
yes	si	*(see)*
yogurt	yogurt	*(yoh-goohrt)*
you	tu/usted	*(too/oos-tehd)*
you	ellos/ellas/ustedes	*(eh-yohs/eh-yahs/oos-teh-dehs)*
young	jovenes	*(hoh-beh-nehs)*
your	su/sus	*(soo/soos)*

Z	z	*(seh-tah)*
zero	cero	*(seh-roh)*
zinc	cinc	*(seenk)*
zip code	código postal	*(koh-dee-goh pohs-tahl)*
zipper	cierre	*(see-eh-reh)*
zone	zona	*(soh-nah)*
zoo	zoológico	*(soh-oh-loh-hee-koh)*
zoology	zoología	*(soh-oh-loh-hee-ah)*
zoom	sumbido	*(soom-bee-doh)*
zucchini	calabacita	*(kah-lah-bah-see-tah)*
zygomatic	cigomático	*(see-goh-mah-tee-koh)*

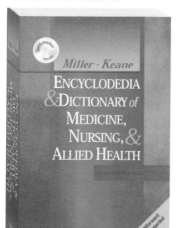

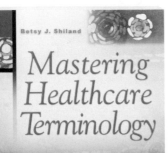